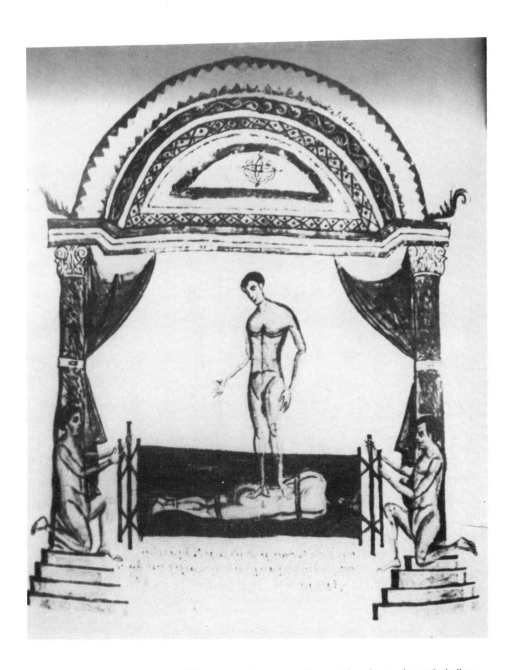

Spinal manipulation, according to Hippocrates. Reduction of the vertebrae by traction and windlass, and a man standing on the patient's back, from a commentary on Hippocrates by Apollonius of Kition. (Reproduced by kind permission of the Biblioteca Medicea Laurenziana, Florence.)

Manipulative Therapy in Rehabilitation of the Locomotor System

Dedicated to my wife

Manipulative Therapy in Rehabilitation of the Locomotor System

Karel Lewit, MUDr, Doc., DSc
Consultant to the Central Railway Health Institute, Prague

Butterworths
London   Boston   Singapore   Sydney   Toronto   Wellington

First published, 1985
Reprinted 1987
Reprinted 1988

© Butterworth & Co (Publishers) Ltd, 1985
Line drawings: © Gerda Istler 1985
Photographs: © Jaroslav Cmíral 1985

British Library Cataloguing in Publication Data

Lewit, Karel
  Manipulative therapy in rehabilitation of the motor system.
  1. Nervous system–Diseases–Treatment
  I. Title   II. Manuelle medizin in Rahmen der medizinischen
  Rehabilitation. *English*
  616.8'046   RC346

  ISBN 0-407-0025209

Library of Congress Cataloging in Publication Data

Lewit, Karel
  Manipulative therapy in rehabilitation of the motor system.
  "Updated English version (not a mere translation) of a textbook which appeared successively in Czech . . . in German . . . in Bulgarian . . .in Dutch, and in Polish"
Pref.
  Bibliography: p.
  Includes index.
  1. Manipulation (Therapeutics)   2. Musculoskeletal system–Diseases–Treatment   3. Pain–Treatment.
  I. Title.   [DNLM: 1. Osteopathy. 2. Reflexotherapy.
  WB 940 L677m]

  RM724.L49   1985   616.7'0622   83-26159

  ISBN 0-407-00252-9

Printed and bound in Great Britain by
Hartnolls Ltd., Bodmin, Cornwall

Preface

This book is the updated English version (not a mere translation) of a textbook which appeared successively in Czech (1966 and 1975), in German (1973, 1977, 1978 and 1983), in Bulgarian (1981), in Dutch (1981) and in Polish (1984). This English version is shorter, more concise and includes the latest techniques.

This book was conceived at a time when the lack of proper textbooks on impaired function of the motor system was a major obstacle to teaching. Now there are a good many manuals dealing with techniques of manipulation, remedial exercise, massage, and so forth, all aspects of the subject which are dealt with in detail in this publication. However, the role of manipulation is limited to passive mobility and an important part of this book deals with active mobility. I would also emphasize that this is a textbook and not a manual of techniques: the latter deals with individual techniques, while my purpose is to show that it can be disastrous to confine one's interest in this manner and to remain unaware of both the broader context of treatment and of the possible alternatives. From this point of view the content of the body of the book (chapters 3–10) becomes clear. There are chapters on functional anatomy, the diagnosis and treatment of disturbed locomotor system function, including indications of appropriate treatment and the place of manipulation, and finally a long chapter on the clinical aspects of impaired function of the locomotor system.

To put my subject in its widest context, I thought it appropriate to begin the book by discussing the major role played by impaired function in the vast majority of patients suffering from pain arising in the locomotor system. This type of pain is altogether the most frequent from which patients suffer, and the first two (theoretical) chapters of this book are mainly concerned with the origin of this pain. It is traditionally associated with rheumatism, but unfortunately rheumatologists are insufficiently aware of locomotor function and leave this field largely to neurologists and orthopaedic surgeons. I believe that the speciality which is principally concerned with impaired function and its restoration to normal is rehabilitation medicine, a term which includes physical therapy, and it is in this framework that the future of manipulation lies.

Acknowledgements

This English version would have been impossible without the devoted care and critical help of my English wife. Next to her my greatest debt is to my friend John Ebbetts, OBE, MRCS, LRCP, for his scrupulous revision of the whole text, his advice on terminology, and his most valuable comments. At the same time it is a pleasure to thank the publishers not only for the opportunity they have provided, but also for forcing me to greater conciseness and brevity.

The book in this form is the result of more than 30 years' consistent work in the field of painful disorders stemming from impaired locomotor function. To have been able to devote myself to this I am indebted first to the late Professor Henner, at whose Neurological Clinic I was encouraged to break new ground in an unorthodox direction. I owe thanks in particular to my first teacher both in neuroradiology and in scientific research, Professor Jirout, whose friendship I cherish to this day. My second great tutor was Professor Starý. To Professor Macek I owe the opportunity to teach systematically at the Post-Graduate Medical Institute for many years. Further progress in my work I owe to my closest collaborators, Professor Janda and Dr Velé, with whom I still enjoy fruitful co-operation. Nor should K. Stein be omitted, the author of most of the techniques of remedial exercise given here. The late Professor J. Wolf gave me valuable scientific guidance.

I owe much, too, to friends and teachers in other countries: Dr G. Gutmann, Dr H.-D. Wolff and the late Dr F. Biedermann of West Germany, Professor Krauss of East Germany, Dr Alan Stoddard of England, Professor F. Kaltenborn of Norway, and in particular Dr F. Gaymans of Holland. It is a special pleasure to acknowledge my debt to many of those it has been my good fortune to teach, and particularly to Dr L. Zbojan, to the late Dr Kubis and to Dr Sachse of East Germany; the latter gave me valuable help with the German editions of the book. Recently Dr M. Berger of Austria has contributed much to my research with his technical vision and inventiveness.

To have been able to continue my work I owe thanks to the Central Railway Health Institute in Prague, in particular to the successive directors, Dr Vostatek and Dr Okres, and for many of the best illustrations in this book I have to thank Dr Stejskal and his X-ray laboratory at the Institute.

This brings me to pay special tribute to my illustrators, to Gerda Istler for her drawings and to J. Cmíral for his photography.

Karel Lewit

Contents

Nociceptive: Painful

Introduction

Pain – especially in the locomotor system – is a curse mankind has always suffered. It has been the commonest reason for his calls for help, answered by a bewildering multitude of diverse treatments. To the orthodox the cure, it seems, can often be 'left to nature', sometimes assisted by rest in bed and the doubtful boon of pharmacotherapy, but there are many other methods (all sincerely held by some to be singularly effective) which belong mainly although not exclusively to the realm of physical therapy. These include local anaesthesia, massage, electrotherapy, needling, manipulation, local cold or hot applications, remedial exercise, hypnotherapy, counter-irritative poultices and even leeches. All of them are used for more or less the same type of disorder, and we may ask if any one of them should be preferred, especially since in practice we very often find that the therapist uses the method he or she knows best.

The common feature of all these methods is that they act reflexly, that is they act on sensory receptors – usually in the region where the pain is felt, or even better where it originates – to produce a reflex response. They may thus be termed 'methods of reflex therapy'. Assuming the reflex nature of the action of this type of treatment, we may then ask what receptors are acted upon and what structures are subserved by those receptors. As nervous control is based largely on reflex action, precise information about where, how and why we should apply one or the other method may be very useful and give us better insight into the various methods, as well as more reliable practical results. As these methods are most frequently applied in painful conditions, it may be useful to begin with the reflex response to nociceptive (painful) stimulation.

Any localized painful stimulation will act in the segment to which the stimulated structure belongs. In this segment there is usually a hyperalgesic zone in the skin,

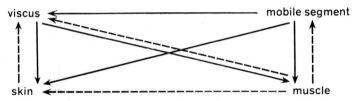

Figure 1.1 Reflex relations within the segment

visceroviseral Reflex
Suprasegmental "

chain Reaction

LimiTus of

muscle spasm, painful periosteal points, movement restriction of the spinal segment and (perhaps) some dysfunction of a visceral organ (*Figure 1.1*). This provides a means both of recognizing clinically which of these changes is present and of using some of the methods available either upon the skin, the muscles (periosteal points), the spinal segment or the visceral organ involved. We may also try to find out which of these structures is the source of the painful stimulus, in which structure the changes are more intense, and so on.

However, these reflex changes are not confined to a single segment. A visceral disturbance is accompanied by visceroviseral reflexes: pain in the region of the gall bladder, for example, causes anorexia; pain in the region of the heart a sense of oppression, etc. These suprasegmental reflexes are most prominent in the locomotor system: acute segmental pain in the lumbar region causes spasm of the whole lumbar erector spinae; any local movement restriction in the spinal column acts upon distant segments, causing what may be called a chain reaction. Any serious painful disorder at the periphery will also cause a central response: the motor pattern will change in order to spare the painful structure. In this way altered motor patterns may be formed which can become permanent and so persist after the painful lesion has disappeared (*Figure 1.2*).

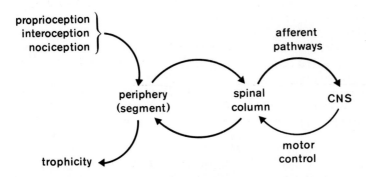

Figure 1.2 Afferent and efferent connections between the periphery and the central nervous system

It is useful to note that at all these levels there are both somatic and autonomic responses to painful afferents. The somatic response consists mainly of muscle spasm (tension) or muscular inhibition, and at the central level of a changed motor pattern. The autonomic response is much more varied: it is manifested by the appearance of hyperalgesic zones and pain spots, vasomotor reaction (mainly vasoconstriction in the relevant segment), and at the central level may affect respiration, the cardiovascular or the digestive system. These central effects are understandable, for pain is also a stress factor.

Once we know the source of nociceptive stimulation, for example movement restriction of a spinal motor segment, and can assess its severity, then the intensity of these reflex responses may give us relevant information about the reaction of the patient to this type of stimulation, particularly in that segment. The subjective assessment of pain allows us to correlate the nociceptive stimulation, the reflex reaction and the (central, psychological) susceptibility of the patient to pain.

This schematic outline shows some possible lines of action to take in painful disorders, using the same orderly approach a neurologist would employ in disorders of mobility. This approach is essential if we are to act specifically, that is if we are to know why, when and where we should use one or other of the methods we call reflex therapy. Precisely for this reason we must first determine clinically the source of pain as well as the reflex reactions in the segment and on the suprasegmental and central levels. I believe that the key to this difficult task lies in the function of the locomotor system and its possible disturbance. As this constitutes one of the main themes of this book, I shall do no more in this introduction than point out that the locomotor system is by far the most frequent source of pain in an organism. This is readily understandable, because not only does the locomotor system constitute about three-quarters of the body weight, but even more important it is under the control of our will – at the mercy of our whims – and has no other way of protecting itself against misuse other than by causing pain. This further implies that pain warns us mainly against harmful *functioning*, and it is disturbance of function that is the most common cause of pain originating in the locomotor system. Movement restriction (blockage) at the segmental level and disturbed motor patterns at the central level may serve as examples. It is therefore no coincidence that pain of any origin (for example, visceral pain) as a rule causes painful muscle spasm in the relevant segment and is usually felt in the locomotor system (like the heart causing pain in the left arm and shoulder, the gall bladder in the shoulder tip, etc.).

Hence specific therapy can be effectively applied only on the basis of a sound knowledge of the function of the locomotor system, and this constitutes one of the most important and difficult subjects in this book.

Obviously, the means of therapy must vary according to the structure upon which we wish to act. There is certainly a great variety of methods available to us if we want to act on a hyperalgesic skin zone, as skin receptors may be reached by most types of physical therapy (massage, electrotherapy, needling or even simple skin stretching). Muscles in tension may be treated by massage, more effectively by post-isometric relaxation, by warmth or by infiltration. Periosteal points may be reached by deep massage, by needling, or – if they are the insertion points of muscles – by post-isometric relaxation of the muscle. The most adequate treatment of joint or spinal segment movement restriction is manipulation; the most adequate treatment of disturbed motor patterns is remedial exercise.

Furthermore, we must decide which of the affected structures is important and which less so, which is likely to be primary and which secondary. The severity of the change may be significant. Even at the segmental level, however, there is a sort of hierarchy: there may be a primary visceral disorder and there may be blockage of a spinal segment. Changes in muscle can be secondary and in the skin this is the rule. But in the locomotor system itself, and in the spinal column, there are regions of greater and of lesser importance, regions in which a primary lesion occurs more readily than in others. It is vital to recognize those faulty central motor patterns which, if significant, will cause relapses at the periphery. In this connection psychological factors play a great role, as motor patterns *are* to a certain degree expressions of the state of mind: anxiety, depression and an inability to relax will greatly influence motor patterns; no less important is the subject's psychological attitude to pain, since it is the most frequent symptom in our patients.

In addition to the importance of the changes diagnosed there is also a practical or technical aspect to be considered, as not all of the methods used are equally effective or 'economical'. Thus needling of a periosteal pain spot (or infiltration) is usually more economical than periosteal massage (deep friction), but wherever possible it is preferable to use post-isometric relaxation of the muscle (if the

relapse: recurrence of illness after a period of important.

periosteal point is a point of muscle insertion) because this method is painless and the patient can usually be taught to do it himself. The attractiveness of manipulation techniques lies mainly in the fact that they are effective and not time consuming.

We can see from this that the choice of treatment is very broad. We can decide which to use by diagnosing each lesion in turn, and from this make what Gutmann (1975) calls the '*Aktualitätsdiagnose*', the diagnosis of the lesion which is the most important link in the chain of pathology at a given moment. We must do this, otherwise we may, for example, apply a method which acts on skin receptors when there are no signs of a hyperalgesic zone; or act on a muscle when there is no change in tension; or manipulate a spinal segment with normal mobility; or give remedial exercise for normal movement patterns. Such very varied methods of treatment should be applied only after full clinical examination and analysis, and with careful testing of the results of treatment. We must act in a systematic fashion and, as we would do when making a neurological examination, start at the peripheral level and work up to the central, applying treatment according to our findings.

At times, however, the results fall far below what we might expect from our premises. One of the chief reasons why this happens in this type of therapy is the presence of a lesion which causes intense nociceptive stimulation and so dominates the clinical picture without the patient being aware of it. The German literature uses the term '*Störungsfeld*', focus of disturbance. This is frequently an old scar after injury or operation, often a tonsillectomy scar. This focus-scar is usually tender on examination, with pain spots, and surrounded by a hyperalgesic zone. If the 'normal' therapy fails, the existence of such a scar acting like a 'saboteur' must be considered; treatment by local anaesthesia or by simply needling the pain spots within the scar can be most rewarding. Another reason for poor results in patients treated for pain may be undiagnosed masked depression, which must then be treated as such.

The most important functional changes in the locomotor system, together with the reflex changes they produce, may aptly be called the 'functional pathology of the locomotor system'. In this connection the unfortunate but frequent use of the term 'functional' as a synonym or euphemism for 'psychological' is most regrettable – it implies a grave underestimation of the importance of function and changes of function consequent on pathological changes. In rehabilitation we are primarily concerned with the restoration of impaired function even in those conditions where there is underlying structural pathology. This is understandable because structural lesions necessarily produce disturbances of function.

The greatest obstacle to the practical application of these apparently simple principles is a general lack of clinical understanding of functional disorders of the locomotor system or even of their reflex manifestations, which are in fact the most typical clinical manifestations of pain. The lesions which are both the most frequent as well as being the object of manipulative therapy are those affecting the spinal column; the term vertebrogenic lesion is often used to describe them, but this is now believed to be not quite appropriate; vertebrogenic disorders also include such pathological states as ankylosing spondylitis, osteoporosis, tumours, etc., while our main concern is with disturbed function. However, function is not confined to the spinal column but involves muscles, nervous control and very frequently the extremities. It is therefore more appropriate to speak of disturbed function of the locomotor system, rather than of vertebrogenic disturbance.

What is the present place of reflex therapy? This question is as difficult to answer as the question of the place of pharmacotherapy. Whereas pharmacotherapy has developed into an exact and sophisticated science, methods of reflex (physical) therapy have for the most part remained empirical, with largely overlapping and even chaotic indications. From what has already been said it is possible to formulate one important principle: we do not prescribe treatment for a particular disease, but for those changes which are of pathogenetic significance in the disease. If, for example, headache is due to muscular tension alone, then muscular relaxation by whatever may be the most effective method is the correct treatment. However, if this muscular tension is due to blockage of a motor segment of the cervical spine, manipulation will be more suitable; if faulty posture is the cause, remedial exercise may be the answer. However, the great advantages of this type of therapy over pharmacotherapy are that (1) the mainly physiological methods used cause a minimum of side-effects if properly applied; and (2) as most methods of reflex therapy act immediately, their effectiveness can be checked immediately.

It is worth saying a few words here about the role of pharmacotherapy in lesions which mainly affect the functioning of the locomotor system. It would be difficult to conceive of a drug that could restore a specific motor function, but drugs may alleviate spasm, influence pain and damp down some of the reflex changes involved, and thus facilitate the restoration of function. Additionally, they are of course necessary for the treatment of depression and anxiety symptoms.

To sum up, neither the clinical diagnosis nor our findings in themselves suffice as the basis for deciding the most appropriate therapy. Only an analysis of pathogenesis enables us to determine the lesion that is the most important at a given moment. After treatment the patient must be re-examined to gauge any immediate effect, and from this we can see at once whether our hypothesis about the pathology was correct and can adjust treatment accordingly. If treatment has been effective, then at the next examination the picture should have changed and again we have to determine which lesion has become the most important. Thus therapy is never a monotonous routine; at the same time it is always verifiable, which encourages the therapist to take an objective scientific approach.

Manipulative therapy, which is one of the most effective and important of the various methods of reflex therapy, is concerned with impaired function of the locomotor system. Because we can define its purpose (treatment of blockage) it serves to show that methods of reflex therapy are more effective if we know exactly on which type of lesion they act, and that they are improperly used if this is not known. This is fundamental to our approach, and it should be applied to all other methods of reflex therapy.

History

It might be as well to say something of the history of manipulative therapy in order to explain the anomalous position it holds in present-day medicine. I will also consider its prospects and take the opportunity to warn against some of the worst pitfalls.

It seems that some forms of manipulative therapy are as old as the history of mankind, and it was and is to this day part of folk healing in Europe and elsewhere in the world. However, it is noteworthy that the father of European medicine, Hippocrates, saw 'rhachiotherapy' as one of the cornerstones of medicine, on a par with surgery and drug therapy. According to Waerland (1950), Hippocrates repeatedly pointed out the importance of knowing all about the spinal column, since so many disorders are related to it. Hippocrates is quoted as saying that manipulation of the spinal column was an old art, and that he thought highly of those who first discovered its importance and who would follow him in furthering the art of natural healing. Writing about articulations, Hippocrates described 'pararthremata', similar to slight dislocation or subluxation, in which the vertebrae are only slightly shifted, and went on to say that the 'eyes and hands of the experienced physician should not miss anything which could be helpful in adjusting the shifted vertebra without harming the patient . . . if treatment is performed *lege artis*, the patient can come to no harm'.

There are numerous relief carvings and other illustrations showing manipulative therapy and traction as performed in classical antiquity. The patient was usually prone on a specially constructed table while traction was applied to both the head and the feet. The physician then dealt with a specific vertebra. Galen, too, knew that nerves originated from the spinal column and could be damaged at this site, as we see from the description of his treatment of the philosopher Pausanius. But while treatment with herbs developed into modern pharmacotherapy, and surgery became the field of specialized practitioners, manipulation remained unchanged throughout the centuries. In England the layman performing manipulations was a 'bonesetter'; in France he was '*le raboteur*'.

The first important school teaching manipulation on a professional basis in modern times was the osteopathic school founded by Andrew Still (born 1824); he served as a surgeon in the American Civil War and then worked as a general practitioner. He founded his school in Kirksville in 1897, and trained lay manipulators. Initially, courses at the school lasted for 2 years, but later the curriculum was extended to 4 years, in line with medical schools, and is now the same length as that of study in university faculties of medicine. For a long time osteopathic schools were private institutions, but in recent years Colleges of Osteopathic Medicine have been established at some American universities, the first being that of the Michigan State University at East Lansing. In addition to osteopathic techniques these colleges give full medical training and graduates are recognized in most of the states of the USA as DO (doctor of osteopathy) by the state administration; this entitles them to carry on medical practice.

Soon after Still founded his osteopathic school, a grocer (D. D. Palmer) founded a school of 'chiropractic'. Born in 1845, he founded his Palmer College of Chiropractic in 1905; his son B. J. Palmer wrote that it was a 'business' where chiropractors were trained. At first the courses were very short indeed – only a fortnight – but the fee was 500 dollars! By 1911 courses lasted 1 year, and now American chiropractic schools also give their students a 4-year course of training.

There are important differences between osteopaths and chiropractors. While the former would like to become integrated into the medical establishment, chiropractors remain a lay sect at variance with official medicine. They maintain their hostility to drug treatment and to surgery. While osteopathy tries to explain the effects its practitioners achieve in accordance with modern medical theory, chiropractors still cling to the 'subluxation' theory, and talk of the 'impingement of the spinal nerves' in the intervertebral foramina, which are freed by manipulation. Even their technique is cruder, using mainly high-velocity thrusts without any of the gentler mobilization techniques.

There is, however, one important point that osteopathy and chiropractic have in common: both are taught in institutions outside the medical faculties, which are apt to perpetuate the great rift between the medical profession and these schools of 'manipulative medicine'. For about a century dialogue was practically impossible, and it is still difficult today. To quote a typical example: 'Chiropractic flourishes where ignorance prevails. Chiropractic will disappear because its time has come. Chiropractic defies logic and common sense . . . . Testimonials are but hypnotic multiples of zero in an empty vacuum . . . .' (Angrist, 1973). Needless to say, such attitudes do more harm to official medicine than to osteopathy or chiropractic, as is borne out by the ever-growing numbers of DOs and DCs in the USA, which now run into tens of thousands. The medical profession thus deprives itself of a very effective tool of therapy as well as of diagnosis, and even of an important field of medical research.

The development of modern medicine in Europe, in particular, has shown that this uncompromisingly negative attitude to manipulation is not shared by the whole of the medical profession. The discovery of the mechanical role of disc prolapse in root syndromes made doctors aware of the possibilities of traction and even of other methods of mechanical treatment, including manipulation. In this way a somewhat paradoxical situation developed: while the osteopaths and chiropractors, who were regarded by the medical profession as quacks, were elaborating sophisticated manipulation techniques, qualified doctors began to use very crude methods of manipulation, even employing anaesthesia.

It is no coincidence that the first medical men who devoted themselves to the art of manipulation were Europeans. One of the first was a Swiss doctor, Naegeli, who used very effective traction manipulation on the cervical spine which was particularly effective in the treatment of headache. His book *Nervenleiden und Nervenschmerzen* (1903, republished 1954, 1979) makes good reading to this day. The most important pioneer of medical manipulation, however, was Mennell, an outspoken protagonist of osteopathic techniques which he also taught, mainly to physiotherapists. It is in a way paradoxical that his famous disciple Cyriax, whose *Orthopaedic Medicine* remains the classic textbook for clinical assessment of motor function, did not follow his predecessor in developing these techniques further.

This gap was later filled by Stoddard, a DO who also graduated in medicine and whose *Manual of Osteopathic Techniques* remains the classic in its field. The London College of Osteopathy (now the London College of Osteopathic Medicine) was the first institution where osteopathic techniques were taught to qualified doctors, originally by osteopaths. Graduates of this College have played an important role in the development of manipulative medicine throughout Europe and particularly in France, where Maigne is the most prominent. Working under De Sèze he succeeded in giving courses in manipulation at the Medical Faculty of the University of Paris, attended by medical practitioners (mainly specialists in physical medicine) but not by physiotherapists.

At the same time, i.e. shortly after 1945, a group of German doctors became interested in manipulation, mainly under the influence of American-trained chiropractors (Illi and Sandberg). Unlike Maigne, these were mainly doctors in private practice; in the early fifties two groups were formed with the aim of promoting and teaching manipulation (exclusively to doctors): the MWE headed by Sell and the FAC with Biedermann, Cramer, Gutmann and H.-D. Wolff. Unlike France and Great Britain, where courses for doctors lasted months or even a year, in Germany doctors were given weekly courses at intervals, arranged in a series of at first 4 and later 8 separate weeks. With this system it has been possible to teach manipulation techniques to far more doctors in Germany, and also in Switzerland, Austria, Holland and Scandinavia. Their numbers run into hundreds. Meanwhile the two German groups united to found the German Association of Manual Medicine, and similar associations have been formed in other countries.

Unlike the USA, where manipulation developed outside the medical profession and aroused a predominantly hostile reaction which is only slowly being overcome, in many countries of Western Europe important groups of medical men have promoted the idea that manipulation should be performed by qualified doctors only. With the exception of Maigne in France they have not, however, succeeded in adding manipulative techniques to the medical curriculum at universities and teaching hospitals. They thus belong to what we may call 'unofficial' trends in medicine; manipulation remains rather an 'outsider's' method, despite the support of some renowned German professors (Nonnenbruch, Gutzeit, Zuckschwerdt, Junghanns, Schuler and others).

The development of manipulative medicine in some of the socialist countries has followed different lines. The first country where manipulation was used and taught on a large scale was Czechoslovakia, where the model that was created has since been adopted by East Germany, Bulgaria, Poland and Hungary. For obvious reasons a cleavage between lay and professional medicine, or between an 'outsider' and an 'official' school of thought, is not likely to develop in an exclusively State-run medical service. Professor Henner encouraged the interest of some members of his staff at the Neurological Clinic of Prague University in the broad field of rehabilitation of the locomotor system, and in the potentialities of 'unconventional' methods, among them manipulation. Švehla, Obrda, Starý, Miřatský, Jirout and the present author, and later Janda and Véle, worked on these lines. Here the impulse came from one of the most prominent university hospitals in the country, and it is in Czechoslovakia that major team-work in research in this field is continuously in progress.

Once the effectiveness and economy of manipulative medicine was recognized, the Czechoslovak Ministry of Health decided to incorporate it in the curriculum of the Institutes of Postgraduate Training which run refresher courses for specialists in all fields of medicine. Doctors are thus trained in each of the provinces, the 'teachers' receiving additional preparation. The policy aims at providing manipulative treatment throughout the State health service. Teaching began in Czechoslovakia in 1961, and on the same lines in East Germany in 1965, in Bulgaria in 1971 and in Poland in 1974 (three courses of 2 weeks each, at 6-month intervals).

There is another striking feature of the development of manipulative medicine in Czechoslovakia – it remains closely bound up with rehabilitation of the locomotor system, in particular with techniques of remedial exercise. As the simpler chiropractic techniques based exclusively on high-velocity thrusts were gradually superseded by gentler osteopathic techniques, and as these were in turn greatly improved in the seventies by the addition of neuromuscular facilitation and inhibition techniques, it became obvious that team-work by qualified doctors together with trained physiotherapists was a practical necessity for maximum effectiveness. Therefore, with the exception of high-velocity thrusts, manipulative techniques are now being taught ever more widely to physiotherapists, who work with doctors.

As in other fields of medicine, doctors in different countries who were interested in manipulation began to work together. The first international meeting took place in Switzerland in 1958. At the next meeting, in Nice in 1962, it was decided to form an international body; this came about in 1965, when the International Federation of Manual Medicine (FIMM) was founded in London, with Terrier of Switzerland as the first President. At present there are 21 national associations affiliated to FIMM, mainly from Europe. However, co-operation with American osteopaths has been growing since 1977, when the Fifth Congress of FIMM was held in Copenhagen.

The harmful effects of leaving manipulation entirely in the hands of non-medical practitioners were only too obvious, and naturally enough, doctors interested in manipulative therapy on the Continent jealously tried to keep the monopoly for the profession. They have only been partially successful in getting manipulative techniques accepted by the profession as a whole, so that they could be taught in medical faculties and teaching hospitals. Very often manipulation has remained an outsider's method, although there are leading universities where it is taught and countries where it is recognized as a part of postgraduate medical specialization, with a view to creating a more comprehensive medical service. As manipulation concerns mainly the locomotor system, such a service is most appropriately accommodated within specialities like Physical Medicine and Rehabilitation. The vast number of patients who can be effectively treated by these methods makes it imperative that such a service should be organised on the basis of team-work between doctors and physiotherapists.

2

Theoretical considerations

abandoned: morally unrestrained.

Morphological aspects

Chapter 1 showed clearly that manipulation and most of the methods of reflex therapy are used in a vast number of cases of pain in the locomotor system, including back pain, even though the cause and therefore the therapy remain *clash of* controversial. For a long time these pains were generally considered to be of *opposing view* inflammatory origin, for the simple reason that this aetiology could best explain the main symptom, the pain itself. For the same reason they were sometimes called 'rheumatic pains'. The many terms ending in '-itis' bear witness to this attitude (spondylitis, arthritis, radiculitis, neuritis, fibrositis, myositis, panniculitis, etc.) as does 'soft-tissue rheumatism'. Since, however, inflammation is a well-defined pathological condition, it has to be proved – or disproved – by the objective methods of pathological anatomy, and this in the long run was fatal for the inflammation theory. It had to be abandoned for lack of evidence. → *outward sign.*

Pathological anatomy and 'pathology *in vivo*' (X-rays) generously compensated clinicians for the loss of this simple theory by demonstrating in abundance what are called 'degenerative changes'. Instead of terms ending in '-itis' we were then *vis-* offered spondylosis, arthrosis, 'discopathy' and the like. There were apparently *a* even theoretical reasons for degeneration, in particular of the disc: its vascularization is reduced early in the ontogenesis and its water content decreases rather rapidly during the first three decades of life (from 90 per cent to 70 per cent). According to Schmorland Junghanns (1953), 60 per cent of women and 80 per cent of men show evidence of degenerative changes at 50 while by the age of 70 the figure is 95 per cent for both sexes. No wonder that under the dominating influence of the pathological anatomist the term 'degenerative disease' is frequently heard.

It is, however, the very abundance of what are called 'degenerative changes' that makes it difficult to define their relation to pain. Degenerative changes increase with age, but back pain, in particular, occurs most often between the fourth and sixth decade, to become less common in old age. Not only do we find subjects in perfect health but showing considerable degenerative changes; a person with these changes *and* severe pain may recover completely from the latter, while his degenerative changes continue to increase with advancing age. On the other hand, there can be severe pain symptoms in young patients with no degenerative changes at all. Even more important, the significance of what are known as degenerative changes appears to be very ill defined. On the one hand there are destructive lesions in extremity joints, e.g. coxarthrosis and gonarthrosis, whose great clinical significance nobody will doubt. On the other hand there are changes that probably correspond to what may be called inevitable 'wear and tear'; then again there may be merely a compensatory process, or adaptation, as in scoliosis and hypermobility. In spondylolisthesis a big osteophyte may give the spinal column better stability than an orthopaedic operation. Changes resulting from trauma can be very similar to what is otherwise termed degenerative. One should therefore ask specifically in each case of degenerative change whether this change is relevant or not. It is therefore ill advised to draw clinical conclusions from the mere existence of degenerative changes in an X-ray picture.

There is, however, some correlation between degenerative change and disc prolapse which may be of clinical importance, for with a few exceptions prolapse occurs mainly in discs already showing some degenerative change. The discovery that disc prolapse could cause root syndromes was undoubtedly a landmark. It made the medical public aware of the importance of the spinal column and of the possibility of mechanical disturbance there. On the other hand, the striking success of surgical treatment meant that for some time disc lesions and disc prolapse were held responsible for almost every disturbance related to the spinal column. The reasoning was straightforward: if root compression in the lower lumbar region was found to be due to disc prolapse, then lumbago which is prior to root compression is likely to have the same cause. If root compression in the lumbar region is due to the disc, the same should apply to the cervical spine, and by analogy to neck pain; and as neck pain is frequently associated with headache, root compression may even be the cause of cervical headache. 'Discopathy' was the fashionable word then, not vertebrogenic or spondylogenic disease.

Surgical practice soon corrected this view, though by default. While disc surgery for lumbar root syndromes became a routine procedure, it remained the exception in simple lumbago, as well as in cervical root syndromes, and is practically never used in the treatment of pain in the neck or other non-radicular cervical syndromes. Nor can disc prolapse be the only cause of root syndromes in the lumbar region: in operation statistics no disc herniation is found in about 10 per cent of the cases; the large majority of root syndromes resolve without operation, and this is true even of cases with typical findings at myelography. If in such cases the X-ray is repeated after clinical recovery (and the myelography is made with non-resorbable contrast oil), it has repeatedly been found that the disc prolapse remains unchanged, just as it was at the time of maximum pain. Reviewing these morphological changes that are usually related to back pain and associated conditions, we can readily see that they do not explain the complaints of the vast majority of our patients. This is also the reason why this type of patient is sometimes vaguely described as suffering from 'back pain' or just 'pain without any pathology' or even 'without any diagnosis' (Jayson's (1970) 'non-specific back pain'); in view of the numerical importance of this group of patients this is little to the credit of clinical medicine.

Theoretical implications of manipulation

If manipulative treatment is successful it usually produces immediate relief of pain. We may therefore infer that an understanding of how manipulation works will give us some clues as to what causes pain in the locomotor system when there is no definite pathology.

The first, naïve explanation of manipulative therapy was 're-positioning', and therefore something like a dislocation or 'subluxation' has to be assumed. This 'theory' is held by chiropractors to this day; Still must have believed in it, as did Hippocrates, and probably all lay manipulators down the ages – just 'putting right something that was out of place'. In fact, if a patient with an acute wry neck or lumbago, unable to straighten up, is successfully manipulated so that he immediately stands erect, there is little wonder that something like 're-positioning' seemed the likely explanation. The reason why this theory has been abandoned by physicians as well as by modern osteopaths, is that with few exceptions neither dislocation ('malalignment', 'subluxation') nor re-positioning ('adjustment') after manipulation can be proved. One of the merits of routine X-ray examination is that the subluxation theory has had to be given up for lack of evidence.

Fascination with the disc also provided an explanation for the effect of manipulation (Cyriax, 1977; Maigne, 1968; Stoddard, 1961) although it is difficult to see how manipulation could achieve re-positioning of a prolapse whose exact position cannot be known. The great weakness of this approach is that manipulation is not applied only to the spinal column; it is also effective in the treatment of extremity joints, and particularly so at the craniocervical junction, on the ribs and at the sacroiliac joint, where there is no question of discs. Clinical experience also shows quite clearly that manipulation is most effective in conditions where we do *not* expect to find disc lesions, and least effective in true disc prolapse.

The sophisticated diagnostic techniques developed by the osteopaths have provided what we believe to be relevant clinical evidence of how manipulation really works: we apply manipulation where we find signs of movement restriction, whether in an extremity joint, a rib, or a vertebral movement segment, and if manipulation is successful, mobility is always restored. In other words, manipulation does not achieve a change of structure, as Still thought, but normalization of *function*. This is even true in cases of wry neck or acute lumbago: the crooked position of the neck or the back in such cases is itself physiological, and it is only the fact that the patient is *fixed* in this position (head rotation plus inclination in wry neck) that is pathological. Manipulation merely frees mobility and thus enables the patient to *return* to the neutral position. In this, wry neck and lumbago are the exception to the rule; in the vast majority of cases movement restriction is found where joints are in the neutral position and there is difficulty in proceeding through the whole range of movement.

Functional aspects

The most important theoretical inference from clinical experience with manipulation can be formulated thus: if one applies manipulation only after adequate clinical examination of mobility and is careful to re-examine after treatment, then one regularly finds that successful manipulation achieves normalization of restricted motor function, and that this goes hand in hand with relief of symptoms. This theoretical inference should then logically be valid not only for passive mobility, but also for active muscle function. We owe to Janda (1967) the proof that this is true in particular for faulty motor patterns (motor stereotypes) producing overstrain in the motor system. This is in keeping with the simple observation that excessive strain causes symptoms, whatever the cause of the strain.

In addition to active motor patterns there is another important function whose disturbance frequently causes symptoms: this is body statics. In fact, in modern society static overstrain may be at least as frequent as faulty mobility, and again we find that correction of faulty statics frequently brings relief. Thus manipulation pioneered our involvement with faulty functioning of the locomotor system and with its normalization, as we shall see throughout this book. Indeed, faulty function *alone* is the cause of frequent symptoms; this can be shown in children. Morphological changes, on the other hand, do not exclude changes in function. This is particularly true for disc lesions and may explain spontaneous recovery and recovery after conservative treatment (including manipulation). This is of great importance for rehabilitation in traumatology, where our primary aim is to improve function *despite* morphological changes, in order to achieve compensation.

As will be shown later, function and its disturbances are rarely confined to one site or structure, and therefore diagnosis must take in the locomotor system as a whole. The term 'vertebrogenic' or 'spondylogenic' is thus no longer appropriate, as even in back pain we must take into account muscle function and its nervous control as well as the function of the pelvis and the extremities. As 'vertebrogenic' diseases or lesions include such well-defined pathological conditions as ankylosing spondylitis or osteoporosis, the decisive criterion for the application of manipulation and other measures aimed at restoring function is whether the patient's complaint is due (mainly or exclusively) to changes of function, or to changes of structure (pathology).

This is a more difficult matter than it may seem: it requires a systematic assessment and a technique of examination that has not yet been formulated. It is the great weakness of manipulative therapy, remedial exercise, etc. – methods concerned with improving the functioning of the motor system – that they have been and for the most part still are mainly concerned with therapy and far too little with clinical diagnosis of the conditions they are supposed to remedy. This is perhaps the main reason for the paradox that in many fields of medicine the importance of changes in function is now well recognized; whereas in the motor system, where function is paramount, this fundamental aspect is rarely considered. However, the functioning of the locomotor system is extremely complex, as we shall see, and diagnosis of disturbed function is a highly sophisticated proceeding carried out, as it were, in a clinical no man's land. There is an additional disadvantage in that it can only be investigated by clinical methods, for the most part, and these are at present regarded as 'subjective', while 'modern' research puts its faith mainly in the laboratory.

The clinical phenomenon of segmental movement restriction

We may now turn back to the intervertebral motor segment and disturbances in its functioning (*Figure 2.1*). These consist in (1) hypermobility and (2) movement restriction; obviously manipulative therapy is concerned only with the latter. The principal (clinical) characteristics are of the utmost importance; they include changes in quantity as well as in quality, of which the former – taking the form of restricted mobility – is certainly the more straightforward. It is easily diagnosed in an extremity joint, while diagnosis of restriction is much more difficult in a single motor segment of the spinal column. Changes in *quality* are therefore of great diagnostic value. They take the form of increased resistance during movement (Stoddard's 'binding'); the most striking change is probably the lack of springing in the end position of a restricted joint or motor segment: in a normal joint the extreme position is never reached abruptly, and a slight increase of pressure

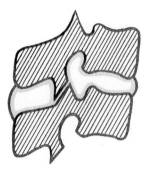

Figure 2.1 The mobile segment (After Junghans, 1955.)

increases the range of movement. There is thus no absolute limit. In a joint with restricted mobility, this springing or giving way has been lost, and we come up abruptly against a barrier. This has given rise to the term 'blocking', or blockage. This is perhaps the most easily diagnosed sign.

Joint play and movement restriction

There are two types of passive mobility that are affected by movement restriction (blocking); the first is 'functional movement', i.e. movement carried out by the subject. Joint play is passive movement, which cannot be carried out by the subject. It comprises a shifting or sliding movement of one joint surface against the other, or even rotation, and also distraction (*Figure 2.2*). Thus we can actively flex, extend or side-bend a finger, whereas passively it may be shifted against the metacarpal in any direction, rotated, or distracted by axial pull. These movements are not only felt, but can be demonstrated by X-ray (including distraction, *Figure 2.2*). Joint play is by no means of academic interest only; its practical clinical importance lies (1) in that it shows blockage at a stage when functional mobility is still normal, which is particularly valuable if we use springing techniques; and (2) in that, as is well illustrated by Mennell's diagram (*Figure 2.3*), these shifting movements as well as distraction are a most effective and gentle way of restoring normal mobility (*Figure 2.4*). It can thus be clinically inferred that normal joint play is the prerequisite of normal joint movement; its disturbance can be likened to a drawer that has stuck, and needs to be eased out.

Movement restriction and reflex changes

Blockage in an articulation and particularly in a vertebral motor segment goes hand in hand with reflex changes mainly in the same spinal segment. These affect the dermatome as well as the muscles, etc. Korr (1975) coined the term 'segmental

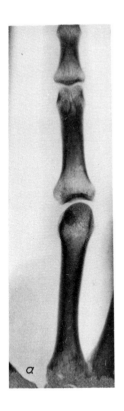
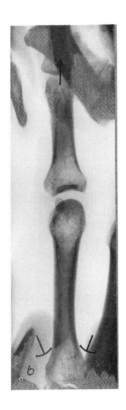

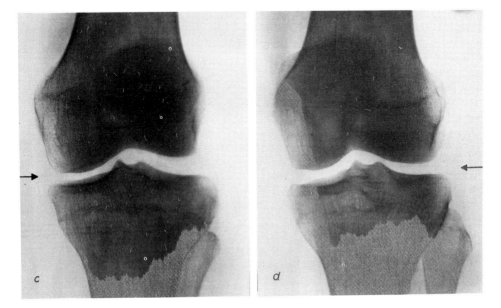

Figure 2.2 Joint play in the knee joint, visualized by X-ray (medial and lateral gapping of the joint)

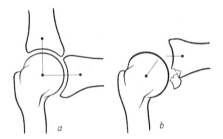

Figure 2.3 Importance of joint play. (*a*) Gliding movement is essential for joint function; if gliding is disturbed (*b*), forceful movement may injure the joint

facilitation'. In movement restriction, muscular tension or spasm is most important, because it may fix the joint and may be a very significant factor causing restriction; this can readily be seen from a positive straight leg raising test. The same goes for the typical antalgesic posture in acute root syndromes, when anteflexion and side-bending of the whole lumbar spine prevent any attempt by the patient to straighten up.

To quote Korr (1975), who has devoted most of his work to the implications of manipulative therapy: 'While usually thinking of muscles as the motors of the body, producing motion by their contraction, it is important to remember that the same contractile forces are also used to *oppose* motion . . . . It is therefore proposed that it is in its capacity as a brake that a muscle may become a major and highly variable impediment to mobility of a lesioned "joint".' After giving a thorough explanation of the role of the muscle spindle and the gamma system, Korr goes on: 'The high gain hypothesis is consistent with, and offers an explanation for, the steeply rising resistance to motion ("bind") in one direction . . . . They [the muscles] would also be provoked into stronger and stronger contraction by the exaggerated spindle discharges as motions that tend to lengthen the affected muscles occur.' To put it briefly, the phenomena found clinically in movement restriction might be explained not by the structure that is usually held responsible for passive mobility, i.e. the joint, but by the organ of active movement, the muscle. That is why osteopaths do

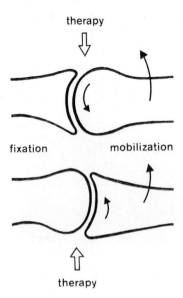

therapy

fixation   mobilization

therapy

Figure 2.4 The direction of gliding movement and joint mobilization, showing how this depends on whether the proximal or distal partner is concave or convex (After Kaltenborn, 1976.)

not use the term 'blockage' for movement restriction, but so as not to commit themselves speak of 'osteopathic lesions', or more recently of 'somatic dysfunction' (Greenman, 1978).

The role of shortened muscles in movement restriction has been demonstrated by Janda (1967). Muscle relaxation techniques are widely used in order to mobilize joints. The question must therefore be put: what is the role of the joint in passive movement restriction?

Blockage as an articular phenomenon

The naïve conception that passive movement is entirely or mainly an articular phenomenon has evidently to be dropped. In fact, as Korr has shown, most clinical phenomena by which we recognize movement restriction in a joint or vertebral motor segment might be explained by muscle activity induced by the muscle proprioceptors and the gamma system. What evidence remains to show that the joint plays a role of any importance?

There is one evident weakness in the purely 'muscular' theory: it does not explain what stimulates the receptors; in other words, if muscle activity is a reflex response, which nobody doubts, where does the stimulus come from? The purely empirical techniques of manipulation are based on joint anatomy. It is surprising that osteopaths, who are the originators of most of these very carefully worked out and exactly taught techniques, appear very little aware of their theoretical implications. More indirect evidence lies in the importance of joint play as a prerequisite of normal joint function: there is no doubt that muscles have a far stronger, direct influence on functional movement which is in fact induced by muscles and can for the same reason be inhibited by muscles, than on the movements of joint play. If therefore the muscular factor was the decisive one, functional movement would be affected first, and not joint play. We know, however, that the reverse is the case. Further evidence comes from analysis of the high-velocity thrust techniques producing gapping of the joint surfaces, together with a popping sound, or 'click'. There are distraction high-velocity thrusts which cause hardly any distension of the muscles, the joint remaining in the neutral position, and the click itself is certainly an articular phenomenon. But there is even direct evidence:

1. There are three joints that are not moved by muscles, nor can their movement be opposed by them: these are the sacroiliac, the acromioclavicular and the tibiofibular joints. Yet these joints show typical signs of blockage and their treatment by manipulation is particularly effective.
2. In order to prove (or disprove) the role of the articulation we made the following experiment: in 10 patients the cervical spine was examined prior to operation (mainly abdominal surgery) and re-examined under anaesthesia with myorelaxants and intubation with artificial respiration. In all cases movement restriction remained unchanged and was even more easily recognizable during narcosis, as the patient was completely relaxed.

Possible mechanism of joint blockage and manipulation

The importance of the experiment just referred to lies not only in proving that movement restriction is an articular phenomenon, but also in that it proved that we have to deal with a mechanical obstacle in the joint. It was Emminger (1967) who first suggested that such an obstacle might be attributed to the meniscoids previously described by Töndury (1948) in intervertebral joints, and later found by Kos (1968) even in extremity joints; the meniscoids may get caught between the moving joint facets. Indeed most joints have very incongruous facets and smooth mobility is possible only if some additional tissue can fill the redundant space. To do this the meniscoid must move freely between the joint facets, and may meet with difficulties. Kos and Wolf (1972) have further elaborated this theory, showing why the mechanism is easily disturbed: (1) the meniscoid has a soft base and a hard edge, which cannot be easily compressed; (2) joint cartilage is hard and elastic only if the force that acts on it does so rapidly. If, however, we subject the cartilage to constant pressure, it adapts to the material exerting that pressure as though it were fluid. If, therefore, the meniscoid is caught between the gliding surfaces of the joint facets, the hard edge produces a cavity in the cartilage and is trapped in it (*Figure 2.5*).

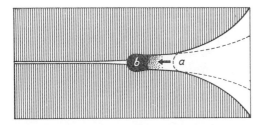

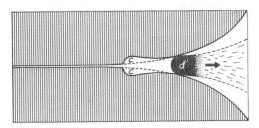

Figure 2.5 Entrapment of a meniscoid at the edge of a joint space, according to the joint blockage theory of Wolf (1975). Top, the meniscoid normally lying in position (a) has moved between the joint facets and its hard edge has impinged (b); bottom, it has returned to normal position after treatment. A groove (c–d) remains for a short time, but being flat it offers only minor resistance to slipping back

The implications for the theory of manipulation are clear: if we separate the joint facets by high-velocity thrust techniques, the meniscoid can slip out. *Figure 2.5* shows that the trapped edge of the meniscoid has only a very slight resistance to overcome, consisting of two very shallow grooves that open smoothly into the wedge-shaped space between the cartilage surfaces. In repetitive mobilization a back-and-forth movement takes place, meeting greater resistance in the direction of incarceration that in that of liberation. After the last resistance has been gradually overcome, the meniscoid slips back into its original position. *Figure 2.6* also illustrates how resistance becomes less with each movement that increases the space between the dotted lines.

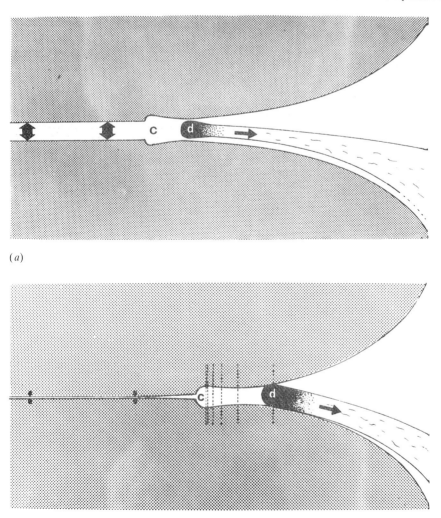

(a)

(b)

Figure 2.6 The effect of therapy. (*a*) Gapping of the joint by high-velocity thrust, making it possible for the meniscoid to slip back. (*b*) Repetitive mobilization enabling the meniscoid to move back into its original position, first by small degrees and then more rapidly

The effect of manipulation

The effect of successful manipulation is two-fold: (1) it restores mobility, including joint play; and (2) it has a very intense reflex effect upon all structures where changes have been found prior to manipulation. This is most striking in the musculature, where increased tension (spasm) is followed by hypotonia. But the skin in the corresponding dermatomes, too, is more easily folded and more easily stretched. There are also, frequently, palpable changes at periosteal points. In all these structures tissue tension diminishes. The effect is not, however, limited only to one segment. According to the importance of the vertebral motor segment concerned, or the joint, the effect spreads to neighbouring motor segments or even to distant ones, as we shall see later. All these changes can and should be assessed clinically, and can also be shown by physiological methods (*see Figures 2.7–2.9, 4.23*).

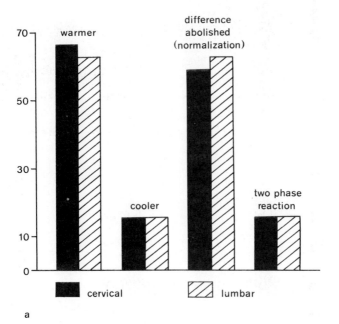

a

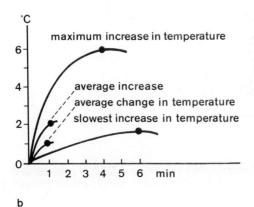

b

Figure 2.7 Changes in skin temperature after traction therapy in root syndromes. (*a*) The statistics for various types of reaction. (*b*) The course of the reaction expressed as a curve

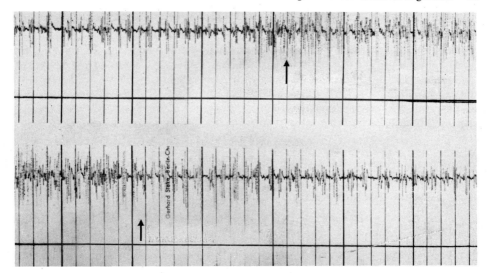

Figure 2.8 Electromyogram showing an increase in muscle activity (force) in the triceps brachia during cervical traction

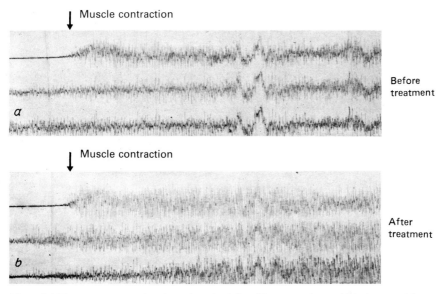

Figure 2.9 Electromyogram taken from three leads in a C8 root syndrome (*a*) before and (*b*) after cervical manipulation

Probable causes of blockage in vertebral motor segments

Faulty movement patterns

In the preceding paragraph I pointed out the effect of blockage of one motor segment on the neighbouring or even distant parts of the spinal column. In fact, blockage in one segment can be caused by blockage in another which has altered the functioning of the spinal column as a whole. This is an important feature of disturbed function in the locomotor system: it rarely remains localized to one region or one structure. The most important factor in spinal and locomotor function is obviously the musculature and its nervous control. This control is expressed by motor patterns and posture, formed in a highly characteristic way in every individual. As Janda has shown (1967), there is a certain balance between various muscle groups (*see* page 33f) that move joints or vertebral motor segments, and if this balance is disturbed the normal functioning of the joint suffers. Modern civilization brings with it very one-sided, forced movements, causing muscular imbalance, and this is no less true of posture – in fact, one of the characteristic features of modern life is lack of movement accompanying static or postural overstrain. Therefore the *first* and most frequent cause of blockage is a faulty movement pattern due to muscular imbalance and postural overstrain.

Trauma

The second cause of disturbed locomotor function is trauma. It is important to point out that there are border-line cases between this group and that of faulty movement patterns, because it is not always easy to say what is and what is not an injury for the spinal column. Usually trauma is defined as an exogenous force acting on the body for a short time and capable of damaging structure or function. Even under normal conditions the forces acting on the spinal column are considerable. If these forces are suddenly increased because of sharp, ill-balanced movement, the line between the two groups of causes appears to be rather arbitrarily drawn.

Reflex action

Blockage may be of reflex origin due to changes in a segment. As said in Chapter 1, the spinal column is involved in disease wherever it occurs in the organism. Visceral disease causing nociceptive stimuli is followed by reflex spasm in the relevant segment (muscular defence) and in particular in the deep layers of the erector spinae muscle. This is likely to fix the vertebral motor segment as well as to interfere with normal mobility of the trunk. If such a spasm is of sufficiently long duration, blockage is likely to occur. Hansen and Schliack (1962) describe characteristic scoliosis in visceral disease. As will be shown in Chapter 7 (page 336), we recognize a number of characteristic 'spinal patterns' in visceral disease, showing that there are certain pathogenetic rules. A striking feature of this type of blockage is its recurrence if the internal disease relapses or exacerbates. In fact, we seem to know more about visceral influence upon the spinal column than about the influence of the spinal column on visceral disease.

The spinal column and its function

Three types of function performed by the spine appear to be particularly pertinent:

1. Giving support and protection.
2. Being the motor axis of the body.
3. Maintaining equilibrium (body statics).

Motor and protective function

Obviously, there is an inherent antinomy between the first two basic functions; as Gutmann (1981) put it: 'The spinal column should be as mobile as possible and as firm as necessary'. If we consider the remarkable mobility of the craniocervical junction in all planes and its relation to the vital centres of the medulla, we can see the complexity of the question. It is easily understood that if motor function is disturbed, this also affects the protective function of the spine. Faulty functioning causes tension which is a stimulus for the receptors producing muscle spasm, which in turn may interfere with nerve structures originating in the spinal column; hypermobility may be a strain even for the structures inside ᵗhe vertebral canal.

The role of balance – the spinal column as a functional unit

The role of the spinal column in the maintenance of balance is usually underrated. Its importance here is largely due to the role of the craniocervical junction, the site of the deep neck reflexes. It is important to remember that under normal conditions the labyrinth is not necessary for the maintenance of equilibrium, while proprioception is. Thus it is no coincidence that vertigo and dizziness are very frequently of cervical origin (*see* Chapter 7) and can be effectively treated by manipulation, whereas auditory disturbances are not as a rule related to cervical lesions, although the labyrinth and the cochlea are supplied by the vertebral artery and the vertebral nerve. There is strong evidence that the great importance of the craniocervical junction for equilibrium lies in the proprioceptors originating in this region. Not only are there important papers in the physiological literature (Frederickson *et al.*, 1976; McCouch, Deering and Ling, 1951) demonstrating the importance of afferents from spinal proprioceptors but there is also direct clinical evidence of cervical nystagmus provided by authors using Greiner's chair. This chair rotates the experimental subject (patient) rhythmically from right to left and back again, while the head remains fixed, in this way stimulating exclusively the cervical proprioceptors while the labyrinth and the eyes are protected from stimulation (Greiner *et al.*, 1967; Moser, 1974; Norré, Stevens and Degeyter, 1976; Simon *et al.*, 1975).

However important the craniocervical junction, proprioceptors are active throughout the spinal column, as Komendatov (1945) has shown in rabbits: on side-bending of the trunk with the head fixed, the eyes move in the opposite direction from the trunk. On side-bending of the head and trunk in opposite directions, neck and trunk reflexes compete, and as a rule the neck reflexes are the stronger. The degree of side-bending also plays a part, however, and these reflexes apparently enable the animal to keep the visual field constant during locomotion; they are therefore very fast: changes in the activity of the eye muscles were registered at a rate as high as 200 side-bends per minute.

I have quoted these experiments in some detail because they show how rapidly certain changes in one part of the body axis are felt at the far end of the body. In man, with his vertical axis, the position of the head is held constant by the plane of the eyes (the visual field), and every change in the position of the pelvis as he walks must immediately be compensated if equilibrium is not to suffer. This is clearly seen if the subject is told to mark time before an X-ray screen. Therefore any disturbance of even a single motor segment may cause important changes throughout the vertebral column. Ushio *et al.* (1973) have shown the deleterious effect of lumbago on vertiginous patients and by laboratory methods proved the good effect of immobilization of the lumbar spine.

In a paper read recently (Potsdam, 1984) I showed that in a group of 106 patients examined on two scales over 5 months, 50 cases where the weight distribution showed a difference of 5 kg or over also had (a) a positive Hautant's test in at least one head position, and (b) movement restriction in the craniocervical junction 49 times; there were only 5 cases without any restriction. Of the 56 cases with a difference in weight distribution of up to 4 kg only 5 had a positive Hautant's test; there was movement restriction in the craniocervical junction 24 times, and normal conditions 41 times.

Not all vertebral segments have the same importance for the functioning of the spinal column, however, and of the motor system as a whole. We therefore speak of 'key segments' or 'key regions'. These are mostly transition areas where the function of the spinal column changes: the two ends of the column, the craniocervical (1) and the lumbosacral (2); and then the cervicothoracic (3) and the thoracolumbar (4) junctions.

1. The craniocervical junction shows extensive mobility in all three planes and balances the heavy head on the fragile cervical spine. Physiologically, this is the site of the tonic neck reflexes, and influences muscle tone throughout the postural trunk musculature. If function here is disturbed, there is most frequently hypertonus of the postural muscles, disturbances of equilibrium and locomotor deficit which has to be compensated by the cervical spine. This is most important for rotation, as only the atlantoaxial joint is ideally adapted for rotation, and the rest of the cervical spine is thus forced to take over a function for which it is poorly fitted.
2. The lumbosacroiliac junction forms the base of the spinal column and therefore determines body statics. At the same time it transmits movement from the legs to the spinal column and acts as a shock absorber.
3. The cervicothoracic junction is the region in which the most mobile section of the spinal column is joined to the relatively rigid thoracic spine and where the powerful muscles of the upper extremities and shoulder girdle insert.
4. The great strain on the thoracolumbar junction is well seen in the transition vertebra T12, where the upper apophyseal joints retain the thoracic pattern while the lower joints have the lumbar pattern, i.e. where one type of function changes abruptly to another. If during walking the pelvis tilts from one side to the other, the lumbar spine side-bends so that the scoliotic curve is broadest at the level of L3, the thoracolumbar junction remaining in line with the sacrum; this, too, can be seen if the subject marks time before an X-ray screen. Disturbance of function causes intense spasm not only of back muscles, but in particular of the psoas muscle (Kubis, 1969); this is of great clinical importance.

In view of their importance and their great vulnerability, these key regions are usually the place where the spinal column suffers first, as can best be observed in children. Disturbance of function at such points jeopardizes the functioning of the spinal column as a whole, causing secondary lesions. Therefore such a disturbance should never be overlooked even if the symptoms are manifest at the other end of the spinal column, or even in the extremities. To leave such a lesion untreated is risking therapeutic failure and relapse.

The importance of nerve control

The spinal column could not act as a functional unit unless all its reactions were co-ordinated by muscles under nerve control. We have already pointed out the role of movement patterns and their disturbance, since this is the most significant cause of blockage in a vertebral motor segment. Janda (1979) has recently shown that the quality of movement patterns varies from one individual to another, and this goes hand in hand with varying susceptibility to vertebrogenic disturbance. On the other hand, any disturbance of function in a single motor segment will have its repercussions throughout the body axis and must be compensated. Here again, nervous control plays a decisive role. This is no less the case with pain, once the lesion becomes painful, for it is the nervous system that determines how intensely the segment will react, and where the threshold of pain lies. In other words, it is the nervous system that determines whether disturbed function will manifest itself clinically. If reaction to nociceptive stimulus is intense, disturbed function in one motor segment will produce an antalgesic response and alter the normal motor pattern, hence producing fixation of a change in function.

Control by the nervous system thus has two aspects: it subserves normal function by the maintenance of correct motor patterns, and it compensates disturbed function. On the other hand, an intense and chronic painful stimulus disturbs normal motor patterns and thus may cause altered, pathological motor patterns to become fixed, thus perpetuating the disease process.

It is therefore no coincidence that disturbed function of the motor system is more likely to be found in subjects with labile nervous regulation, who are as a rule psychologically labile as well. In this connection it is of interest that Starý (1970) and Figar (1970) were able to show that patients with severe radicular syndromes very easily formed conditioned reflexes to additional pain stimuli, and that these reflexes were more difficult to extinguish than in healthy controls. Furthermore, Kunc, Starý and Šetlík (1955) showed that the mental condition of patients plays a great part in recovery after disc operation. Gutzeit (1951) found that a prominent psychological factor is characteristic for vertebrogenic pain patients. Šráček and Škrabal (1975) compared two types of mental patients: 50 cases of neurosis with signs of anxiety and depression, and 25 schizophrenics with low emotivity. Blockage, most frequently in the cervical spine, was absent in only five neurotics, but in 16 schizophrenics. The segment most frequently affected was the atlanto-occipital; the difference was significant at the $p = 0.01$ level.

Again the latest observations by Janda (1978) are of great relevance: in patients with poor motor patterns, inclined to imbalance of the muscle groups, he found (1) minor neurological disturbances which he termed 'microspasticity', in which movements were not fully co-ordinated and appeared clumsy; (2) slight sensory impairment, in particular of proprioception; (3) worse adaptation to stress situations as a result of poorly co-ordinated behaviour. All this corresponds to a (relatively) new clinical entity, minimal brain dysfunction, which is found in 10–15 per cent of the child population. Janda (1979) compared the somatic and psychological findings in these children with the findings in adult patients who had very unfavourable motor patterns that produced relapsing vertebrogenic disorders, and concluded that such children are those patients who present themselves in adult life with the principal symptom of pain, because of small neurological changes which do not disappear during adolescence but instead take the form of disturbed function of the motor system, with resulting pain.

Yet, however important motor imbalance may be, it is not identical with impaired joint function or blockage of a vertebral motor segment. Such lesions do appear even in subjects with perfect motor patterns, while they may be missing in patients with severe neurological disease. In 1420 patients with disseminated sclerosis Schaltenbrand (1938) found 22.3 per cent suffering from back ache. In our experience back ache is the rule in Parkinson's disease, understandably if we bear in mind the muscle rigidity in this condition. However, no matter how severe the neurological disorder, it is not tantamount to pain due to disturbance of a specific function of the motor system and the vertebral column, such as increased or (more frequently) restricted mobility of a joint or spinal motor segment.

Disturbance of function (blockage) in childhood

From what has been said it follows that disturbances of function may (1) by themselves cause symptoms and (2) appear much sooner than structural (morphological) changes. For this reason I have been particularly interested in disturbances of function in childhood. Schön (1956) and later Gutmann and Wolff (1959) have shown that clinical symptoms as well as changes in function visible in X-ray motion studies appear about 10 years earlier than degenerative changes.

The most typical vertebrogenic lesion in children is acute wry neck. Although it is a self-limiting affection, traction and mobilization techniques, if well applied, should give immediate relief. This is particularly true for the new techniques which utilize muscular facilitation and inhibition.

The most numerous child patients, presenting a real problem, are those who suffer from headache, the cervical spine being one of the most frequent causative sites. This is true of various types of headache, including migraine. In a group of 30 children suffering from non-migrainous headache, manipulation gave excellent results, with only two failures, while in a group of 27 children suffering from migraine there were three failures, and excellent results in 24 cases. These findings were confirmed by Kabátníková and Kabátník (1966). A particularly important type of headache in children, known as 'school headache', formerly believed to be of psychological origin, was proved by Gutmann (1968) to be due to head anteflexion during school hours, when patients were bent over horizontal desks. This was confirmed by Lewit and Kuncová (1971). One clinical manifestation of disturbed function in the lumbosacral region is dysmenorrhoea or algomenorrhoea with negative gynaecological findings in young girls, frequently starting at the menarche. Pain is usually felt in the low back and in the abdomen. Not only is this type of pain amenable to manipulative treatment; it is frequently the first sign of disturbed function in the lumbosacral region in women.

True lumbago is much less frequent in childhood, but there exist rare cases of true disc herniation as early as puberty. With the exception of acute wry neck, disturbance of function in the spinal column manifests itself indirectly, for the most part as headache, and in young girls as algomenorrhoea.

For this reason we were interested to see how frequently disturbances of function could be found in children of different age groups. The most striking phenomenon found especially frequently in children and adolescents is pelvic distortion which will be dealt with in later chapters. I found it in 11 of 80 children (14–41 months old) examined in crèches; in 81 out of 181 children (aged 3–6 years) in nursery school and in 199 out of 459 schoolchildren between the ages of 9 and 15. Statistical evaluation showed no significant difference between boys and girls. From nursery school age onwards, pelvic distortion is found in about one-third to one-half of the children. In contrast, I found movement restriction in the cervical spine (mainly at the craniocervical junction) in none of the infants in crèches, in only eight out of 181 nursery-school children, and in 73 out of 459 schoolchildren over the age of 9.

These investigations date from 20 years ago, when the technique of examination for the upper cervical spine was much less sophisticated than it is today. Our current clinical experience, using subtler techniques, has shown that pelvic distortion in children goes hand in hand with blockage, mainly at the atlanto-occipital joint, and also that after manipulation of this joint, pelvic distortion disappears. In 1982 I therefore examined a group of 75 nursery-school children (aged 3–6 years) and found pelvic distortion in 24, of whom 23 had movement restriction at the atlanto-occipital joint! In 12 of these manipulation was carried out (atlas–occiput); the pelvic distortion disappeared simultaneously. There is thus good reason to believe that most of the children in whom we found pelvic distortion 20 years ago also suffered from blockage at the craniocervical junction. Some scoliotic deformity was found in 175 of the 459 schoolchildren then examined, in 15 out of the 181 nursery-school children, and only in one of the 80 children in crèches.

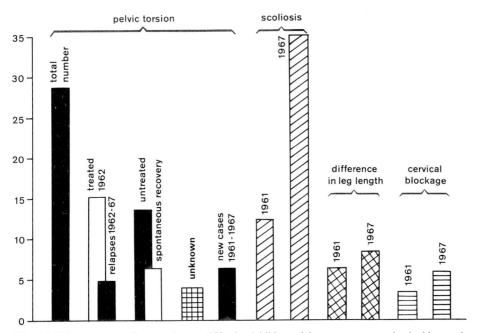

Figure 2.10 Follow-up studies over 6 years of 72 schoolchildren of the same age, covering incidence of pelvic torsion, scoliosis, difference in leg length and cervical blockage

The primary importance of the craniocervical junction is in keeping with important observations by Kubis, confirmed in 1093 new-born babies by Seifert (1975). Postural neck reflexes can be examined in the new-born: on turning the head to one side, the pelvis turns to the opposite side if the craniocervical junction functions normally. It was abnormal in 298 of the 1093 examined. In 58 per cent of this group, using the normal techniques, she diagnosed blockage at the craniocervical junction, between the ages of 4 and 9 months. Another important group of children of all ages who showed blockage mainly of the atlanto-occipital joint are those with relapsing or chronic tonsillitis: in a group of 76 such cases examined and followed up by Lewit and Abrahamovič (1976), 70 (92 per cent) had movement restriction at the craniocervical junction, mainly at the CO–Cl level.

In order to establish whether these findings in children are fortuitous or fairly constant, a group of children who started school attendance in 1960 were systematically followed up for 8 years; half the number showing some impaired function were treated, and the other half left as controls. In addition to the spinal column the extremities and particularly the musculature was thoroughly tested. The results are given in *Figure 2.10,* the most important finding being that with few exceptions changes in the function of the pelvis and of the craniocervical region remained constant if not treated. On the other hand, there were only a few relapses after treatment.

From this it follows that changes in the functioning of the spinal column and the locomotor system cause symptoms far more frequently than is generally assumed even in children. Much more frequently, however, these lesions are clinically latent. Pelvic distortion plus upper cervical lesions are found in almost half of all schoolchildren. Muscular imbalance is even more frequent, although less constant. It can further be inferred that:

1. Disturbance of function appears much earlier in the locomotor system than do degenerative morphological changes.
2. This disturbance, alone, can cause symptoms without structural changes.

Possible consequences of blockage in the vertebral motor segment

If blockage occurs in the spinal column of a child or an adolescent, at first sight the consequences may seem relatively insignificant; there may be some transitory pain – as in wry neck – but in the spine, unlike the extremity joints, function is readily compensated by neighbouring or even distant motor segments, and the lesion remains masked for a very long time. There is, however, a price to be paid for that compensation: increased demands on the compensating structures, with possible dysfunction. A good example is head rotation when there is blockage between atlas and axis. While the joints between the atlas and the axis are admirably suited to rotation, the rest of the cervical spine is not. Therefore head rotation carried out with a blocked atlas–axis movement can be deemed a dysfunction, and even more so when the restricted movement is not symmetrical. Quite obviously, movement restriction in one segment produces hypermobility in another, and in general, as we have seen, the consequences of dysfunction will be most marked if function is disturbed in key regions.

Osteophytes are the typical consequence of long-lasting overstrain, nor is blockage without consequences; for as we well know, much of the little vascularized tissue of cartilage and discs depends on movement for its nutrition. Radiology supplies ample evidence of regular osteophyte formation in the motor segment adjacent to a congenital block. Functional blockage in ante- and retroflexion, as seen in X-ray pictures, is as a rule accompanied by degenerative changes – narrowing of the disc – in the restricted segment, and by osteophytes in the neighbouring hypermobile segment (Jirout, 1956). Müller (1960) has shown that this hypermobile segment eventually becomes blocked, and the process spreads to neighbouring segments. This is understandable, for osteophytes are ring shaped and have a stabilizing function, as can best be seen in stabilized spondylolisthesis.

Degenerative changes in themselves need not produce manifest clinical symptoms. They do, however, make the spinal column more susceptible to further damage. It is again disturbed function that establishes itself more easily in a structure already marked by degenerative changes; in other words, if function remains compensated in a spinal column with degenerative changes, as a rule no symptoms will arise. Such a spinal column, however, is more liable to decompensation. That is why, for instance, the sequelae of trauma are usually more severe in structures with degenerative changes. Indeed, quite frequently what are called degenerative changes are in reality an attempt to compensate dysfunction. They are then testimomy to previous damage. One important complication of degeneration can be disc prolapse, but here again we find a complicated relationship between structural change and altered function: we know that even disc prolapse may be compatible with absence of symptoms, and it may be a disturbance of function on top of that which makes the lesion manifest. On the other hand, restoring correct function in a blocked joint, for example, may produce compensation.

That altered function may be important in nerve compression (entrapment syndromes) we have seen in the carpal tunnel syndrome (*see* page 320), particularly in the initial stages. On thorough examination we regularly find increased resistance to joint play of the carpal bones. When joint play is restored, the symptoms disappear. In other words, only if there is free mobility between the bones forming that tunnel can the walls adapt themselves to the contents of the tunnel under varying conditions of strain and movement. We should not forget that part of the wall of the intervertebral canal where root compression occurs is also the apophyseal joint.

Figure 2.11 summarizes the mechanical factor in pathogenesis.

The significance of disturbed movement patterns (stereotypes)

I consider disturbed movement patterns as the most important cause of blockage, and remedial exercise as the therapy of choice. Remedial exercise is widely recommended in painful vertebrogenic conditions, but what is meant by the term is much less clear, since we are not dealing here with obvious paresis, deformity or well-defined locomotor lesion (with the exception of blockage, where self-treatment exercises can be taught to the patient).

We have Janda (1975) to thank for shedding light on this problem. The main object of remedial exercise in disturbed function of the locomotor system is the correction of faulty patterning (faulty locomotor stereotypes), i.e. faulty co-ordination of muscle function due to disturbed central nervous control. Unfortunately for the systematically minded, movement patterns are highly individual, formed by each subject in the course of his life as a chain of

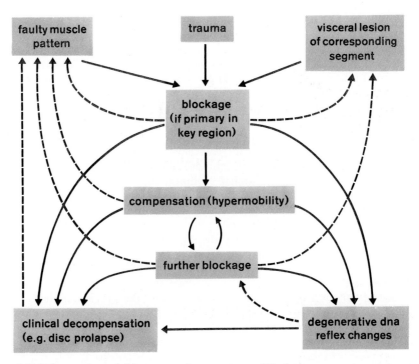

Figure 2.11 Pathogenesis: probable causes and consequences of blockage

unconditioned and acquired (conditioned) reflexes. There is therefore great variability, and the limits of the norm are very broad. In fact, the way each individual moves is so characteristic that we can recognize him by his gait, his gestures, the way he writes, and so on. Ideally, locomotor patterns should allow movement to be as economical as possible, i.e. to consume the smallest possible quantity of energy.

Here, as in many other situations, it is abnormality that provides the relevant clues; even a layman will recognize an awkward performance, which more often than not is tantamount to an uneconomical one. The layman will often be able to correct what he sees – for instance, sports trainers do so during their work.

In patients with chronic vertebrogenic pain and awkward movements, Janda (1972) applied the classic muscle test to individual muscles. This revealed two significant facts. First, the simple test movements believed to be characteristic for a specific muscle group are more often than not patterns in which a greater number of muscles take part than is commonly thought. Examining hip extension by polyelectromyography, Janda showed that hip extension is not only a test for the gluteus maximus muscle but that the prime movers in hip extension are the hamstrings, and that in addition to these two muscle groups the lumbar erector spinae also takes part. The characteristic disturbance of hip extension is the decreased and belated activity of the gluteus maximus (*Figure 2.12*). We have now learned to recognize clinically which muscles take part in simple test movements, thus using the test to assess not only muscle weakness but also quality of performance. This quality may be considerably altered without much change in

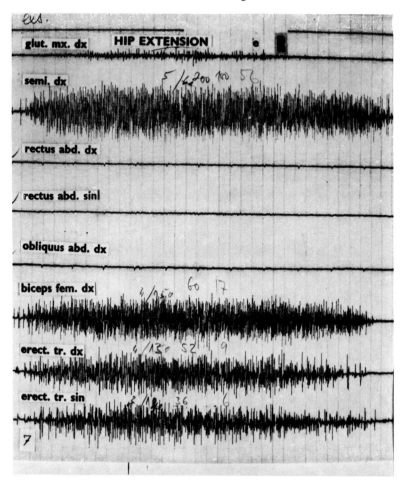

Figure 2.12 Electromyogram of right hip extension: the right gluteus maximus is brought into action late and little; marked activity in the hamstrings on the right and the erectores spinae on both sides; inhibition of the right gluteus maximus (From Janda, personal communication.)

force; the strength of hip extension with the aid of the hamstrings and the erector spinae may remain normal, while the pattern is greatly changed, with important consequences for locomotor function, as we shall see later.

Secondly, in testing these simple movements, a surprisingly constant pattern emerged. Certain muscles always showed a tendency to lesser activity (weakness) and hypotonia, while others tended to hyperactivity, increased tension and even tautness, which caused a typical motor imbalance. This is so characteristic that we can now determine syndromes that are of clinical importance. They are characteristic for individual patients; in some cases there is a preponderance of weakness, flabbiness going hand in hand with hypermobility, while in others tautness with increased muscle tension prevails. It is thus possible to draw up useful lists of muscles (muscle groups) that show a tendency to hyperactivity, and of those that tend to inhibition (*Table 2.1*).

TABLE 2.1. Muscle groups that show a tendency to hyperactivity or inhibition

Hyperactivity	*Inhibition*
On the dorsal aspect of the body	
Triceps surae	The gluteal muscles
Hamstrings	Lower part of the trapezius
Lumbar section of the erector spinae	Serratus lateralis
Quadratus lumborum	Supra- and infra-spinati
Middle and upper trapezius	Deltoid
Levator scapulae	
On the ventral aspect of the body	
Thigh adductors	Tibialis anterior
Rectus femoris	Extensors of the toes
Tensor fasciae latae	Peronei
Iliopsoas	Vasti
Oblique abdominal muscles	Rectus abdominis
Pectorales subscapulares	Deep neck flexors
Scalenes	
Sternocleidomastoid	
On the arms	
Flexors	Extensors

This difference in the behaviour of muscles can be seen under various clinical conditions and is particularly characteristic in common painful states: in a painful hip it is always the flexors and adductors that are tense and the glutei weak; in shoulder pain the pectoralis and subscapularis are taut while the supraspinati, infraspinati and deltoids are weak; in chronic painful conditions of the knee the vasti are weak, the rectus femoris remaining like a tight band.

Conditions are very similar in fatigue: again the same type of muscle will be inhibited and frequently superseded by muscles with a tendency to hyperactivity and tautness. On closer scrutiny we find that muscles with a tendency to inhibition are those that are also inhibited (flabby) in upper motor neurone lesions, while those with a tendency to hyperactivity become spastic. Neurologically, the typical imbalance in faulty movement patterns, enhanced by pain and fatigue, may be interpreted as 'microspasticity'.

Those muscles with a tendency to inhibition are called by Janda 'predominantly phasic', while he calls muscles with a tendency to hyperactivity 'predominantly postural'. These terms, which are still provisional, indicate that the real physiological basis for the difference, which is clinically very striking, is not yet known. Without going too deeply into the question here, it should be stressed that these groups do not correspond to the types of muscle fibre distinguished by modern neurophysiology, histology and biochemistry. Clinical diagnosis and therapy will be dealt with in the relevant chapters. It is important to point out, however, that trigger points may occur in both types of muscle, one type being painfully tense, the other painfully flabby (inhibited). In both, however, these trigger points are most effectively treated by postisometric relaxation.

Examination of simple movements by applying the muscle test is only our first step; our habitual movements are individually acquired patterns or stereotypes with a degree of plasticity, so that they are capable of being trained. However, this training is very tiring, particularly at first, the fatigue seeming out of all proportion to the energy required for the movement for which the subject is being trained. This is true even for healthy subjects, and all the more so for the sick; it is something that must never be forgotten in planning remedial exercise (rehabilitation).

The concept of patterning is a very important one, and can change our view of the difference between agonists and antagonists quite decisively. For example, the hamstrings and the quadriceps can be considered as antagonists if we are thinking of the simple movement of knee flexion. However, the movement of walking is much more complex than simple bending and stretching of the knee; during walking both these muscles have to contract and to co-ordinate as stabilizers of the knee. This is equally true of the abdominal and back muscles, and of the flexors and extensors of the neck. In fact, in well-coordinated straightening up from a stooping position it is the abdominal muscles that play the decisive role. It is therefore a grave mistake in remedial exercise to train these muscles simply according to the results of the muscle test, and not with regard to their function in the vital stereotype concerned.

In training correct movement patterns it is important to remember that they function like a 'chain reaction' which can be readily facilitated or triggered if the correct afferent impulses are employed. For extremity movements, most receptors are on the periphery, i.e. the fingers and toes. To facilitate walking it is important for the patient to think about lifting his big toe; he will then automatically dorsiflex the foot, and bend the knee and hip. Similarly, flexion of the fingers will trigger flexion in the elbow and shoulder. What the fingers and toes are for the extremities, the eyes are for the trunk: looking up facilitates straightening of the body, looking down facilitates stooping, while looking to the side facilitates rotation or inhibits movement in the opposite direction. Furthermore, as straightening of the body is connected with inspiration, and stooping with expiration, it is enough for the patient to look up to facilitate inspiration and inhibit expiration, and vice versa. This, as we shall see, plays a crucial role in the modern techniques of muscular facilitation and inhibition that we use for mobilization.

Returning to the question of imbalance of muscle groups, with the predominantly phasic muscles inhibited and the predominantly postural muscles over-active, it is easy to see that this must seriously interfere with co-ordinated locomotor patterns. This is particularly so as in many instances they are antagonists, the hyperactive muscle therefore having an inhibitory effect on its weak antagonist. Hyperactive lumbar erectores spinae will therefore unfavourably affect weak abdominal muscles, and hyperactive hip flexors will influence weak glutei.

The pathogenic mechanism of disturbed movement patterns

Having explained what movement patterns are and how they can be disturbed by imbalance of specific muscle groups, I will now trace the mechanisms by which disturbances of the most important muscle patterns (stereotypes) will have a deleterious effect on the locomotor system.

Walking and standing

Here the most important imbalance is between weak gluteal muscles with hyperactive hip flexors, and hyperactive lumbar erectores spinae with weak abdominal muscles. In standing we see increased pelvic tilt and a protruding abdomen.

The pathogenic mechanism is this: standing places an increased load on the lumbar spine, as even while standing at ease there is hyperactivity of the back muscles; when walking, hip extension is not performed by the inhibited glutei maximi, but by the lumbar erectores spinae, causing hyperlordosis instead of extension of the hip joint – that is, there is increased strain on the lumbar spine, due to hypermobility in the sagittal plane. This is greatly enhanced by the weak glutei medii; when the patient stands on one leg these muscles stabilize the pelvis in the coronal plane; if these muscles are weak, there is increased swaying of the pelvis, causing lumbar hypermobility in the coronal plane.

Straightening up from a stooping position (weight lifting)

If the trunk is conceived as a straight lever during weight lifting and the L5–S1 disc as the fulcrum, forces acting on it of up to about 1000 kPa have been calculated (Matthiasch, 1956; Morris, 1973). Such a force would crush the disc. Nachemson (1959) measured intradiscal pressure in various positions of the body and found that the maximum pressure during weight lifting was about 275 per cent of that in the upright position, i.e. 340 kPa

The reason for this lies in the co-ordinated activity of back and abdominal muscles during straightening up from a stooping position or while lifting an object that is not heavy. The function of the abdominal recti is to bring the sternum towards the pubic symphysis, thus bending the trunk forward. While straightening up from a stooping position the lumbar and thoracic spine form an arch; with correct muscular co-ordination a curling-up movement occurs, so that the erector spinae acts like a rope over a pulley, this pulley being first at L5, then at L4, and so on, and no leverage takes place. If, however, the abdominal muscles are weak and the back muscles hyperactive, then there is danger of leverage, with its deleterious effect on the disc. This curling-up movement enables us to sit up from the supine position even with legs bent, without the feet being fixed to the floor, so long as the abdominal muscles are normal.

Lifting the arms

Here the decisive factor is correct fixation of the shoulder girdle; this is the function of the upper part of the trapezius muscle and the levator scapulae from above, and of the lower part of the trapezius muscle and the serratus lateralis from below, the first two muscles being attached to the cervical spine and the last two to the thoracic spine.

The muscular imbalance found here is weakness of the lower part of the trapezius and serratus lateralis, with hyperactivity of the upper part of the trapezius and of the levator scapulae, resulting in overstrain of the cervical spine.

Weight carrying

Here the position of the shoulder joint is crucial: if the shoulder of the weight-bearing arm is behind the line of gravity of the body, the shoulder girdle is fixed in such a way that very little or no weight is borne by the upper fixators of the shoulder girdle (the upper part of the trapezius and the levator scapulae). If the shoulder is drawn forward, on the other hand, weight is immediately transmitted to the upper fixators and to the cervical spine, which then carries the brunt. The muscular imbalance causing this situation is a hyperactive pectoralis muscle, in particular the subclavicular part, a weak lower trapezius and perhaps the rhomboids.

This same imbalance also causes a forward-drawn position of the head, resulting not only in overstrain of the cervical spine as a whole, but even in compensatory lordosis of the craniocervical junction, producing relapsing lesions in the region.

These are some of the most obviously pathogenic examples of faulty movement patterns due to muscular imbalance. The most important locomotor stereotype and therefore the most pathogenic disturbance, however, is faulty breathing.

The role of respiration in locomotor disturbance

Thinking of breathing, one naturally has in mind the respiratory system. Yet it is the locomotor system that makes the lungs work, and the locomotor system that has to co-ordinate the specific respiratory movements with the rest of the body's locomotor activity. This task is so complex that it would be a miracle if disturbances did not occur.

It is widely held that muscular activity is facilitated during inspiration and inhibited during expiration, but this is an oversimplification. The abdominal muscles may be activated by expiration, especially expiration against resistance. I have already mentioned the close connection between looking up, inspiration and straightening of the body, and between looking down, expiration and stooping. This, however, applies only to the cervical and lumbar spine (which are decisive in view of their great mobility) and not to the thoracic spine. Here it is maximum inspiration that facilitates flexion and maximum expiration that facilitates extension, i.e. the thoracic extensor spinae, and this to such an extent that deep inspiration is probably the most effective method of mobilizing the thoracic spine into flexion, with maximum expiration most effective for extension.

The most surprising effect of inspiration and expiration, however, is the alternating facilitation and inhibition of individual segments of the spinal column during side-bending, discovered by Gaymans (1980). It can be regularly shown that during side-bending resistance increases in the cervical as well as in the thoracic spine in the even segments (occiput–atlas, C2, etc., and again in T2, T4, etc.) during inspiration; during expiration we obtain a mobilizing effect in these segments. Conversely, resistance increases in the odd segments (C1, C3, T3, T5, etc.) during expiration, while we obtain mobilization during inspiration. There is a 'neutral' zone between C7 and T1. An important feature of the atlas–occiput segment is that here inspiration increases resistance not only against side-bending but in all directions, while expiration facilitates mobility. This effect is most marked at the craniocervical junction and decreases in a caudal direction; in particular the mobilizing effect of inspiration (in the odd segments) diminishes in the lower thoracic region.

A well-known yet no less striking phenomenon is that we breathe in and hold our breath in situations in which maximum muscle activity is desired, for instance when delivering a blow, lifting a heavy weight, or sprinting; that is, when oxygen consumption can be expected to be very high. If we have not time to take a breath, as when we are forced to brake suddenly while driving, we hold our breath without breathing in.

Morris, Lucas and Bressler (1961) showed that the spinal column is supported by the diaphragm, the abdominal cavity being a fluid-filled space and therefore not compressible so long as the abdominal muscles and the muscles of the perineum are contracted; in fact Morris (1973) showed electromyographic activity of the abdominal muscles during weight lifting (*Figure 2.13*). Skládal *et al.* (1970) made the important observation that the diaphragm contracts when the patient stands on his toes, and rightly interpreted this as a postural reaction. Indeed, we stand on our toes as a start reaction before running, jumping, etc. He therefore rightly described the diaphragm as a 'respiratory muscle with a postural function' and the abdominal muscles as 'postural muscles with a respiratory function'. The significance of holding the breath during maximum muscle activity (the Valsalva manoeuvre) lies in the fact that postural stability is achieved at the cost of the vital function of respiration, which is (momentarily) sacrificed to it.

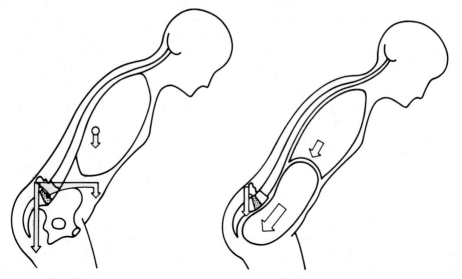

Figure 2.13 Loading of the lumbosacral junction without (*a*) and with (*b*) the support of the abdominal wall (From Kapandji, 1974. Reproduced by kind permission of author and publishers.)

Obviously, the postural role of respiration is not confined to Valsalva's manoeuvre, and persists in all phases of respiration so long as we are in the vertical position. This is most obvious during expiration; all respiration against resistance activates the abdominal muscles, and the shouts of judo wrestlers and ski jumpers are examples.

The situation is more complicated during inspiration; the clue to what happens must be sought in the fact that the thorax widens in the horizontal plane as we breathe in. Anatomists like to explain this phenomenon by the activity of the external oblique intercostal muscles, but a more significant factor is the contraction of the muscular diaphragm, which lifts the lower ribs so long as the central tendon is supported by counterpressure from the abdominal muscles (Campbell, Agostoni and Newsom Davies, 1970; Kapandji, 1974). This is borne out by the activity of the abdominal muscles during inspiration in the erect position (Basmajan, 1978; Campbell *et al.*, 1970). This is the only explanation of the widening of the thorax from below, a phenomenon which is an important criterion of correct respiration (Parow, 1953; Gaymans, 1980).

It can therefore be concluded that respiration guarantees postural stability in all its phases; this can be considerably enhanced by Valsalva's manoeuvre, but only if the stereotype of respiration is that described by Parow (1953) and Gaymans (1980): the thorax widening from below, from the waist-line; it must not be lifted. The shoulders are relaxed, the clavicles and upper ribs are not lifted but rotate slightly to allow widening of the thorax. It is this type of respiration that has a strong mobilizing effect on the spinal column (Gaymans respiration type A). If, however, the subject is supine or on all fours, no postural reaction is required; pure abdominal respiration is then physiological, the abdomen bulging, its wall completely relaxed. Under these conditions the thorax need not widen at all (Gaymans type B).

The close relationship between respiration and the motor system is shown in what may be called respiratory synkinesis', i.e. a certain type of movement is linked either with inspiration or with expiration. One such example is the Gayman's effect during side-bending, described above. Another example is the close link between trunk and head extension and inspiration, and between flexion and expiration. Since under physiological conditions trunk (head) extension goes hand-in-hand with looking up, and flexion with looking down, in itself looking up facilitates inspiration, looking down expiration, and vice versa. Trunk rotation in the upright (sitting) position, from neutral position to the side, is linked with inspiration and can be inhibited by expiration. Resistance against traction of the neck increases during inspiration and disappears during expiration; in the lumbar spine, on the other hand, resistance (prone) against traction increases during expiration and ceases during inspiration. There is even a link between inspiration and opening the mouth, and between expiration and closing the mouth. It is evident that these natural reactions can be very usefully applied.

What are the relevant mechanisms of disturbance of respiration patterns? The first is insufficient or no activity in the abdominal muscles, the spinal column thus losing the support of the diaphragm (*see* also 'Straightening up from the stooping position', page 164).

The second mechanism is insufficient widening of the thorax during inspiration and in particular the patient's inability to breathe into the posterior wall of the thorax even when prone, although no blockage has been found in the thoracic spine. The thoracic spine shows no respiratory wave. In such cases we find relapsing movement restriction of the thoracic spine owing to the absence of the mobilizing effect of respiration.

The most important respirational fault is lifting the thorax with auxiliary cervical muscles instead of widening it in the horizontal plane. Not only is this type of breathing ineffective from the point of view of ventilation, but it also overstrains the cervical musculature and the cervical spine (*see Figure 4.66*), causing recurrent cervical syndromes. When this fault is slight, it is demonstrable only if the patient is asked to take a deep breath. When it is severe, the faulty position of the thorax during inspiration and the absence of abdominal respiration are evident even at rest in the erect position; in very severe cases it can be seen in a supine patient. In some cases the fault is asymmetrical, one shoulder being raised higher than the other, causing unilateral cervical lesions.

The immense importance of faulty movement patterns for pathogenesis should now be clear. Things are all the more serious because modern industrialized civilization encourages this imbalance between predominantly phasic and predominantly postural muscles in favour of the latter; while mobility is increasingly limited, the locomotor system is overburdened by ever more static performance.

The practical consequences of faulty movement patterns will be shown in the chapters on diagnosis and therapy and training techniques suggested. The patient can often be trained adequately to correct the predominating fault in a relatively short time, often resulting in permanent relief. However, it is also important to be aware of certain limitations (Janda, 1978).

The significance of constitutional hypermobility

The importance of movement restriction (blockage) and of short muscles restricting mobility has been dealt with. The experienced clinician, however, is well aware that hypermobility is frequently an even more difficult problem, with considerable significance for pathogenesis. Where this problem concerns disturbed function of the locomotor system we owe a major contribution to Sachse (1969). He distinguishes the following:

1. Local pathological hypermobility, which may be primary or secondary (compensatory, in the vicinity of a restricted joint); the latter is particularly characteristic of the spinal column.
2. Pathological generalized hypermobility, frequent in certain congenital and neurological conditions.
3. Constitutional hypermobility, which is most important from our point of view. In itself it is a variant of the norm, but under conditions of strain its pathogenic importance becomes evident. Overall mobility is greatest in childhood and decreases with age, being generally greater in women than in men.

There are conditions in which hypermobility may even be an advantage, for instance in certain sports, in gymnastics, etc. and in employment where mobility is a requirement. It is accompanied by decreased stability, however, and since in most occupations today static posture predominates, these individuals are less able to adapt to static overstrain. As ligamentous laxity is usually accompanied by weakness of the postural muscles, the consequence is overstrain, resulting in pain. Some jobs are particularly unsuitable for such patients: they should not be dentists, for instance, or telephonists, or have to spend long periods bent over a desk or a machine. In some very pronounced cases there is a tendency to general instability, to a lack of co-ordination which can be interpreted as a type of 'minimal brain dysfunction'; this will be dealt with below.

There are patients in whom it appears impossible to achieve motor stereotypes of the desired efficiency even if patient and physiotherapist do their utmost. Analysing a hundred such 'hopeless' cases, Janda (1978) found that detailed neurological examination revealed changes which can be classified in three distinct types: one might be called 'microspasticity', i.e. very discreet signs of upper motor neurone lesions with some asymmetry between right and left; the second comprised a degree of hypotonia, asymmetrically irregular tendon reflexes and some signs of instability suggesting choreoathetosis; the third type presented slight changes in proprioception, for example when the patient stood on one leg with eyes closed – findings that gave a general impression of clumsiness. There were also slight psychological disorders: poorly sustained attention, low tolerance of stress, increased tension and difficulty in coping with the problems of daily life.

On close scrutiny the clinical picture corresponds exactly to what is known as 'minimal brain dysfunction' in child neurology. The incidence of this clinical picture is estimated at about 10–15 per cent of the child population, but it is usually believed to disappear in adolescence. It is very likely that in fact these subjects constitute the core of that group of patients who are unable to adjust or adapt themselves adequately to altered conditions, in their locomotor system as well as psychologically, and whom we find in adult life suffering from relapsing pain due to disturbed function of the locomotor system because they are unable to form movement patterns that would guarantee adequate function for any length of time, while their nervous system is also less capable of dealing with painful stimuli.

The reflex factor in the pathogenesis of pain in disturbed function

In the preceding paragraphs I have tried to show the importance of disturbed function in the locomotor system and the spinal column. Nevertheless disturbed function in itself is not identical with clinical disease. Indeed, the patient does not as a rule seek medical advice, nor does he complain because of disturbed mobility, but because he feels pain in the back, or in the head, the extremities, or even perhaps the viscera. On the other hand, there are people with disturbed functioning of the locomotor system who are not particularly conscious of pain and who do not consider themselves ill. In fact, disturbance of locomotor function is only the nociceptive stimulus acting on the nervous system, and it is the reaction of the nervous system that now plays the decisive role. The question that now arises is: in what way can disturbed function produce nociceptive stimulation and pain?

Before presenting an explanation I should stress that it is not the purpose of this book to deal with the theoretical aspects of the physiology of pain; nevertheless some pertinent theoretical conclusions should be drawn from clinical observation. As I have already pointed out, observation before and after manipulation has given us important clues, for not only does clinical examination show that mobility is improved after manipulation; it reveals that *tension* has disappeared from affected muscles, and even from other tissues. It is interesting to note that the same effect on tension can be observed after local anaesthesia, needling, massage, etc., if pain has been relieved. Similarly, in many other situations pain subsides if harmful functioning is corrected. If we are forced to maintain an uncomfortable position for long, we feel discomfort at first, but after a time we are forced by *pain* to change that position. The same is true of dynamic work that exceeds our strength: the moment we desist, pain diminishes and will soon subside. The common denominator in all this is the close correlation between tension and pain in the locomotor system. This is particularly evident in postisometric muscle relaxation with its immediate analgesic effect not only in the muscle itself, but also in its attachments (*see* Chapter 6).

Any harmful or disturbed functioning is bound to create tension: blockage, whenever the patient tries to move in the restricted direction; hypermobility due to excess movement; uncomfortable position resulting in static overstrain; etc. This makes good sense, and is in keeping with the biological role of pain as a warning sign of impending danger – warning of the onset of harmful functioning. As the locomotor system is under voluntary control, it is ours to damage as we will, and has no other way of protecting itself than by causing pain. If pain were merely the consequence of morphological change it would not play this significant role. In this way the voluntary activity of the locomotor system is kept within due bounds by pain. The locomotor system is thus by far the most frequent source of pain in the human organism, nor is it mere coincidence that referred pain from other organs or systems is, as a rule, perceived in parts of the locomotor system.

The close connection between physical and mental factors can also be inferred: pain itself is both a physical and a psychological phenomenon. The same is true of relaxation; it would be difficult to imagine psychological relaxation without relaxed muscles. This should be borne in mind when dealing with patients suffering from pain in the locomotor system.

What is the reaction to nociceptive stimuli due to disturbed function? First, the changes in the segment, which we have already mentioned. This reaction may be of lesser or greater intensity, which is of great clinical significance; it allows us to correlate the degree of changed function to the reflex changes, and in this way to establish the patient's lability or stability. It is by no means only a matter of autonomic functions, as is frequently thought, but also concerns muscle spasm or muscle inhibition, etc. There may be considerable differences between individual patients, but reactions may also change considerably in the same individual. If, for instance, acute vertebrogenic pain has been provoked by a draught, it cannot be due to the cold air alone, for in such patients we find acute blockage in at least one segment, with severe muscle spasm. This blockage is clinically latent, but produces a hyperalgesic zone in the segment. The cold draught striking this hyperalgesic zone is an additional stimulus which intensifies the patient's reaction and causes severe muscle spasm which makes the lesion manifest.

Thus there is no need to explain pain by mechanical irritation of nervous structures, as is frequently suggested, under the obvious influence of the root-compression model. It would indeed be a peculiar conception of the nervous system (a system dealing with information) that would have it reacting, as a rule, not to stimulation of its receptors but to mechanical damage to its own structures. Referred pain from the viscera can serve as an example as can the experimental infiltration of hypertonic saline solution into ligamentous structures of the spinal column, which was first performed by Kellgren (1939) and confirmed by Hockaday and Whitty (1969) and Piťha and Drobný (1972), Feinstein etc. (1954).

Just as in these experiments, pain arising from deep structures (joints, ligaments, etc.) frequently radiates in the segment and is accompanied by changes in skin sensitivity (hyperalgesic zones), sometimes with dysaesthesia, muscle spasm, etc., thus imitating radicular pain. Brügger (1960, 1962) therefore called it 'pseudoradicular'. Since muscular spasm is a prominent feature with concomitant pain in tendons and insertions as well as in fasciae, the term 'myofascial pain' ('myotendinosis' in the German literature) is frequently used.

I have dwelt most upon the segmental reaction as this can most readily be examined clinically. However, it should not be forgotten that whatever this reaction, it is perceived as pain only if it passes the threshold of pain perception which is under central nervous control. On examination, indeed, we very frequently find changes in many segments that patients are entirely unaware of.

Impaired function, as we have seen, is closely connected to the reflex changes typical for nociceptive stimulation. They therefore constitute an entity that we propose to term 'functional pathology of the motor system'.

Radicular pain

After showing that pain in the motor system is due to nociceptive stimulation of pain receptors, what is our explanation of pain in cases of true mechanical root compression such as disc prolapse? First it should be pointed out that nerve compression alone causes paresis and anaesthesia, but no pain. What is then the most likely mechanism by which, for example, disc prolapse causes pain? Quite obviously, disc prolapse cannot impinge on the nerve root before acting on the dura and the dural sheaths. It is precisely these structures that are richly supplied with pain receptors, and we should be aware that at every movement of the legs and trunk the dural sheaths are being rubbed over the prolapse. It should not be forgotten that Lasègue's sign indicates meningeal involvement. This is in keeping with the effect of epidural anaesthesia in disc lesions.

Another clinical observation also indicates that pain is primarily due to stimulation of pain receptors, even if there are clear neurological signs of nerve root involvement. Černý (1948) registered the radiating pain in patients with radicular syndromes, using autodermography of the pain, and found that this was more exact and reliable in dermatome localization than the typical neurological signs, in particular more so than hypoaesthesia. This is because a nerve root does not contain fibres from one segment only, but transitory fibres from neighbouring segments are usually also present. This is not only a fact well known to anatomists; it explains the overlap thanks to which radicotomy is not, as a rule, followed by hypoaesthesia in the corresponding segments. This rule, however, is only partially valid; there are frequent exceptions. Hanraets (1959) explained it thus: during operation he frequently found that nerve roots vary considerably in thickness: if a root is very thick on one side its neighbour is likely to be much thinner, because the transitory fibres belonging to this neighbouring segment can be very numerous; in the thin (neighbouring segment) root, transitory fibres are consequently very few, or may be absent altogether. Conditions on the other side may be quite different, for example if the L5 root is thick on the right, this need not be so on the left. If a very thin root is compressed or cut, there will be very little or no sensory change, but if a very thick root is involved there will be hardly any transitory fibres in the neighbouring root or roots, hence there will be marked hypoaesthesia and some dysaesthesia originating in the transitory fibres which will affect neighbouring dermatomes as well and produce some changes of sensitivity in them. When Hanraets (1959) stimulated such a thick root during operation, his patients also felt dysaesthesia in the neighbouring dermatomes. Hence, a nerve root is not necessarily mono-segmental! Starý and I found something very similar (Starý and Lewit, 1958) after radicotomy in patients operated on for root syndrome, in whom no disc prolapse was found (there was a time when radicotomy was carried out in such cases). Most of these patients had little or no complaints, but there were some in whom permanent hypoaesthesia followed, and was resented. Here, apparently, a thick root with most of the transitory fibres of the neighbouring segments had been cut.

Pain coming from receptors, however (i.e. from dural sheaths), is felt in one segment only and therefore radiates only in the dermatome corresponding exactly to the compressed root. In other words, what we call a radicular syndrome is a combination of pain originating from pain receptors with irradiation in the segment, and of neurological signs of root compression (hypaesthesia, dysaesthesia and paresis).

There is yet another very interesting feature that shows the role of the functional component: this is the frequent immediate improvement of muscle strength in weak muscles and even of tendon reflexes (*see Figures 2.8* and *2.9*) after manipulation. This agrees with the electromyographical findings of Drechsler (1970) and Hanák (1970), showing that in true radicular syndromes with clinical signs of muscle weakness, nerve conduction velocity may be normal. This may be interpreted as mere reflex inhibition. Drechsler insisted that the clinical prognosis was worse in those radicular syndromes in which he found decreased conduction velocity.

The term 'vertebrogenic'

After terms like 'degenerative disease' and 'discopathy' had been abandoned, the non-committal term 'vertebrogenic' seemed useful and has been widely adopted. I have already touched on its shortcomings: it includes structural disease of the spinal column but does not cover changes in the functioning of the locomotor system outside the spinal column. However, in the sense that the spinal column is used as a *pars pro toto*, the term is acceptable. As long as it is used for back pain and (closely) related disorders, it is hardly controversial. It became and still is controversial when applied to disorders, mainly pain, usually ascribed to internal organs. This controversy became particularly heated because of some of the therapeutic consequences of manipulation.

There is little room for controversy if our present knowledge about referred and radiating pain is taken into account. Melzack and Wall (1965) and Milne *et al.* (1981) have shown that nociceptive stimuli from all structures in a segment converge to cells in the lamina V of the basal spinal nucleus. This of course also applies to pain coming from receptors in the joint capsules of apophyseal intervertebral joints as well as from internal organs. It is therefore easy to see that the locomotor system can readily *simulate* visceral pain, and vice versa, and that this constitutes an important aspect to be taken into account in differential diagnosis. If this is clear the therapeutic consequences should not cause much controversy.

Yet, as will be seen in further chapters, vertebrovisceral relations are more complex, and for this reason some circumspection is desirable when using the term 'vertebrogenic'. There are many disorders that are caused by more than one factor, and the spinal column may be only one of several factors causing a pathological condition. In such a case it would be better to speak of disease with a vertebrogenic factor, rather than vertebrogenic disease. A typical instance is migraine; we should reserve the term vertebrogenic for those conditions in which the spinal column (the locomotor system) is the sole or decisive factor, as in cervicocranial syndrome.

But, as Junghanns has pointed out (1957), the role of the vertebrogenic factor may change in the course of a single disorder. It may trigger the disease process, but once this has started it may develop independently. It was Gutzeit (1953) who very aptly characterized the spinal column according to its various roles in the pathogenesis of some diseases, as 'initiator, provocator, multiplicator, localisator'.

Conclusions

1. Morphological changes cannot explain the great majority of pains arising from the locomotor system. These changes may, however, play the role of a *locus minoris resistentiae*.
2. By far the most frequent cause of pain is disturbed function. This may concern passive mobility (joints), active movement patterns, or body statics. Manipulative treatment is directed to movement restriction of joints or motor segments of the spinal column – blockage.
3. The most important cause of blockage is overstrain due to faulty movement patterns or body statics, trauma or visceral disease. It is frequently found even in early childhood.
4. Its consequences are disturbed function, hypermobility and again blockage in the neighbouring or even in more distant parts of the locomotor system. In the long run, by disturbed function or compensatory hypermobility, they cause degenerative changes.
5. The locomotor system and the spinal column act as a functional unit which adapts itself to and compensates for disturbed function, so that equilibrium is always maintained.
6. Changes of mechanical function alone do not cause clinical symptoms (pain). They constitute, however, the nociceptive stimulus which produces reflex changes in the segment (muscle spasm, hyperalgesic zones, etc.). If these are of sufficient intensity to pass the pain threshold, pain is felt. The most likely nociceptive stimulus is increased tension.
7. Pain in the locomotor system is therefore a warning sign of harmful functioning which should be corrected in time before it causes permanent damage. It is probably the most frequent type of pain throughout the organism.
8. If the patient is able to describe and localize the pain, and we find some of the typical reflex changes in a corresponding area and have excluded gross pathology, then it is our task to find the disturbance of function that is the most likely cause. Undiagnosed impairment of motor function is – in our view – the most frequent type of pain without a specific diagnosis, and treatment of the pain as such, without a thorough clinical understanding of the functioning of the locomotor system, is courting failure.

3

Functional anatomy and radiology of the spinal column

Without a good understanding of functional anatomy as presented by X-rays it is almost impossible to understand impaired function and therefore to interpret correctly what we have felt with our hands during examination. It is of course not the purpose of this chapter to give a complete and detailed anatomy, but to present those features that are essential for an understanding both of the way in which function may be impaired, and of the mechanisms involved.

Diagnosis of structural changes

Classic X-ray diagnosis is concerned mainly with changes in structure, and this type of diagnosis is essential in order to avoid serious error; methods aimed at correcting function are out of place in cases where the underlying condition is structural pathology. Our special interest in this field, however, lies in such changes of structure as may have a direct influence on function, such as various anomalies, in particular in the shape of joints, asymmetry of the vertebrae, spinal curvature etc. Not only is the shape or deformity of some vertebrae the cause of asymmetrical function (e.g. in scoliosis), but it can itself be the result of asymmetrical function (e.g. rotation of the lower cervical spine owing to dominance of one hemisphere and asymmetrical loading of the upper extremities, as Jirout has shown (1980)). Diagnosis of structural change can be found in the classic textbooks both of anatomy and of radiology, and therefore need not be dealt with in detail here.

Diagnosis of disturbed function (mobility studies)

The X-ray examination of disturbed function involves examination of the spinal column in various, usually extreme, positions such as ante- and retroflexion (extension), side-bending or even rotation. This type of examination undoubtedly provides some direct information about mobility; as a routine examination, however, it is very time consuming and uneconomical, and its practical value is thus limited to complicated cases where special information is required, or to cases involving litigation. It is advisable to use X-ray examination in clinically relevant positions, e.g. in retroflexion in cases of vertigo caused by bending the head back.

Doctors familiar with manual diagnosis of disturbed function are accustomed to assessing mobility by clinical examination; nevertheless X-ray examination of mobility is extremely important for research purposes, as it gives insight into the mechanisms underlying mobility and its disturbance, an insight no other method can provide.

Diagnosis of disturbed static function (spinal curvature and 'malalignment')

Mobility is what is usually meant by 'spinal function', yet static function is no less important, and X-rays of the spinal column with the patient standing or sitting (taken under standard conditions) can and should be evaluated for static function. As will be shown in more detail below, spinal curvature should be such as not to upset balance. This goes not only for the sagittal but also for the coronal plane, in which every obliquity (e.g. in walking) produces a scoliotic curvature with the corresponding rotation. Curvature may be smooth, or less so; in certain segments there may be a sharp bend (scoliotic, kyphotic, lordotic) or even some rotation or shift ('offset').

The importance of these signs of malalignment is highly controversial, especially in view of the discredited subluxation theory. The controversy is fuelled by the doubtful importance of asymmetry, as, in fact, asymmetry is the rule rather than the exception. Yet Jirout (1978) has shown that although asymmetry of the position of the atlas in relation to the axis is the rule, its incidence increases with age. This is equally true for the asymmetrical shape of the spinous processes. He concluded that this is probably the result of asymmetrical pull due to the dominance of one cerebral hemisphere.

From this it appears reasonable to deduce that asymmetry and irregularity of 'alignment', while not in themselves pathological, can be the expression of asymmetry or anomaly in function. If, for example, the axis is rotated in neutral position, not only will it rotate asymmetrically during side-bending, but the rest of the cervical spine will follow suit (see page 81). Without jumping to conclusions, marked asymmetry or 'malalignment' in the X-ray picture should be correlated to the clinical findings. Marked irregularity of the relative position of vertebrae in the X-ray can be regarded as a warning signal that there may also be some functional anomaly or at least susceptibility to disturbed function.

One obvious advantage of the examination of static function is its economy; only two X-rays are required, the anteroposterior (AP) view and the side view. Standard conditions must be adhered to. As individual posture is highly characteristic, i.e. constant, comparable pictures can be expected on repetition. Gutmann (1978) has very aptly summed up the importance of static function: 'The dominating principle of the spinal column is body statics'. All other functions are subordinate to the requirements of upright posture on two legs. Loss of mobility and painful impingement of nerves roots is preferred to sacrifice of the erect posture.

Technical requirements

The X-ray should be taken in a position that corresponds to the patient's natural posture, either standing or sitting (with the exception of the AP view of the cervical spine, which is taken with the patient supine). There should therefore be no artificial correction of the patient's posture. Distortion must be avoided and focusing must be scrupulous to obtain clear pictures which can be used successively for comparison. To achieve this, some correction is unavoidable, for instance to prevent distortion or tilt, but the natural posture must be registered. It is also essential to visualize a sufficiently long section of the spinal column to make it possible to assess posture. To determine the position of the cervical spine, the base of the skull must be visible, as well as the whole of the cervical spine down to about T1; to assess the shape of the lumbar spine we need to see at least the thoracolumbar junction, the ilia, the pubic symphysis and both hip joints on a single AP picture. This gives a sufficient number of landmarks by which to assess correct focusing and to compare successive pictures if a standard technique is used.

The ideal method for X-ray examination of the spinal column is to show the whole column on a single picture. An AP and a lateral view with the patient standing are required; the only condition to be observed for the AP view is that both feet must be placed symmetrically in relation to the X-ray screen, and that the patient be requested to distribute his weight equally between his two feet, keeping his legs straight. In the lateral view, the feet should be placed so that the ankles are about a finger's breadth behind the vertical to the floor, from the mid-point of the horizontal edge of the cassette; the head should be neither bent to the side nor rotated, the patient fixing some object at eye-level in order to avoid anteflexion or retroflexion of the head; the patient holds his arms crossed over the chest and his hands on his shoulders.

X-ray of the lumbar spine and the pelvis

The patient must be standing if X-ray pictures that can be evaluated for static function are to be obtained. He is therefore placed before the X-ray screen as when pictures are taken of the whole spinal column. To acquire information about the statics of the spinal column as a whole, a device described by Gutmann (1970) is used, in which a plumb-line indicates the vertical line from the head. A line which corresponds to the centre of the screen is drawn on the floor; for the AP view the patient places one foot symmetrically on each side of the line. A moveable plumb-line of metal wire is attached to the screen. The screen is first raised to the level of the patient's occiput and the metal wire moved to a point corresponding to the outer occipital protuberance. In this way the plumb-line shows the head position. The screen is then adjusted to the height required to take a picture of the lumbar spine and the pelvis (with the central beam and the centre of the screen roughly at the height of the navel). The wire should now be taped to the lower edge of the screen and the patient leans against the screen so as not to blur the picture (*Figure 3.1*).

For the lateral view the patient puts his feet as described for the X-ray of the whole spine; the screen with the plumb-line is raised to the level of the head so as to place the plumb-line at a point corresponding to the outer meatus acousticus, and with the plumb-line in place the screen is then lowered to the level required for the lateral view of the lumbar spine (the centre of the screen at the level of the navel or slightly above). The plumb-line must again be taped to the lower edge of the screen and the patient must lean against the screen to avoid blurring. In the lateral view it is an advantage not to focus the central beam on the middle of the picture but

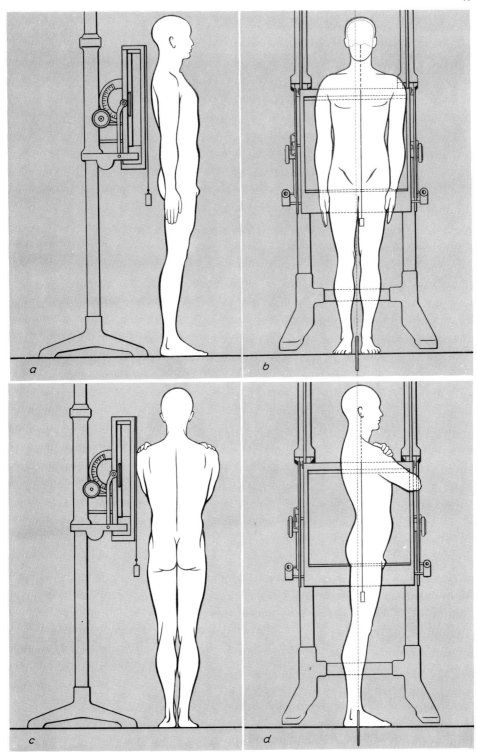

Figure 3.1 X-ray technique of the lumbar spine with the patient standing. AP view: (*a*) Positioning of the movable plumb-line; (*b*) the device prepared for X-ray, lateral view; (*c*) positioning of plumb-line; (*d*) the device prepared for X-ray (After Gutmann, 1970.)

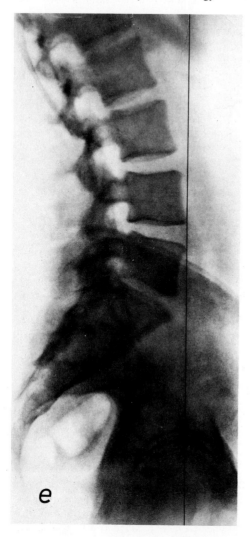

Figure 3.2 Lateral view of the lumbar spine using the technique illustrated in *Figure 3.1*: perfect visualization of the innominate and the femoral heads, and of the lumbosacral junction. The rest of the lumbar spine is neither over-exposed nor distorted

eccentrically midway between the iliac crest and the greater trochanter, i.e. roughly at the level of the sacral promontory. The advantage of this technique is that it gives an undistorted view of the pelvis and the hip joints and correct exposure of both the lumbar spine and the lumbosacral junction, and yet there is no distortion of the lumbar spine (*Figure 3.2*). With the normal technique, either the lumbar spine is over-exposed or the lumbosacral junction is under-exposed. The distance of the X-ray tube to the film should be as great as possible, depending on the power of the apparatus and the corpulence of the patient, the ideal distance being 2 m.

X-ray evaluation of lumbar spinal statics

As we have already seen, X-ray examination of the patient standing serves mainly for diagnosis of static function and its disturbance. It should be borne in mind that clinical examination alone can ascertain the position of the outer occipital protuberance, the spinous processes, the intergluteal line and the mid-point between the heels in relation to a plumb-line. In the sagittal plane clinical examination can show the position of the shoulders, the great trochanters and the heels in relation to a plumb-line from the external auditory meatus. Clinical examination, however, cannot provide information about the position of the sacrum and L5, i.e. the true base of the spinal column, information which is essential for the understanding and evaluation of spinal statics.

This explains why clinicians interested in body statics have devoted their attention mainly to the question of body equilibrium as a whole, studying deviation of the head and deviation from the line of gravity by means of statovectography. Rash and Burke (1971) pointed out that 'in stationary posture the centre of gravity of each body segment should be vertically above the area of the supporting base, preferably near its centre. If persistent gravitational torques are being borne by ligaments, or if excessive muscular contraction is required to maintain balance, this principle is being violated'. X-ray examination under static conditions provides pertinent information on this type of static disturbance.

The mechanism of balance differs in the coronal and the sagittal planes. This is readily understood if the effect of a heel-pad is considered: an artificial difference of more than 1 cm in leg length changes the balance in the coronal plane; it is immediately felt and resented by the subject, whereas raising (or lowering) *both* heels is hardly noticed. This is because in the coronal plane the line of gravity lies between the two hip joints and the heels, guaranteeing (relatively) stable equilibrium. Purely mechanical static changes are therefore much more readily felt in the coronal than in the sagittal plane. In the latter the trunk is in a state of labile equilibrium above the two perfectly round surfaces of the hip joints. Balance in this plane cannot be maintained by static forces alone; dynamic muscular forces must be brought into play, but should be kept at a minimum.

Lumbar spinal statics in the coronal plane

Under 'ideal' conditions the pelvis and sacrum in the AP view are straight and all vertebrae are symmetrical; the outer occipital protruberance is in the mid-line and so are all the spinous processes down to the sacrum, as well as the coccyx and the pubic symphysis. Not only is such a spinal column the exception but it is of little interest. Nobody ever stands naturally symmetrically on both feet, and during movement the pelvis constantly swings from one side to the other. The problem is thus not obliquity in itself but correct or faulty reaction to obliquity, and the criteria by which this reaction can be judged.

This can be studied physiologically if one creates obliquity of the base in a healthy subject by lengthening one leg (*Figure 3.3*). The pelvis shifts to the higher side while the lumbar spine bends to the same side, if both legs are straight and the patient relaxes.

In X-rays the same shift to the side, scoliosis *and* rotation to the lower side can be observed. The summit of the scoliotic curve is usually at the mid-lumbar region, so that the thoracolumbar junction comes to stand above the sacrum. The degree of rotation in lumbar scoliosis depends on lordosis; if this is present, rotation is normally found. If there is no lordosis – as in acute lumbago or sciatica, for example – there is also no rotation; if there is kyphosis there may even be rotation to the opposite side.

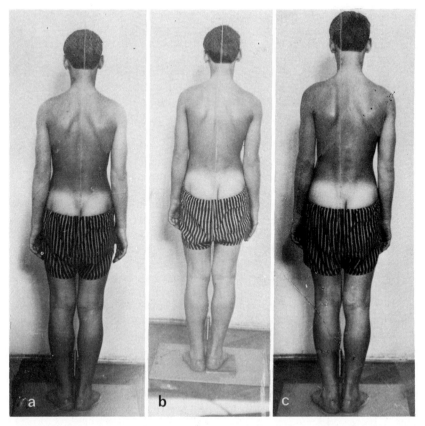

Figure 3.3 Body statics with the subject standing: (*a*) with his weight equally on both feet, the body axis corresponds to the plumb-line between the heels; (*b*) with a heel-pad, the weight again equally on both feet; the pelvis shifts to the higher side; (*c*) with the weight on the right foot the whole body deviates to the right, the head deviating furthest

The criterion of normal static function of the lumbar spine must therefore be its reaction to obliquity at the base – this base not necessarily being only the sacrum but also the lower lumbar vertebrae up to L3. If the obliquity is not due to a short leg (pelvic inclination) but only to inclination of the base of the spine, it will persist when the patient is seated, and therefore correction of the sitting position should also be considered.

Reaction to obliquity at the base is normal if: (1) there is scoliosis to the lower side; (2) there is rotation to the same side, provided that lordosis is present; (3) the thoracolumbar junction stands vertically above the sacrum; and (4) the pelvis shifts to the higher side. Thoracic scoliosis is always in the opposite direction to lumbar scoliosis (*Figure 3.4*).

These facts reflect the physiology of balance and affect the whole question of difference in leg length. This in itself is of no significance if it does not cause obliquity of the base of the spinal column. Therefore, the age-old dispute over how to measure this difference is beside the point. What is important is that while clinically we determine pelvic tilt, we cannot determine the position of the sacrum

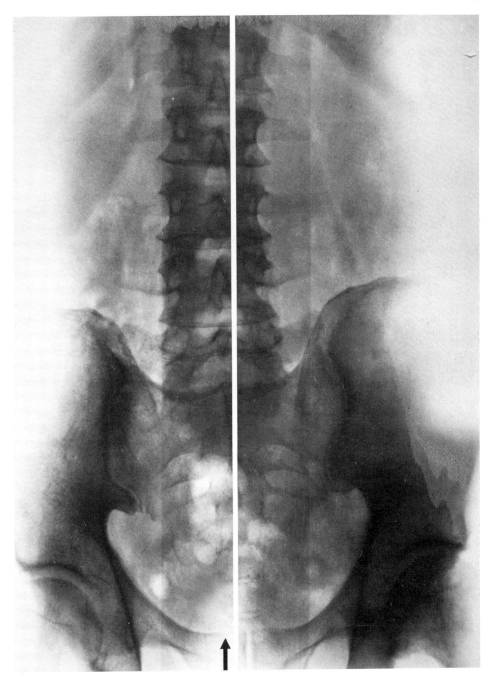

Figure 3.4 Normal reaction of the lumbar spine and pelvis to a short right leg (pelvic obliquity): static dextroscoliosis with dextrorotation of the lumbar spine, deviation of the pelvis to the left from the mid-line (arrow)

nor that of the lumbar vertebrae that constitute the base of the spinal column, since the pelvis may be straight while the sacrum is tilted, and vice versa. Only by X-ray examination can the true base of the spinal column and the reaction of the spinal column to inclination be determined (*Figure 3.5*).

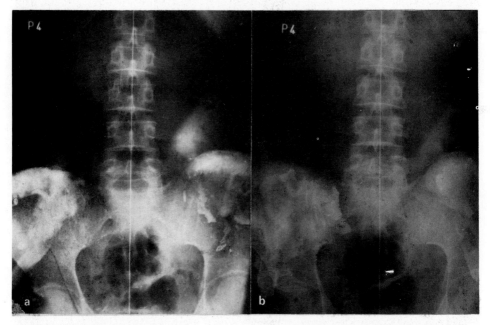

Figure 3.5 Pelvic obliquity. (*a*) Pelvis lower on the right (short right leg) with a horizontal sacrum, the lumbar spine straight; (*b*) with a right heel-pad sacral obliquity appears, with deviation of the lumbar spine to the left and slight dextroscoliosis

The principal pathological findings are:

1. Obliquity *without* scoliosis or with *insufficient* scoliosis, so that the thoracolumbar junction is not above the lumbosacral.
2. No pelvic shift to the higher side.
3. No rotation when there is scoliosis and lordosis or rotation in the opposite direction from the scoliosis, or even scoliosis to the higher side.

Correcting disturbance of statics by means of a heel-pad is the practical application of these criteria. This is of course always a clinical question which can never be decided by X-ray alone. Nevertheless it is X-ray examination that provides the most important information.

What do we expect to achieve by using a heel-pad to reduce obliquity?

1. If scoliosis is not sufficient to bring the thoracolumbar junction above the lumbosacral, or if scoliosis is absent, the thoracolumbar junction will be brought to stand above the lumbosacral, or to approach this position.
2. If the pelvis is shifted, usually to the higher side, it will return to the mid-line.
3. Even if the scoliosis (scoliotic curve) has been balanced, it will decrease after one heel has been raised.

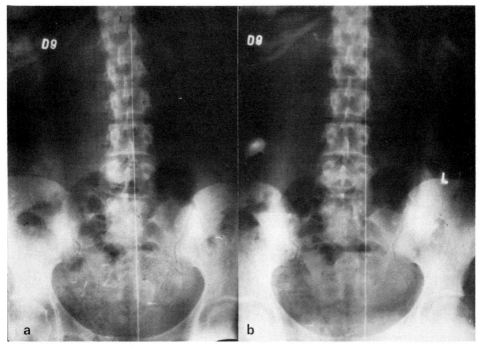

Figure 3.6 Pelvic and sacral obliquity due to a short left leg. (*a*) Left scoliosis with deviation of the thoracolumbar junction to the right; (*b*) normal lumbar statics after application of a left heel-pad

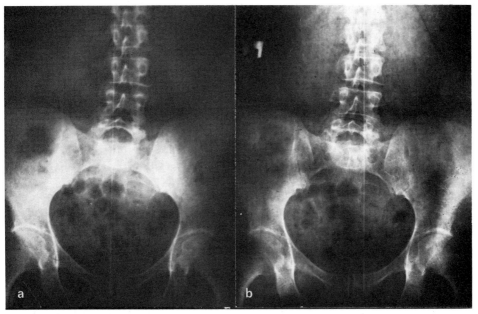

Figure 3.7 Pelvic and sacral obliquity due to a short left leg. (*a*) Left scoliosis with deviation of the thoracolumbar junction to the left; (*b*) less pelvic obliquity after application of a left heel-pad, but no improvement in lumbar statics

All this must be checked again by X-ray. With each of these possibilities we observe a positive or a negative reaction, the spinal column either 'accepting' or 'rejecting' the correction. In cases of 'rejection' it would be wrong to 'force' correction upon the patient, because this would only increase the strain at the base (*Figures 3.6* and *3.7*).

Deviation from the plumb-line can usually be interpreted as a sign that the patient puts more weight on the leg towards which the plumb-line is shifted.

The traditional reaction to obliquity has been studied by Illi (1954) and Biedermann and Edinger (1957), with the subject marking time in front of an X-ray screen. At every step obliquity appeared at the base and with it scoliosis to the opposite side; the summit of the scoliotic curve appeared at L3 and the thoracolumbar junction was brought above the sacrum. Above T12 the thoracic spine made a (compensatory) scoliosis to the opposite side, but it was less marked, like a damped wave. According to Biedermann and Edinger (1957) the thoracolumbar junction forms a kind of fixed point which should not swing more than 4 cm from one side to the other.

The relation of scoliosis to rotation under the influence of lordosis has been studied by Lovett (1907), according to whom the lumbar spine rotates in the direction of scoliosis if there is lordosis, but to the opposite side in kyphosis. This can be explained by the relative mobility of the vertebral bodies and the arches during side-bending. If there is lordosis the articular processes which are mainly in the sagittal plane are locked, and therefore resist side-bending; the vertebral bodies, however, are free to bend sideways. Hence there will be more lateral flexion of the vertebral bodies than of the arches, and rotation to the side of scoliosis will result, the spinous processes remaining almost in the mid-line.

On the other hand, if there is kyphosis the joints are much freer to move, as the joint facets are in loose apposition. The vertebral bodies, however, are pressed against each other, particularly at their anterior edge, and are therefore not as free to bend as in lordosis. Side-bending of the arches will thus be the same as or even exceed lateral flexion of the vertebral bodies. The result will be either no rotation at all, or rotation in the opposite direction from the scoliosis, as can be seen in X-ray pictures of patients with acute lumbago, taken standing (*Figure 3.8*). This can also be ascertained clinically if a subject with a marked lumbar kyphosis when sitting relaxed is told to side-bend: while in lordosis his lumbar spinous processes will remain almost in mid-line, in kyphosis they will form a perfect scoliotic arch.

Lumbar spinal statics in the sagittal plane

In the sagittal plane we are concerned with what are called 'normal' curvatures, generally held to comprise cervical lordosis, thoracic kyphosis, lumbar lordosis and sacral kyphosis. Sollmann and Breitenbach (1961) have the credit for disproving this widely accepted view, on the basis of 1000 X-rays of the entire spinal column. They came to the conclusion that there is only an 'individual norm'; they do not, however, lay down any criteria.

Cramer wrote in 1958 that there is a constant correlation between the tilt of L5 and that of T12, and more important still, that the T12 vertebra lies 4 cm behind L5 (150 measurements were taken). I myself confirmed this in 200 cases (Lewit, 1973) and also showed that the plumb-line from the external acoustic meatus passes exactly through the scaphoids at its base. The sacral promontory lies 4 mm and the axis of the hip joints lie 4 and 12 mm, respectively, in front of this plumb-line.

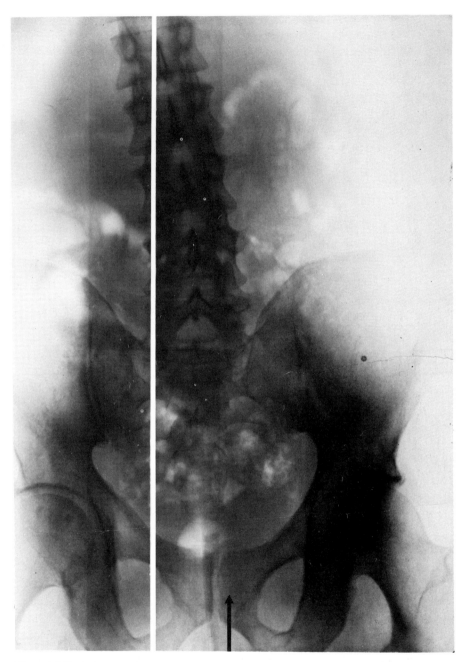

Figure 3.8 Typical posture in acute root lesions with deviation of the plumb-line and the (straight!) pelvis to the side of the unaffected leg; 'paradoxical' scoliosis with slight rotation to the opposite side

These conditions are changed in disturbance of dynamics, i.e. of muscular function. This is most evident in muscle spasm due to acute sciatica or lumbago in disc lesion, when there is a forward thrust posture (*Figure 3.9*) or in flabby posture in which the sacral promontory shifts forward and there is an increased difference between L5 and T12, the latter being more than 4 cm dorsal to L5 (*Figure 3.10*).

'Flabby' posture is the typical reaction to imbalance of the muscles controlling posture of the lumbar spine and pelvis; it may be the result of weak abdominal and gluteal muscles, but equally well of hyperactive back muscles and hip flexors (*see* Chapter 4).

Lumbar spinal curvature is clearly dependent on pelvic tilt which in turn varies according to the 'type' of pelvis, as will be shown in the following section.

It can therefore be concluded that lumbar spinal curvature is adequate if in the sagittal plane the thoracolumbar junction is behind the lumbosacral junction and there is no excessive anteposition of the sacral promontory, and if T12 is not too far behind L5 (not more than 8 cm, which is double the average). In the coronal plane the most important criterion is also that the thoracolumbar junction should be vertically above the lumbosacral. If there is obliquity at the base the normal reaction is adequate scoliosis and rotation (if lordosis is present) and a shift of the pelvis to the higher side.

If curvature of the spinal column subserves these rules, i.e. the rules of body statics, then it is physiological; I am not aware of any other criteria of spinal curvature. Furthermore, it can be inferred that the spinal column not only helps to maintain equilibrium of the whole body but also determines the relationship between the various parts of the body under the influence of gravity. We may therefore speak of 'partial equilibrium' subserved by the spinal column in accordance with the criteria of Rash and Burke (1971) (*see* page 49).

Curvature cannot be evaluated if the patient is recumbent or if the position of the pelvis and the lumbar spine up to at least the thoracolumbar junction cannot be seen on a single radiograph.

It is important to realize that a slight curvature (a 'flat' spine) goes hand in hand with hypermobility and lack of stability, while greater curvature (in both the sagittal and the coronal plane) corresponds to stability and less mobility.

The pelvis

The pelvis and the spinal column constitute a functional entity, the pelvis being the base of the column and the point of connection with the lower extremities. The pelvis transfers motion from the lower extremities and acts as a shock-absorber. From the ilia powerful muscles and ligaments attach themselves to the spine as though to a mast. The sacroiliac joints and the pubic symphysis allow for some mobility (springing) while guaranteeing adequate stability.

Pelvic types

The function of the pelvis and its influence on body statics depend largely on its type. We owe this concept to Erdmann (1956) and Gutmann (1965). There are

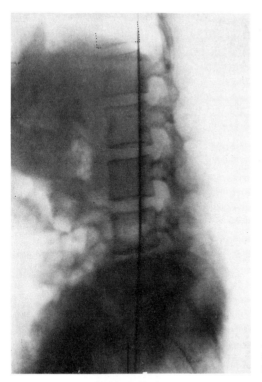

Figure 3.9 Lateral view of the lumbar spine with a forward thrust posture, in an acute radicular syndrome

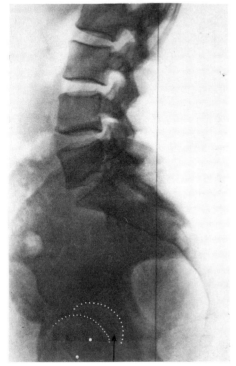

Figure 3.10 Lateral view of the lumbar spine in 'flabby' posture – a forward shift of the pelvic promontory – in this case due to a shortened iliopsoas muscle

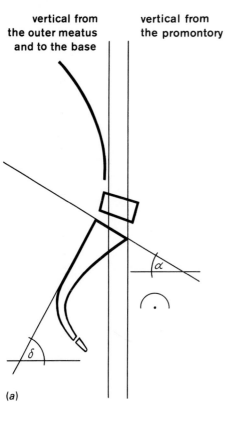

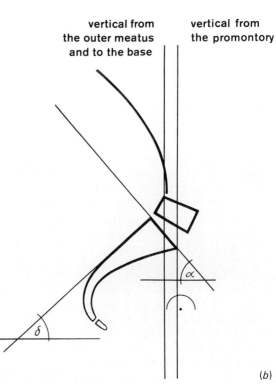

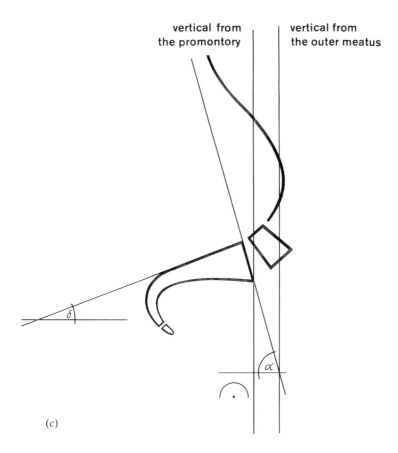

vertical from
the promontory

vertical from
the outer meatus

(*c*)

Figure 3.11 Pelvic types. (*a*) High promontory; (*b*) average type; (*c*) increased pelvic (sacral) inclination
(After Gutmann, 1965.)

frequent anomalies of the lumbosacral region: the last lumbar vertebra is a
'transitional' vertebra and shows by definition that there is hardly any 'norm' and
that variation is the rule. If the variations are asymmetrical, the result may be
obliquity of the sacrum, causing the changes in statics already dealt with. If,
however, there is symmetrical variation, the most important consequence is a
change in the length of the sacrum, affecting the position of the sacral promontory.

Gutmann (1965) and Erdmann (1956) distinguish three pelvic types with
far-reaching differences in function and possible pathology. The first presents a
long sacrum and high sacral promontory, the second the average or intermediate
type, and the third a low promontory and considerable pelvic inclination, which the
authors call 'Hohes Assimiliationsbecken', 'Normal Becken' and
'Überlastungsbecken', respectively. For greater clarity the different criteria are
shown in *Table 3.1* and *Figure 3.11*.

All of this should be borne in mind when evaluating X-ray findings; the type of
pelvis will determine the degree of lordosis to be expected, while the height of the
last intervertebral disc will determine the mobility of the segment.

TABLE 3.1. Pelvic types

Criterion	Type		
	High promontory	*Intermediate*	*Low promontory*
Inclination of sacrum (degrees)	50–70	35–50	15–35
Inclination of upper surface of S1 (degrees)	15–30	30–50	50–70
Position of L4 disc	Above the line of the iliac crests	At the height of the line of the iliac crests	Below the line of the iliac crests
Position of the promontory in the pelvic ring	Eccentric (dorsal)	At the centre	At the centre or even ventral
Shape of L5 vertebra	Rectangular	Wedge shaped	Wedge shaped
Shape of L5 disc	Rectangular and higher than L4	Wedge shaped and lower than L4	Wedge shaped and lower than L4
Level of maximum mobility	L5–S1	L4–L5	L4–L5
Role of iliolumbar ligament	Little fixation of L5	Good fixation of L5	Good fixation of L5 and even of L4
Weight-bearing structure	End-plate of L5	End-plate of L5	Joint surface of S1, sacroiliac joint
Spinal curvature	Flat	Average	Increased
X-ray statics	Hip joints in front of promontory; the plumb-line from the outer acoustic meatus coincides with the vertical from the os naviculare and lies behind the hip joint, slightly behind the promontory	As for high-promontory type	The plumb-line from the outer acoustic meatus lies in front of the promontory, which lies in front of the hip joint
Clinical consequences	Hypermobility, degeneration or prolapse of L5 disc; ligament pain	Blockage, disc lesion of L4 disc	Arthrosis: lumbosacral, sacroiliac and of the hip

The sacroiliac joints

Thanks to the sacroiliac joints and the pubic symphysis there is some mobility of the otherwise firm pelvic girdle, the sacroiliac joints playing the decisive role.

The sacrum is wedge shaped in two directions: (1) the whole structure tapers like a pyramid in the caudal direction; and (2) the upper part (S1–S2) tapers in a dorsal direction (according to Solonen, 1957), while the lower part may taper in either direction. There is a tuberosity on the innominate bone approximately in the middle of the joint surface, fitting into an impression on the joint surface of the sacrum at the level of S2, but there is great variability and this is not the only tuberosity. In the AP X-ray there is a double contour owing to the wedge shape described above, but this varies from case to case and is frequently asymmetrical. It is of some importance that the greater the distance between the two contours of the joint, the greater the divergence (or convergence) and the narrower the joint space appears. Conversely, if there is no convergence and we see only one contour, the joint space appears to be wide.

It is important to point out that despite its unusual shape and the fact that there are no muscles moving the sacrum against the innominate, the sacroiliac joint is a true diarthrosis with its own mobility (Mennell, 1952; Weisl, 1954; Colachis *et al.*, 1963; Duckworth, 1970). According to Duckworth, 'the normal movement that occurs is rotation of the sacrum around the shortest and strongest part of the interosseus sacroiliac ligaments, which run from the iliac tuberosities to the transverse tubercles of the second sacral vertebra'. This movement can be described as nutation, and the weight of the spinal column during walking will tend to rotate the sacrum forward with each step, the sacroiliac joints playing the role of springing shock-absorbers. This rotational movement of the sacrum against the ilium can be palpated and is familiar to gynaecologists in the management of labour. However important it is that there should be some mobility of the sacroiliac joint, it should be very limited and laxity is undesirable.

At the end of this section on the functional anatomy of the pelvis some remarks are required about a clinically very striking phenomenon which may be called 'pelvic distortion'. If the most prominent points of the bony pelvis are palpated, a peculiar apparent discrepancy emerges: whereas the posterior spina iliaca superior (PSIS) is higher on one side, usually the right, the reverse is found on palpating the anterior spina iliaca superior (ASIS). The iliac crest may be laterally at the same level, or there may be a slight difference. On palpation of the posterior part of the iliac crest a similar difference will be felt to that observed on the posterior spinae iliacae, confirming the findings. This might give the impression that one innominate was rotating against the other on a horizontal axis. This cannot be so, because we should then find a considerable shift of the pubic bones at the symphysis.

These clinical facts may best be illustrated anatomically by Cramer's diagram (*Figure 3.12*). This shows a one-sided nutation and therefore also slight rotation of the sacrum between the ilia, producing rotation of one innominate round a horizontal axis and of the other round the vertical.

Although many attempts have been made to visualize by X-ray some of the asymmetrical changes to be expected, X-ray diagnosis of this condition remains unsatisfactory. There is one change, however, that does appear in the X-ray picture, and that is a change in the statics of the lumbar spine, consisting clinically in a shift of the pelvis to the side of the higher posterior iliac spine, which may produce static decompensation of the lumbar spine, visible in the X-ray picture taken standing (*Figure 3.13*).

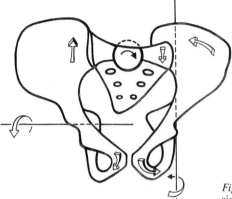

Figure 3.12 The mechanism of pelvic distortion (After Cramer, 1965.)

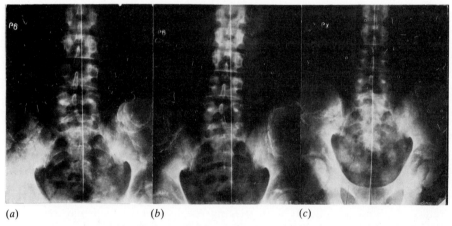

(*a*)   (*b*)   (*c*)

Figure 3.13 Disturbed statics in pelvic distortion. (*a*) Pelvis straight, obliquity at L4 with deviation of the lumbar spine to the left and slight sinistroscoliosis. (*b*) No improvement after applying a left heel-pad. (*c*) After treatment of a blocked atlanto-occipital (!) joint, normal statics and no pelvic distortion

The lumbar spine

Although only a little shorter than the thoracic spine, the lumbar spine is usually formed of five vertebrae. However, mobility in ante- and retroflexion as well as in lateral bending ensures most of the mobility of the trunk. In addition to this important aspect, the lumbar spine has to carry most of the weight of the trunk. The vertebral bodies as well as the arches are therefore more robust.

The apophyseal joints give both mobility and stability. They are vertical, the (larger) lateral part in the sagittal plane and the (smaller) medial part in the coronal plane. The two parts may thus typically form an angle; however, frequently they only form an arch, the lateral part pointing into the sagittal and the medial into the coronal plane. If there is angularity the joint is easily visualized by X-ray, but this is not the case if it is arched. The lumbosacral joint, however, is mainly in the coronal plane. As the final shape of the joint is formed during ontogenesis, anomalies and asymmetry are very frequent.

The shape of the articulation determines the function of the lumbar spine; it allows for much ante- and retroflexion and practically excludes any rotation. It limits lateral flexion as long as lordosis is present, as has already been explained (*see* page 54).

The intervertebral discs are thickest in the lumbar spine and allow great mobility. Their thickness increases from L1 down to L4, hence maximum mobility is usually found at the L4/5 segment. Only in the pelvic type with a high sacral promontory is maximum thickness and mobility found between L5 and S1.

X-ray anatomy

The whole of the vertebral arch may be recognized in *Figure 3.14*; the oval or kidney-shaped pedicles (radix arcus) are most evident. Only the last pedicle projects on to the upper lateral edge of the body of the fifth vertebra and is often less distinct. This is most probably due to the triangular shape of the vertebral canal in the lowest part of the lumbar spine. From the pedicle we may follow the broad shadow of the lamina in the direction of the spinous process. Lateral and above the pedicle we can find the upper articular process; from the lamina downwards and below the pedicle the lower articular process can be traced in a caudal and lateral direction towards the pedicle (and the upper articular process) of the next (caudal) vertebra. Between the arch formed by both lower articular processes and the spinous process of the caudal neighbouring vertebra it is possible to see into the vertebral canal, i.e. the canal is not covered by bone. Where both articular processes meet (close above the pedicle) we can see the joint space (if part of the joint is in the sagittal plane). There is slight divergence of the apophyseal joint in a cranial direction.

The lateral view (*Figure 3.15*) also shows the thick pedicles, from which the articular processes arise. Here, too, we may see the joint space if part of the joint is in the coronal plane. Between the upper and lower articular processes lies the pars isthmica, the site where spondylolysis may be sought. Below the pedicles we see the intervertebral foramina which lie almost exactly in the sagittal plane. Their horizontal diameter almost corresponds to the anteroposterior width of the spinal canal. The lamina is covered by the articular processes, and dorsal to these processes only the broad shadow of the spinous process can be seen. The transverse process projects on to the articular process behind the pedicle, as a small thick shadow.

The last lumbar vertebra differs from the rest in many ways: in the side view it is wedge shaped and with powerfully developed transverse processes it shows a transitional shape in relation to the sacral vertebrae. It is important to bear in mind that the iliolumbar ligament is attached to the transverse process of L5 so that the fifth lumbar vertebra transmits impulses to the lumbar spine both from the sacrum and from the ilia, playing the role of a shock-absorber as well. As the upper surface of the sacrum is usually considerably inclined, the position of the lumbosacral apophyseal joints in a mainly coronal plane may act as a prevention against forward gliding.

Some of the important anomalies encountered have already been dealt with under pelvic types. In cases of transitional lumbosacral vertebrae it may be difficult to determine whether the relevant vertebra is a lumbarized S1 or a sacralized L5. The most reliable reference is to a line drawn between the two iliac crests: if an intervertebral disc lies on that line, the vertebra below this disc is L5. If, however,

64

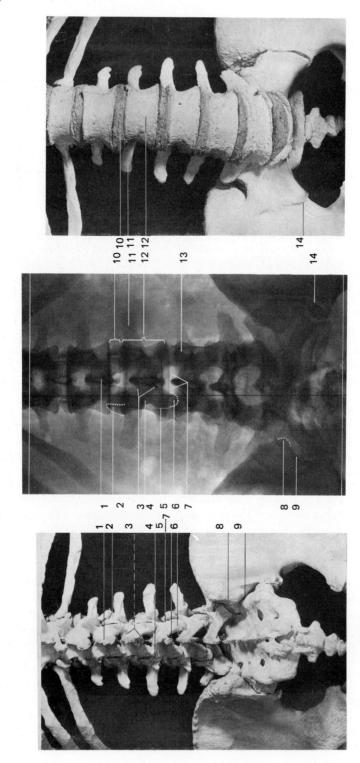

Figure 3.14 Comparison of the anatomical structures in the dorsal aspect of the lumbar spine and the sacrum (left) with the anteroposterior X-ray (centre) and the ventral aspect (right). 1 = Spinous process; 2 = upper articular process; 3 = lamina; 4 = pars interarticularis; 5 = joint space; 6 = lower articular process; 7 = spinal canal; 8 = posterior spina iliaca superior; 9 = dorsal part of the sacroiliac joint; 10 = disc; 11 = transverse process; 12 = vertebral body; 13 = pedicle; 14 = ventral part of the sacroiliac joint

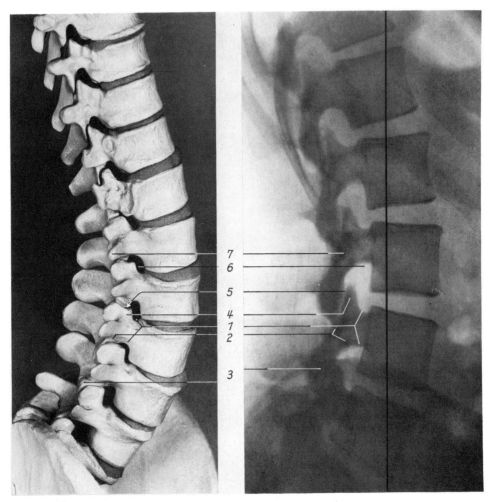

Figure 3.15 Comparison of the anatomical structures in the lateral view of the lumbar spine (model) and the X-ray. 1 = Pedicle; 2 = pars interarticularis; 3 = lower articular process; 4 = upper articular process; 5 = joint space; 6 = intervertebral foramen; 7 = transverse process

this line passes through the middle of a vertebral body, it may be impossible to determine the transitional vertebra, in particular if there appear to be six lumbar vertebrae, without taking an X-ray of the thoracic spine. Instead of a transverse process, a transitional lumbosacral vertebra may have a massa lateralis which forms a pseudoarthrosis with the massa lateralis of the sacrum, and may even cause symptoms.

The most important anomaly, clinically, is probably a narrow spinal canal which may become even narrower as a result of spondylosis. This is relatively easily recognized in the lateral view by the disproportion between the large vertebral body and short thick pedicles, the narrow intervertebral foramina and the steep lower articular processes. In the AP view, although it would appear logical to do so, this condition should never be assessed according to the interpedicular distance,

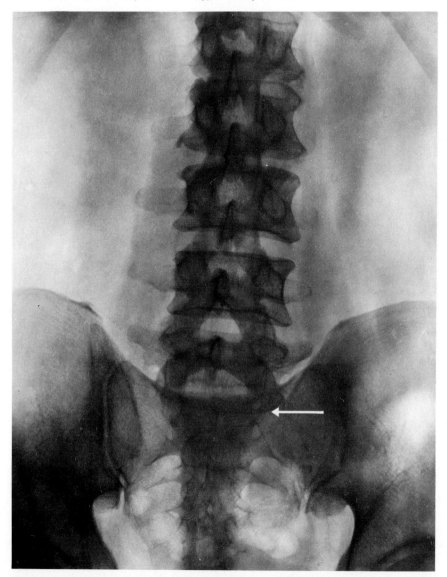

Figure 3.16 The anterior lower edge of the vertebral body of L5 is lower on the left side (arrow) in relation to the sacrum, hence the L5 disc is narrower on the left; compensatory lumbar scoliosis with left rotation

but by the distance between the two lower articular processes, i.e. the width of the translucency corresponding to the spinal canal. In such cases the articular processes present a swallow-tail shape on X-ray. The articular processes are very thick and the joints clearly visible. If a typical picture is seen in both views we may infer that the spinal canal is trefoil in section. (However significant these signs may be in classic radiology, CT scanning visualizes the spinal canal directly.)

It is of course important to establish sound criteria for assessing the thickness of an intervertebral disc; it should be borne in mind that congenital disc hypoplasia is a common anomaly, not to be confused with disc degeneration. The former condition is found particularly frequently at the lumbosacral disc (where anomalies most often occur). Therefore if the last vertebra shows marked signs of being a transitional vertebra and there are no signs of marginal sclerosis, bone spurs or increased laxity (shift), a diagnosis of degeneration is unfounded. A valuable sign of disc hypoplasia is reduced width of both vertebral margins adjacent to the hypoplastic disc. Although we usually rely on lateral views for the assessment of discs, marked asymmetry in the AP view may be of some importance, particularly at the L5–S1 interspace, as here assessment may be difficult in view of the frequency of anomalies. A marked narrowing on one side may then point to disc degeneration (*Figure 3.16*).

Evaluation of function

For evaluation of function and its possible disturbances, pictures must be taken under standard conditions (*see* pages 46–48).

Assessment of rotation is of value, because rotation should be proportionate to scoliosis and can be modified by the degree of lordosis; if rotation is disproportionate, or limited to one or two intervertebral segments only, it can be a sign of disturbed function. Rotation is recognized by a shift of the spinous process and the pedicles in the direction opposite of that to rotation. On the side of rotation the pedicle becomes wider and the articulation is better visualized; the transverse process is shorter (*Figure 3.17*). Rotation should never be evaluated on the basis of one single sign (such as deviation of the spinous process). The assessment of lateral flexion (scoliosis) is carried out according to the principles of body statics.

In the lateral view we assess lordosis or kyphosis as well as a forward or backward shift. A *local* interruption of the lordotic line or of kyphosis, between two vertebrae, can be a sign of disc lesion. A shift (forwards or backwards) may be a sign of increased mobility – laxity. This may be particularly conspicuous during ante- or retroflexion. Very slight, proportional shifts in ante- or retroflexion in young patients, seen at X-ray examination, can be regarded as normal. Two diagnostic pitfalls must be stressed. The first is the incongruous surfaces of two adjacent vertebrae, occurring most frequently between L5 and the sacrum; the upper surface of S1 in such cases is usually slightly longer than the lower surface of L5, and looking at the posterior edge of the adjacent vertebrae one gets the impression of an anterior shift of L5, or (looking at the anterior edge) of a posterior shift of L5. The second pitfall is slight rotation: here the posterior and anterior margins of the vertebrae form a double contour which can be mistaken for a shift.

These shifts due to hypermobility must, of course, be distinguished from true spondylolisthesis (with spondylolysis) and from degenerative spondylolisthesis (the pseudospondylolisthesis of Junghanns, 1930) due to deformity, the bending forward of an upper articular process (most frequently L5) over which the vertebra above glides forward.

X-ray studies of movement

X-ray pictures in the upright position may not provide any clues to disturbed function; those taken in ante- or retroflexion or lateral flexion may then reveal some irregularity. We may distinguish segments of increased or lowered mobility.

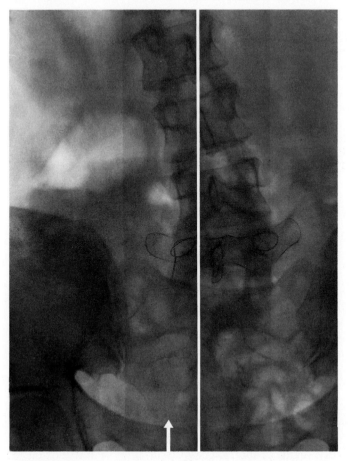

Figure 3.17 Rotation of lumbar vertebrae with lateral shift of the spinous processes and pedicles in relation to the vertebral bodies

In ante- and retroflexion increased mobility may take the form of ventral or dorsal shift respectively ('disc rolling'). As has already been pointed out, very slight proportional shifting movements in all segments may be considered normal, particularly in young subjects (Jirout, 1956). There is one interesting exception: in the lumbosacral segment there sometimes occurs a 'paradoxical' shift, i.e. during anteflexion a dorsal and during retroflexion a ventral shift, which may be described as a sort of leverage (Jirout, 1956).

Narrowing of an intervertebral disc, due to degeneration, may sometimes be visible only in ante- or retroflexion. In such cases we see exaggerated anterior narrowing of the disc (without compensatory posterior widening) in anteflexion and exaggerated posterior narrowing (without compensatory anterior widening) in retroflexion.

Mobility studies are usually made where there is a clinical reason for doing so, i.e. if movement in some specific direction causes symptoms. A condition in which this type of examination is particularly important is spondylolisthesis, because it is advisable to ascertain whether the spondylolisthesis is fixed or mobile; it is the latter that causes symptoms and has a tendency to deteriorate.

In lateral flexion it is most important to correlate the degree of flexion and rotation with regard to the degree of lordosis (*see* page 54).

The thoracic spine

Functional anatomy

The thoracic spine (*Figures 3.18* and *3.19*) is the longest part of the spinal column and that which enjoys the least mobility. The main reason for this is its close relationship to the thorax but it is also explained by the thinness of the intervertebral discs. The apophyseal joints are almost vertical and show a slight tilt in the coronal plane, as if on the periphery of a cylinder whose centre is in front of the vertebral body. This shape would allow for considerable rotation were it not for

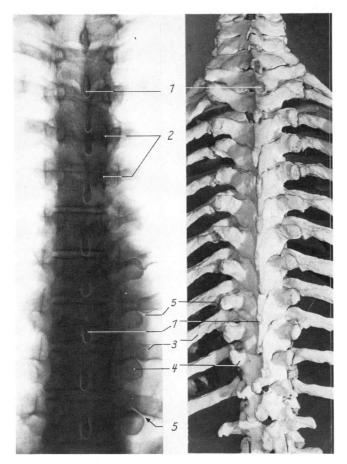

Figure 3.18 Comparison of the anatomical structures in the dorsal view of the thoracic spine (skeleton) with the anteroposterior X-ray. 1 = Spinous process; 2 = pedicles; 3 = ribs; 4 = transverse process; 5 = transversocostal joint

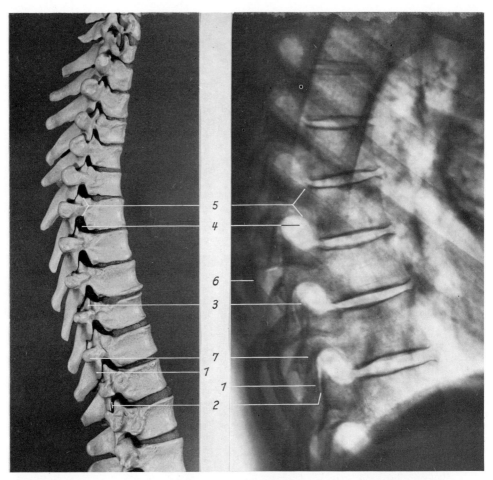

Figure 3.19 Comparison of the anatomical structures in the lateral view of the skeleton of the thoracic spine with the X-ray. 1 = Lower articular process; 2 = joint space; 3 = upper articular process; 4 = intervertebral foramen; 5 = pedicles; 6 = rib; 7 = transverse process

the ribs and the intervertebral discs. Side and forward bending, too, are limited mainly by the ribs, although the latter movement is also held in check by the inter- and supraspinal ligaments. Back bending is limited mainly by apposition locking of the articular and the spinous processes. Due to this relatively limited mobility, trunk rotation takes place mainly in the lowest thoracic segments, those least fixed by the ribs.

Function and its disturbances are of particular significance at the thoracolumbar junction. This may be because in this region movement changes from one type to another within a single segment, as can be deduced from the shape of the apophyseal joints: on a single vertebra the upper articular processes may be in the coronal plane and the lower mostly in the sagittal plane (*Figure 3.18*). Whereas in the lowest thoracic segments axial rotation is the most prominent function, it suddenly ceases between T12 and L1. As we have already seen (*see* page 54), with the patient marking time the thoracolumbar junction forms a relatively fixed point where lumbar scoliosis to one side changes to thoracic scoliosis to the opposite side.

Another region of transition and increased vulnerability is the cervicothoracic junction down to T3–4, because it is here that movements of the head and neck end, as is most clearly seen in maximum ante- and retroflexion. The same is true for side-bending and rotation if the cervicothoracic junction is held upright. This function is particularly vulnerable because here the very mobile cervical spine meets the much less mobile thoracic spine. The shoulder girdle, with its powerful muscles, is also attached to this junction.

All transitional regions are rich in anomalies. There may be a rudimentary twelfth rib or a (rudimentary) lumbar L1; remarkably, a cervical rib (C7) is quite common, while we rarely find a rudimentary first rib.

The ribs

The ribs are attached to the vertebrae at the transversocostal and costovertebral joints. The head of the rib articulates with the upper margin of the body of the corresponding vertebra and with the lower margin of the vertebral body next above. The centre of the head of the rib (crista capituli) is attached to the intervertebral disc by ligaments. The first rib is an exception in that it articulates exclusively with the body of the first thoracic vertebra. The neck of the rib fixed between the costovertebral and costotransversal articulation forms an axis for rib movement. This axis is horizontal in the true (vertebrosternal) ribs and produces a movement by which the sternum is lifted and at the same time the thorax broadens. In the false (vertebrochondral) ribs the axis is oblique, laterodorsocaudal, and produces a wing-like movement.

The X-ray picture

In the AP view visualization of the structures of the vertebral arch is much less detailed than in the lumbar spine. In addition to the vertebral bodies and intervertebral discs we see the spinous processes and the pedicles (*see Figure 3.18*). It should be borne in mind that from about T4 to T10 the tip of the spinous process is seen at the level of the body of the next vertebra below. The characteristic feature is the costovertebral junction, the head of the rib against the intervertebral disc and the overlapping shadow of the costal neck and the transverse process. As the facets of the costotransverse joints are tilted from dorsocranial to ventrocaudal (almost to the vertical plane) the joint is usually poorly visualized in the AP view, with the exception of the lower thoracic ribs, if this tilt is considerable.

In the lateral view (*Figure 3.19*) the vertebral arches are partly overlapped by the ribs. If, however, the pictures are clear, we get a good view of the intervertebral foramen and even of the joint facets (articular processes). The thoracic spine above T3 is unfortunately hidden by the structures of the shoulder girdle and must be visualized either by oblique views or by tomography.

It may be difficult to number the vertebrae in the lateral view, as T1 cannot be seen and it is hard to recognize T12. It is therefore useful to remember that the lower angle of the shoulder blade is usually at the height of T7, the arch of the aorta at T4, the fork of the trachea at T5 and the dome of the diaphragm at T9/10.

Evaluating X-rays

As in all parts of the spinal column, curvature is important here from the point of view of function, the most significant changes being scoliosis and increased kyphosis. Here again it must be pointed out that it is essential for us to know whether the curvature is in static equilibrium. There is yet another important aspect of curvature: the more marked it is, the less mobile that section of the spinal column will be, and conversely, a flat thoracic spine is accompanied by hypermobility, which is of considerable clinical significance.

Changes in function may go hand in hand with signs of sudden rotation of one vertebra to the next, or with a sudden deviation of the spinous processes together with signs of rotation. Again rotation is diagnosed by a shift of both the spinous processes *and* the pedicles in the opposite direction from that of rotation.

Shifts are hardly ever seen in the lateral view of the thoracic spine, nor is kyphotic angulation between two vertebrae which is simply due to changes in function. Angulation may, however, be due to deformity, which is particularly frequent in the thoracic spine as a consequence of juvenile osteochondrosis.

In asymmetrical movement restriction of the ribs there may be asymmetry of the distance between the vertebral arches.

The cervical spine

The cervical spine is the most mobile section of the whole spinal column. It is the site of the tonic neck reflexes with their repercussions throughout the entire postural musculature; disturbances of function in this region are therefore particularly disastrous, and their adequate treatment strikingly effective.

X-ray technique

In order to obtain pictures that can be evaluated for function, adequate standard techniques must be established. The usual technique, which visualizes the craniocervical junction poorly in the side view and not at all in the AP view, is not even adequate to show the anatomical details properly and is completely useless for the evaluation of function.

In the AP view the entire cervical spine should be visible, from the craniocervical junction (foramen magnum with the occipital condyles) to the first thoracic vertebrae. An 18 × 24 cm film is usually sufficient, but 15 × 40 cm can also be used, showing the upper thoracic spine at the same time. The patient is placed as follows (Gutmann, 1956; Sandberg, 1955): first he is seated on the X-ray table so that the extended legs are symmetrically placed one on each side of the mid-line. Only then is he asked to lie down, without using his arms, in the position that is most natural to him (the position may be checked by repeating the procedure). If the head regularly deviates from the mid-line *this must not be corrected*, because to do so would either correct or produce cervical scoliosis, and at the same time induce axis rotation and lateral deviation of the atlas.

It is therefore necessary to shift the film and the X-ray tube accordingly. The patient now opens his mouth as wide as possible and a gag is placed between his teeth; he then draws his chin in until the glabella and the filtrum are on the same horizontal plane. For this a pillow beneath the head is often necessary.

We are now ready to focus the X-ray tube. The central ray must pass through a point one finger below the upper premolars and one finger above the posterior margin of the occipital foramen (*Figure 3.20*). If the patient has no teeth the central ray passes through a point one finger below the upper gums to the posterior margin of the foramen magnum. The distance from focus to film should be 1 m.

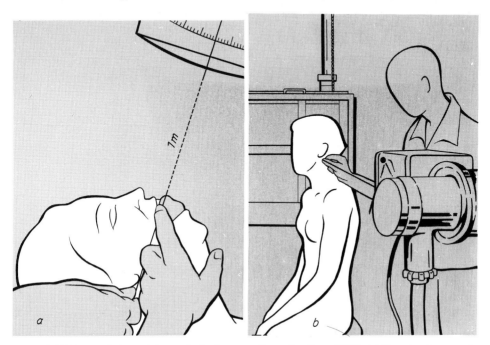

Figure 3.20 X-ray technique of the cervical spine according to Sandberg (1955). (*a*) Focusing the central ray in the anteroposterior view with the aid of a string, the head in a horizontal position; (*b*) focusing the X-ray tube in the lateral view

Finally we correct any rotation of the patient's head, bearing in mind the possibility of asymmetry (the upper teeth are a useful landmark).

It is possible to proceed in an analogous manner with the patient seated, which is more difficult but has the advantage of being performed under the influence of body statics. Nevertheless there can be diagnostic advantage if the side view, which must *always* be taken with the patient seated, reveals discrepancies when compared with the AP view taken with the patient supine. In such cases the AP view can always be repeated in the sitting position.

Some authors dislike the open-mouth technique because the mandible overlaps the mid-cervical spine, and prefer to take the picture while the patient rhythmically opens and shuts his mouth; in this way the shadow of the mandible is blurred. The technique, however, presents the danger of a slight shaking of the head, which will cause blurring of the image of the apophyseal joints of the craniocervical junction.

In the lateral view the patient is seated relaxed in front of a vertical X-ray cassette; no Potter–Bucky diaphragm is needed. The film may be 18 × 24 cm or 24 × 30 cm, and must be placed so that the X-ray shows the base of the skull with the sella turcica, the hard palate and the cervical spine down to C7, if possible with the first two thoracic vertebrae. This is only possible in subjects (usually women) with very tapering shoulders. The patient fixes his eyes on some object at eye-level, to keep the head in a standard position; head rotation or lateral flexion must be corrected.

The central ray is focused *not* at the mid-cervical region (centre of the film) but at the mastoid process. This yields an undistorted view of the base of the skull and yet causes no distortion of the lower cervical spine (because the base of the skull is wide, while the cervical vertebrae are narrow). In addition we achieve correct

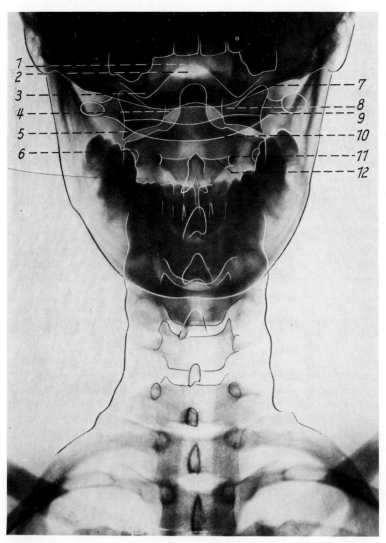

Figure 3.21 Anatomical structures of the craniocervical junction, anteroposterior view. 1 = Lower edge of the clivus; 2 = foramen magnum; 3 = occipital condyle; 4 = lower edge of the anterior arch of the atlas; 5 = lateral triangle; 6 = foramen transversarium of the axis; 7 = lower contour of the squama occipitalis; 8 = medial translucency of the atlas; 9 = transverse process of the atlas; 10 = lower edge of the posterior arch of the atlas; 11 = pedicle of the axis; 12 = lamina of the axis

exposure of both the base of the skull and the craniocervical junction *and* of the cervical vertebrae. The distance from focus to film should be 150 cm or more. With this technique pictures of the craniocervical junction are so clear that tomography is seldom necessary.

Assessment of the quality of X-ray pictures

Before evaluating an X-ray of the cervical spine, particularly where function is concerned, we must assess its quality as a picture (*Figure 3.21*). In the AP view we first make sure that we can see both occipital condyles, the atlas and the axis with both transversocostal foramina (foramina of the vertebral artery), and at the caudal end, the first thoracic vertebra. If the view is correct we see the cleft between the upper and lower front teeth in mid-line, together with the centre of the odontoid process and of the chin. The cervical spine as a whole must lie symmetrically

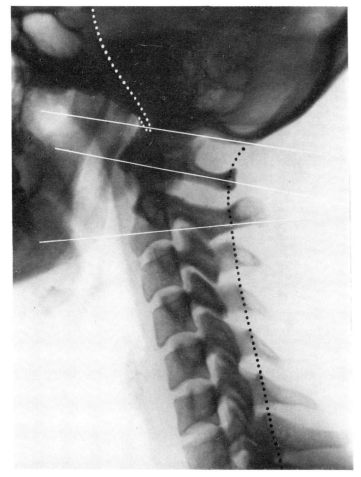

Figure 3.22 Lateral X-ray of the cervical spine with the plane of the foramen magnum, the atlas and the axis indicated; the clivus and the posterior edge of the vertebral canal are also shown

between the two halves of the mandibula. Even if each of these structures is asymmetrical there are sufficient landmarks by which to recognize distortion. A picture without the craniocervical junction and the first thoracic vertebra with the thoracic outlet is insufficient for our purpose.

In the lateral view we need to see the base of the skull with the sella turcica, the clivus down to the basion, the posterior margin of the foramen magnum, the hard palate, the odontoid process and the cervical spine down to C7; if possible even the first thoracic vertebra should be seen, but in heavily built patients it may be impossible to visualize C7 in the lateral view. It is important that the hard palate should be horizontal (for assessment of lordosis or kyphosis) and that the two halves of the mandibula should be exactly overlaid, showing that there is neither side-bending nor rotation (*Figure 3.22*). Fineman *et al.* (1963) showed that a difference of only 10 degrees in inclination of the head is sufficient to change lordotic to linear posture and vice versa.

The oblique view serves mainly to show the intervertebral foramina, which in the cervical spine are not visualized at all in the side view and poorly in the AP view. It should be taken with the patient sitting on a chair turned at 45 degrees to the cassette; the patient usually sits with his back to it, but like Gutmann I prefer the patient to face the cassette and to hold the head in retroflexion, because if the patient faces the cassette it is the foramen nearer to it that is visualized, and narrowing of the foramen is often visible only in retroflexion (*Figure 3.23*).

Oblique views are particularly important in cervical radicular syndromes and in cases of the vertebral artery syndrome, because of the close relationship between the intervertebral foramen, the nerve roots and the vertebral artery.

Functional anatomy of the cervical spine

The cervical spine has two very distinct sections: the craniocervical junction between the occiput and C2, and the section from C2 to C7. Most of the movements it performs start at the craniocervical junction, and the movements of the head and neck are usually initiated by eye movements. I shall therefore begin with a short anatomical description in which the two parts will be treated separately, while the function of the cervical spine will be dealt with as a whole.

Functional anatomy, C2–C7

As in other parts of the spinal column the degree of movement in the cervical spine is determined mainly by the thickness of the intervertebral disc; this is usually the greatest in the segments C4/5 and C5/6, where mobility is also the greatest. The characteristic feature of the cervical vertebral bodies is a lateral ridge, the unciform process. Its significance for cervical function is that the shape of the vertebral body limits lateral flexion while encouraging ante- and retroflexion.

The apophyseal joints are almost parallel on both sides and are tilted from ventrocranial to dorsocaudal in the direction of the eyes. This tilt varies considerably (round about 45 degrees), being greatest at C2/3 as a rule. At this level the joints are frequently not parallel but as if on the surface of a cylinder with its centre behind the spinal column; it is therefore *not* pathological if the articulation of C2/3 is not well visualized in the side view (unlike the other cervical apophyseal joints). This shape of the cervical apophyseal joints is best suited to

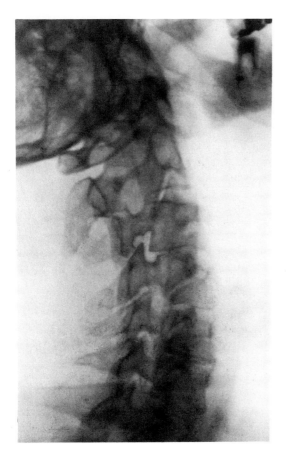

Figure 3.23 Oblique view of the cervical
spine in retroflexion showing a narrowed
intervertebral foramen of C3/4 on the right

ante- and retroflexion. On lateral flexion the tilt of the joints produces rotation to
the side of inclination and during head rotation inclination results for the same
reason.

During anteflexion there is frequently a slight forward shift of the cranial
vertebra, and in retroflexion a slight backward shift which is also in accordance with
the tilt of the articular facets. According to Penning (1968) this forward and
backward movement of the cranial on the caudal vertebra is like a rotation of the
upper vertebra in the sagittal plane round an axis situated in the dorsal part of the
lower vertebral body. It should be pointed out that these shifting movements,
which are the rule in children and young adults, are less frequent and less marked in
higher age groups. It is important to realize that they are physiological if they are
proportionate, and that the shift is greatest in the C2/3 segment (*see Figure 3.29*).

It must also be borne in mind that during anteflexion the cervical vertebral canal
lengthens considerably, shortening during retroflexion. This produces a significant
movement of the meninges with their root sleeves, and also of the spinal cord,
which can be seen in pneumomyelography to get longer and thinner in anteflexion
and shorter and thicker in retroflexion.

Another highly significant feature is the course of the vertebral artery, which
enters its bony canal at the transversocostal foramen of C6 and runs upwards,

crossing the intervertebral canals in close contact with the articular processes and the unciform processes almost at right angles to the course of the nerve roots. Therefore, as the intervertebral foramen (canal) narrows in retroflexion, this may affect both the nerve root *and* the vertebral artery.

Functional anatomy of the craniocervical junction

Study of this most important junction is concerned with the mobility of each of its joints and the bony structures and ligaments that limit it. There are no intravertebral discs.

The upper articular facets of the atlas are oval, with their long axis running obliquely, converging anteriorly and medially like a section of the surface of a sphere with its centre located above both articular surfaces. The main mobility in the atlanto-occipital joints is ante- and retroflexion, about 15 degrees (*Figure 3.24*). There is posterior gliding of the occipital condyles during anteflexion and anterior gliding during retroflexion. Slight rotation is possible, which Jirout (1981) has shown to be a synkinesis during side-bending of the head; there is very limited lateral flexion, rotation being coupled with side-bending to the opposite side.

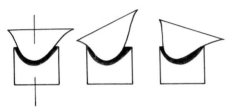

Figure 3.24 Ante- and retroflexion between occiput and atlas

The atlantoaxial joints comprise the atlanto-odontoid as well as the joints between the massae laterales and the axis, and their main function is axial rotation. The joint facets run anteroposteriorly and are concave on the massa lateralis of the atlas and convex on the axis. In addition there is the atlanto-odontoid joint between the anterior arch of the atlas and the odontoid process anteriorly, while the posterior surface of the odontoid process is lined by cartilage and in contact with the transverse ligament.

The possible movements are ante- and retroflexion and rotation. During ante- and retroflexion the anterior arch of the atlas glides up and down on the odontoid and if the transverse ligament is firm the space between these two structures does not widen. The range of movement here is again about 15 degrees.

The most important movement, however, is rotation, in which all joints take part; while there is rotation round the odontoid, the massa lateralis of the atlas glides on the axis posteriorly on the side of rotation and anteriorly on the opposite side. Rotation is limited by the joint capsules and the powerful alar ligaments which are attached to the margins of the foramen magnum. Rotation amounts on average to 25 degrees to each side, the maximum being 40 degrees (*Figures 3.25* and *3.26*).

Kinesiology of the cervical spine as a whole

ROTATION

During rotation, movement starts between the atlas and axis and is limited to these joints until their range is exhausted; i.e. to about 25 degrees to each side, on average. Recently this has been demonstrated by X-ray (Berger, Lewit, Stampfel,

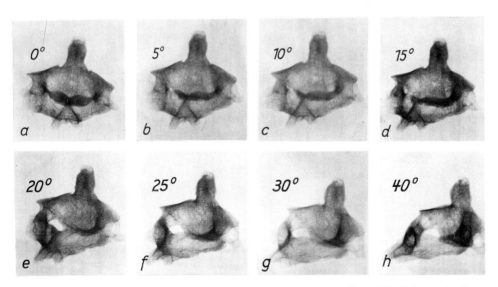

Figure 3.25 Anteroposterior X-rays of an isolated axis: (*a*) in neutral position and (*b–h*) in rotation from 5 to 40 degrees; the pictures are useful for gauging

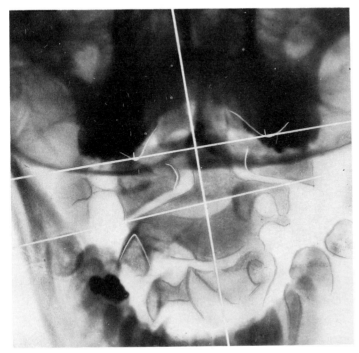

Figure 3.26 Rotation of the axis in relation to the atlas (head): the head is fixed in neutral position, the body in maximum rotation (here at 40 degrees axis rotation; cf. *Figure 3.25(h)*)

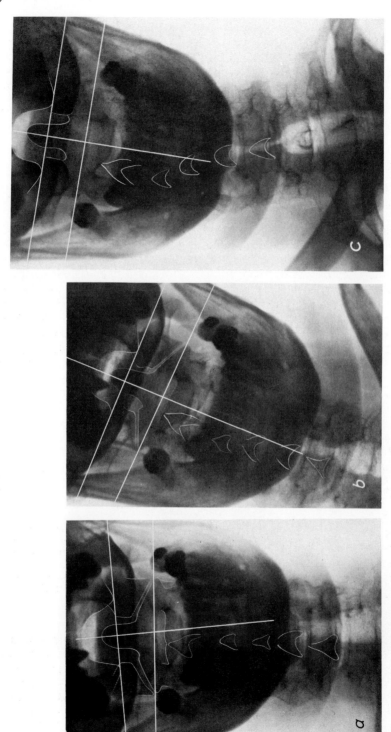

Figure 3.27 Anteroposterior X-ray of the cervical spine of a healthy subject, in neutral position, during active lateral flexion and passive lateral flexion limited to the upper cervical region. (*a*) In neutral position the atlas is to the right in relation to the condyles and the plane of the condyles and the axis converge on the right, the axis being rotated about 5 degrees to the left. (*b*) At active lateral flexion to the left the atlas is still to the right of the condyles and the plane of the condyles and the axis converge a little to the right, the axis now being rotated about 10 degrees to the left. (*c*) Passive lateral flexion of the upper cervical spine to the left: the atlas is now clearly to the left of the condyles and the plane of the condyles is now parallel to the axis which is rotated about 10 degrees

in press). Up to this point there is pure axial rotation in the horizontal plane. From this point onwards rotation takes place from C3 to C7 in succession if there is flexion at the cervicothoracic junction, and as far as T3 if the cervicothoracic junction is straightened up. There is still some additional passive rotation between the occiput and the atlas. The moment rotation is performed in the cervical spine *below* the axis, side-bending automatically takes place at the same time, unless deliberately avoided.

SIDE-BENDING

Side-bending can only be studied by X-ray, and will therefore be dealt with under X-ray mobility studies. Like rotation it begins at the craniocervical junction. This can best be studied during a passive side-tilting movment localizing lateral flexion mainly in the upper cervical area (*Figure 3.27*). This shows that lateral flexion starts with *rotation of the axis* in the direction of side-bending and at the same time there is synkinesis of the atlas, shifting relative both to the occipital condyles and to the axis, in the direction of side-bending.

On lateral flexion of the whole of the cervical spine we see side-bending *and* rotation in the direction of lateral flexion, being greatest at the axis. As Jirout (1968) has shown, this rotation usually ends in the lower cervical spine during flexion to the right, but during bending to the left can be followed down into the upper thoracic region. (This he explains as the result of the stronger pull of the muscles of the shoulder girdle attached to the spinous processes on the right side.)

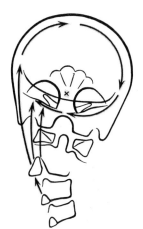

Figure 3.28 Mechanism of lateral flexion of the cervical spine according to Jirout (1971). During side-bending the head rotates round a sagittal axis (x) situated in the anterior cranial fossa. The diagram shows how the base of the skull, with the condyles, shifts in the opposite direction to lateral flexion against the atlas, and how the axis with the lower cervical vertebrae is brought into rotation and the spinous process of the axis is tilted forward by cranial pull

This combination of side-bending and rotation is, of course, in accordance with the tilt of the cervical apophyseal joints but is not a direct consequence of the tilt, as is usually thought, since the movement starts at the craniocervical junction and rotation of the axis comes first, followed by rotation of the lower cervical vertebrae in succession. As will be shown in detail later, if rotation of the axis does not take place, there is no rotation of the rest of the cervical spine. Jirout (1971) has shown the force causing rotation during side-bending in a diagram (*Figure 3.28*). It can easily be seen that some anteflexion might take place with rotation during side-bending, and these synkineses in the sagittal plane have in fact been confirmed by Jirout (1971); they constitute joint play in the cervical spine. Yet the exact mechanism that forces the axis to rotate the moment lateral flexion starts (which can easily be palpated) is still unknown.

ANTEFLEXION AND RETROFLEXION

Anteflexion can be carried out in different ways: we can either draw the chin in; or let the head drop forward; or bring the chin to the chest, which is a combination of the first two movements. In retroflexion there are no such differences. The two mechanisms of anteflexion are somewhat in competition: unless there is hypermobility, if we draw the chin in we cannot drop the head far forward and if we drop it forward we cannot draw the chin in. The explanation lies in the mechanism of atlas tilt, which must be understood in order to assess cervical ante- and retroflexion.

The following changes can be observed in X-ray studies in the sagittal plane (*see Figures 3.29* and *3.30*).

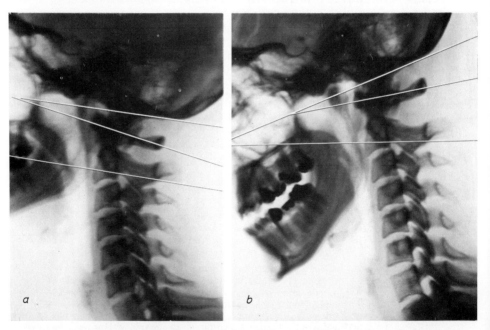

Figure 3.29 Mobility of the cervical spine during ante- and retroflexion. (*a*) Neutral head position with the patient erect; the atlas is in retroflexion with relation to the axis and the head in anteflexion with relation to the atlas. (*b*) With the chin drawn in, anteflexion of the occiput with relation to the atlas increases only very little, while there is now marked anteflexion of the atlas in relation to the axis. (*c*) Anteflexion: while anteflexion of the atlas is now at maximum (anterior tilt of the atlas) the head has moved into retroflexion so that the plane of the foramen magnum and of the atlas now lie almost parallel. (*d*) Retroflexion, sitting: there is both retroflexion of the head against the atlas and of the atlas against the axis, the former being less owing to the tilting of the atlas; as in anteflexion, the plane of the foramen magnum lies parallel to the plane of the atlas. (*e*) Retroflexion with the patient on her side: as the weight of the head no longer plays a role, there is no backward tilt of the atlas and there is thus maximum retroflexion of the head against the atlas and far less retroflexion of the atlas against the axis. Note also the shift of the basion during head anteflexion (forward) and backwards during retroflexion (sitting!)

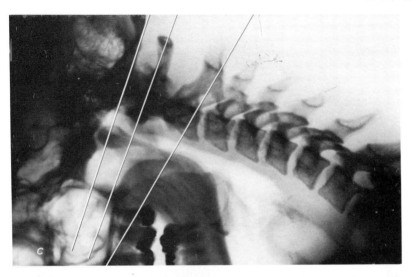

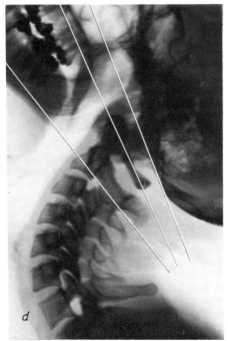

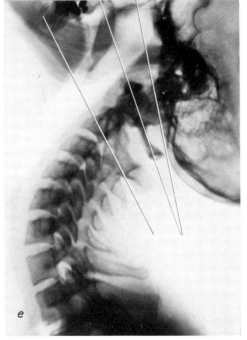

1. With the patient in the erect position the plane of the foramen magnum and the axis run almost parallel, the atlas being tilted backwards at an average angle of about 6 degrees.

2. When the patient draws in the chin, anteflexion between occiput and atlas increases only slightly; the main movement is anteflexion between atlas and axis, the former being now tilted forward while the rest of the cervical spine remains almost straight.

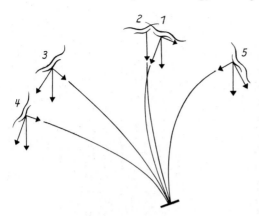

Figure 3.30 The mechanism of atlas tilt

3. In maximum anteflexion the cervical spine is almost horizontal; there is proportionate ventral shift of the cervical vertebrae up to C2/3; there is maximum anteflexion between C1/2, but contrary to positions (1) and (2) anteflexion of the occiput against the atlas has now disappeared, i.e. there is retroflexion of the head against the atlas or forward tilt of the atlas. Consequently, the angle between the clivus and the odontoid, i.e. the measure of kyphosis between the head and the odontoid, remains the same as with the head erect, and is greatest when the chin is drawn in. There is some degree of forward shift of the basion against the tip of the odontoid.
4. In retroflexion with the patient sitting, there is maximum retroflexion of the atlas against the axis (not between the occiput and the atlas!); we see a proportionate backwards shift of the cervical vertebrae and of the basion against the tip of the odontoid.
5. In retroflexion while lying on the side there is now maximum retroflexion of the occiput against the atlas and much less retroflexion of the atlas against the axis. There is no shift of the basion backwards (the subject must *not* force his head back).

The mechanism underlying these phenomena, in particular movement of the atlas, is illustrated in *Figure 3.30*, which shows how the atlas is tilted forward during anteflexion and backwards during retroflexion, with the subject seated, by the weight of the occipital condyles.

X-ray anatomy of the cervical spine

AP VIEW (*Figures 3.31* and *3.32*)

In the AP view we see the arch formed by both occipital condyles and the anterior margin of the foramen magnum. The condyles articulate with the lateral masses of the atlas, the atlanto-occipital joints being visible on both sides, their planes meeting at an angle of about 125–130 degrees. Beneath the condyles we see on both sides of the odontoid process the lateral masses of the atlas, which are wedge shaped, tapering towards the medial border. Close to this border we often see a translucency which should not be taken for osteolysis. Laterally there are the transverse processes. From one transverse process to the other one can follow the

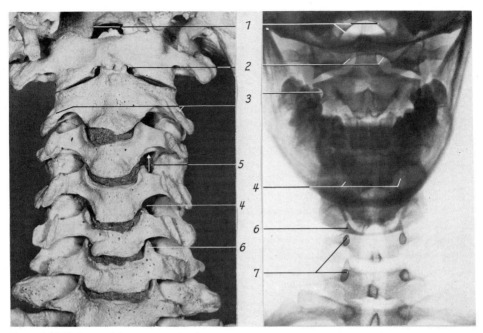

Figure 3.31 Skeleton of the cervical spine (ventral aspect) compared with the anteroposterior X-ray. 1 = Anterior edge of the foramen magnum; 2 = lower edge of the anterior arch of the atlas; 3 = foramen transversarium of the axis; 4 = foramen intervertebrale; 5 = course of the vertebral artery; 6 = unciform process; 7 = pedicle

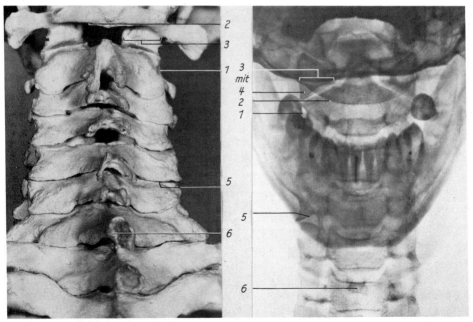

Figure 3.32 Skeleton of the cervical spine (dorsal aspect) compared with the anteroposterior X-ray. 1 = Foramen transversarium of the axis; 2 = lower edge of the posterior arch of the atlas; 3 = massa lateralis of the atlas with (4) the lateral triangle; 5 = joint space; 6 = spinous process

course of the posterior arch which is like a spindle, broadest at its centre. The lateral triangles of the massae laterales project below the shadow of the posterior arch. Sometimes the anterior arch can be seen crossing the tip of the odontoid.

Below the massa lateralis of the atlas we see the atlantoaxial joints and the joint facets of the axis. Medially these facets end in a notch bordering the odontoid process situated between the lateral masses of the atlas and well below the border of the foramen magnum. Close beneath the lateral tip of the axis joint facets we see the foramen costotransversarium of the axis. Medial to this foramen we see the pedicles, while between the pedicles we see the arch of the axis with the spinous process in mid-line. If there is marked lordosis it is possible to see the translucency of the spinal canal at that level.

Below C2 the cervical vertebrae are characterized by the uniform processes on both sides; the intervertebral disc is therefore much higher medially than laterally. The narrow shadow of the pedicles lies below the uniform process and the spinous processes are in mid-line. Lateral to the uniform process the intervertebral foramen can be seen. The lateral contour is formed by the transversocostal process and sometimes the intervertebral joint can be seen.

SIDE VIEW (*Figure 3.33*)

In the side view an undistorted picture of the base of the skull with its relationship to the upper cervical spine is obtained. In particular, the clivus can be followed

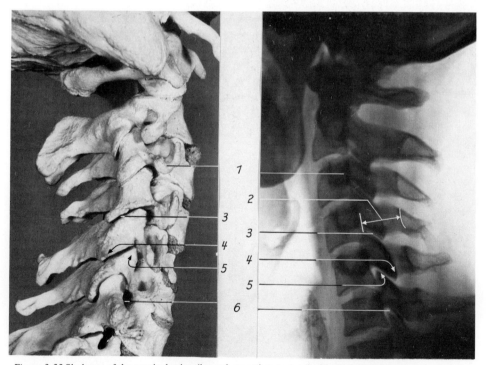

Figure 3.33 Skeleton of the cervical spine (lateral aspect) compared with the lateral X-ray. 1 = Transverse process; 2 = width of the spinal canal; 3 = joint space; 4 = lower articular process; 5 = foramen intervertebrale

down to where it forms the anterior margin of the foramen magnum (basion) which is usually situated above the tip of the odontoid process. The position of the posterior margin of the foramen magnum opisthion is sometimes clearly seen, if the squama occipitalis is followed down to the base of the skull. If not the posterior margin of the cervical spinal canal is followed and where its prolongation meets the base of the skull the position of the opisthion is determined (*see Figure 3.22*).

The mastoid process frequently overshadows part of the massa lateralis of the atlas and therefore the atlanto-occipital joint is not always well visualized in the side view; in some cases, however, it can be seen very well (*Figure 3.34*).

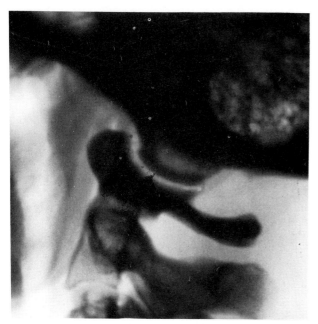

Figure 3.34 Atlanto-occipital joint, lateral view

To determine the plane of the foramen magnum a line is drawn from the basion to the posterior margin of the foramen magnum. The plane of the atlas corresponds to a line connecting the centre of its posterior and anterior arches; the plane of the axis corresponds to a line from the lowest point of the transversocostal process to the lower margin of the arch of the axis. This allows relative ante- or retroflexion of the head, atlas and axis to be assessed.

The shadow of the odontoid process is just behind the anterior arch of the atlas, the tip of the odontoid being usually about the same level as the upper margin of the anterior arch. It should not be much above the palato-occipital line; this is the case in basilar impression.

Unlike the rest of the spinal column, the transversocostal processes with the pedicles project on the vertebral bodies in the side view. The upper margin of the transversocostal process is even slightly above the upper margin of the vertebral bodies, somewhat blurring the lower contour of the intervertebral discs.

The shadows of the articular processes and the translucency of the joints projecting into the spinal canal can be seen behind the vertebral bodies. If the side view has been taken correctly only one line can be seen, showing that the joints are parallel. The posterior margin of the spinal canal is indicated by a shadow at the base of the spinous processes where the laminae meet. This shadow is usually also clearly visible at the level of the atlas; its absence is a clear sign of spina bifida, a frequent anomaly of the arch of the atlas.

X-ray evaluation of function

The most characteristic disturbance of statics in the cervical region is the forward-drawn position (*Figure 3.35*). This is so because even when statics are normal the centre of gravity of the head is slightly in front of its support and therefore there is always some muscular activity in the neck musculature in the erect position. Obviously, in the forward-drawn position this imbalance is greatly enhanced, producing increased activity in the neck muscles and (by counter-pressure) increased strain on the cervical spine.

As Gaizler (1973) has shown, in order to get a true picture it is very important to take the lateral view in a relaxed position, the subject sitting without support, or faulty posture may be overlooked. It is necessary, however, to insist on the patient

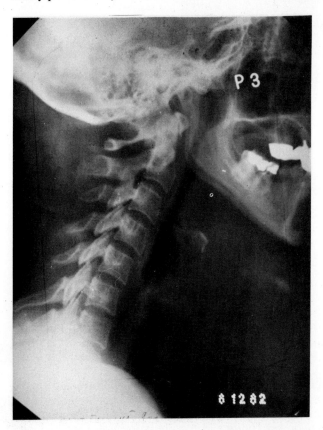

Figure 3.35 Forward-drawn position of the head: the external auditory canal and the odontoid process lie far anterior to the upper and anterior edge of C7; the craniocervical junction is in a position of compensatory hyperlordosis

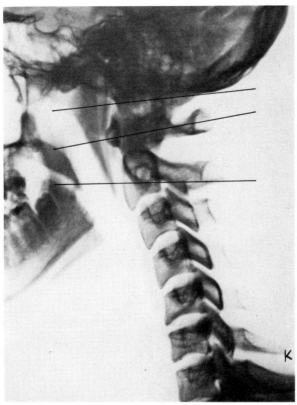

Figure 3.36 Lateral view of the cervical spine with the atlas in anteflexion (relative to the axis)

relaxing while constantly keeping his gaze on an object at eye-level, to avoid head anteflexion. In a group of 50 patients I compared lateral views with the patient sitting erect, standing, and sitting relaxed. Whereas with the subject sitting erect the outer auditory meatus was almost exactly above the anterior upper edge of the C7 vertebra (on average 0.9 mm behind), in standing patients it was 7 mm in front of this edge, and in the relaxed position sitting (i.e. the habitual working posture) it was 16 mm in front. In individual cases there were differences of up to 5 cm! This is particularly so if there is marked lumbar kyphosis in sitting, caused by lumbar hypermobility.

In addition to changes in statics concerning the whole cervical spine, there can be relative forward or backward shift (even in the neutral, erect position) and/or locally increased lordosis or kyphosis. At the craniocervical junction the atlas may be in a position of ante- or retroflexion in relation to the axis and the occiput in ante- or retroflexion towards the axis (the terms 'atlas superior' and 'atlas inferior' used by chiropractors are most confusing and should be avoided). Because of the tilting mechanism of the atlas as described in anteflexion and retroflexion sitting (*see Figure 3.29*) the atlas is usually in a slightly retroflexed position if there is cervical lordosis, the head being consequently in anteflexion; conversely, in a kyphotic, forward-drawn position, the atlas tends to be in anteflexion and the head in retroflexion in relation to the atlas (*Figure 3.36*).

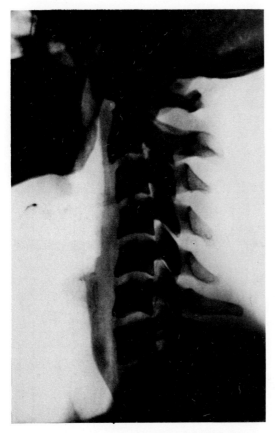

Figure 3.37 Lateral view of the cervical spine with the patient sitting erect: the external auditory canal (centre of gravity of the head) and the odontoid process lie above the anterior and upper edge of the vertebral body of C7. In this case kyphosis of the mid-cervical spine is in keeping with a normal static function, owing to a flat back, C7 being almost horizontal

In addition to rotation in individual segments there is frequent asymmetry of the atlas in relation to the axis, as though the atlas was shifted to one side. At the same time the condyles are shifted, relative to the atlas, in the opposite direction. This is frequently described as a shift of the atlas relative to the axis and the condyles, in the same direction, but this is not quite consistent, as movement in the spinal column should always be described in relation to the lower element (*Figures 3.38, 3.39*). Isolated rotation of the atlas in relation to both the axis and the occiput is uncommon. On the side of rotation there is a narrower articular cleft between atlas and axis and a larger lateral triangle of the atlas, the centre of the posterior atlas arch being shifted in the opposite direction and the massa lateralis being larger on the side opposite to rotation (*Figure 3.40*).

Much more frequent than rotation of the atlas is axis rotation in the neutral position of the head and neck (*see Figures 3.25* and *3.26*). In fact, rotation of the order of 5 degrees is quite common and even of the order of 10 degrees is not

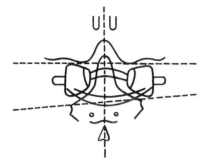

Figure 3.38 Asymmetrical position of the atlas relative to the condyles and the axis

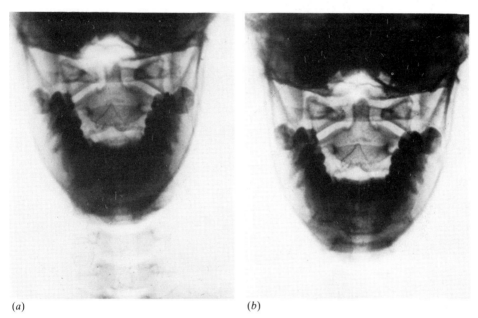

(*a*)   (*b*)

Figure 3.39 (*a*) Anteroposterior X-ray showing asymmetrical position of the atlas against the occipital condyles to the left. (*b*) After treatment the position is symmetrical

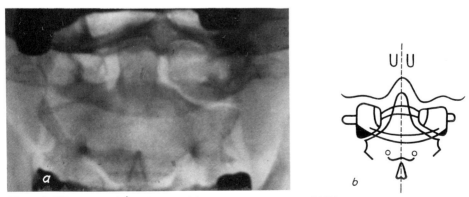

Figure 3.40 Dextrorotation of the atlas. (*a*) Anteroposterior X-ray. (*b*) Diagram

unusual. Interestingly, rotation (and even more asymmetry of the spinous process) of the axis is accompanied by rotation of the cervical vertebrae below the axis, quite frequently down to C7, particularly when rotation is to the left. The mechanism is probably that described during side-bending (*see* Mobility studies, below).

The characteristic features of axis rotation in the AP view are: the spinous process and the pedicles shift in the opposite direction to that of rotation, the transverse foramen opens on the side of rotation and the atlas/axis joint space narrows on the opposite side. In the rest of the cervical spine there is distortion of the unciform processes in addition to the shift of the spinous processes and pedicles. In the side view of rotation of the cervical spine, the structures that normally overlap are separately visualized: joint spaces, articular processes and transverse processes. In fact the transverse process of the axis is projected in front of the body of the axis (*Figure 3.41*).

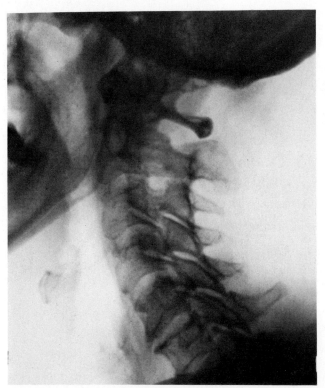

Figure 3.41 Rotation of the cervical spine in the lateral view: the transverse and articular processes as well as the joint spaces are visualized separately, owing to rotatory distortion

An important sign of static disturbance is discrepancy between the AP view taken with the patient supine and the lateral view in sitting, in particular if there is marked rotation in sitting and none at all in the supine position; this is usually due to obliquity *below* the cervical spine.

Mobility studies

X-rays of lateral, ante- and retroflexion can be useful in the diagnosis of movement restriction and of hypermobility; rotations tells us much less because it is more difficult to assess.

LATERAL FLEXION

The physiological reaction of the cervical spine during side-bending has been described under functional anatomy. Lateral flexion is examined mainly in order to detect movement restriction. One of the most interesting observations is that if there is no rotation in the upper cervical spine during side-bending, there will be none in the lower cervical spine (*Figure 3.42*). On the other hand, lack of rotation

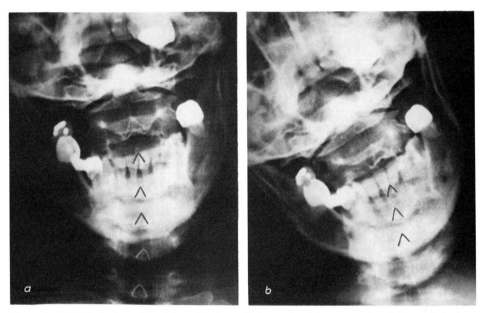

Figure 3.42 (a) Blocked rotation of the axis at lateroflexion to the right: no rotation of the cervical spine below C2 (*b*) After treatment: normal dextrorotation from the axis down to C5, lateral flexion of the entire cervical spine increased compared with (*a*)

in the lower cervical spine will not have any effect on rotation in the upper cervical spine. This is yet further proof that rotation of the cervical spine during side-bending originates at the axis. Jirout (1970) has shown that rotation is transmitted to the lower cervical vertebrae by means of the spinous processes. If, for example, the spinous process of C2 or C3 is asymmetrical without that vertebra being rotated, e.g. pointing to the right, then on side-bending to the right this spinous process will not deviate to the left, but may reach only the mid-line. In such a case the rest of the cervical spine below this vertebra will not rotate, just as though rotation had been restricted in the upper cervical area (*Figure 3.43*).

Though side-shifting of the atlas is the rule in lateral flexion, at times it does not take place without movement restriction, in particular if there is marked asymmetry, and even more important, even in cases of clinically severe movement restriction between atlas and occiput, this side-shift may be seen. On the other hand, if the axis does not rotate there is no side-bending at the craniocervical junction (*Figure 3.44*). This is in keeping with the fact that in cases of atlas assimilation to the occiput, side-bending at the junction may be normal.

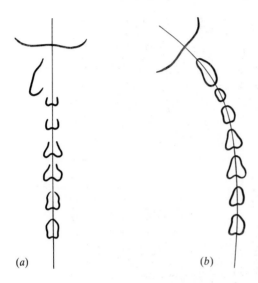

(*a*)   (*b*)

Figure 3.43 The effect of asymmetrical position of a spinous process on rotation of the caudal cervical vertebrae at side-bending. (*a*) At neutral position the spinous process of C2 deviates to the right. (*b*) Side-bending to the right causes dextrorotation of the axis, the spinous process of the axis rotating only into mid-line, however; the caudal cervical vertebrae remain unrotated (After Jirout, 1970.)

The question now arises whether movement restriction between atlas and occiput on side-bending can be visualized by X-ray. We have shown this to be possible (Lewit and Krausova, 1967), but only with the head rotated, i.e. with atlas/axis blocked. This is of great importance for clinical diagnosis.

It is usually easy to see movement restriction between atlas and axis on side-bending: the axis does not rotate (*Figure 3.44*). In the rest of the cervical spine this is much less easy to visualize by X-ray even where it can be clearly diagnosed clinically. According to Jirout (1970) small tilting movements in the sagittal plane take place on side-bending and can be recognized by a change in the position of the spinous process. These synkineses in the sagittal plane are apparently more prone to movement restriction than is lateral bending (as can be seen from comparison of X-rays taken before and after manipulation).

We may therefore conclude that lateral flexion of the head against the cervical spine in the coronal plane is mainly the result of axis rotation, and conversely if we restore blocked side-bending at the craniocervical junction we restore rotation between atlas and axis.

Lateral flexion between occiput and atlas can be established clinically or by X-ray only if the atlas and axis are locked, i.e. if the head is rotated. Movement restriction of the occiput on the atlas does not interfere with side-bending in the coronal plane, nor with a shifting synkinesis of the atlas against the occiput during axis rotation.

ANTEFLEXION

Anteflexion is the most usual test for mobility. For the clinician interested in manual therapy, however, this particular examination has one great disadvantage:

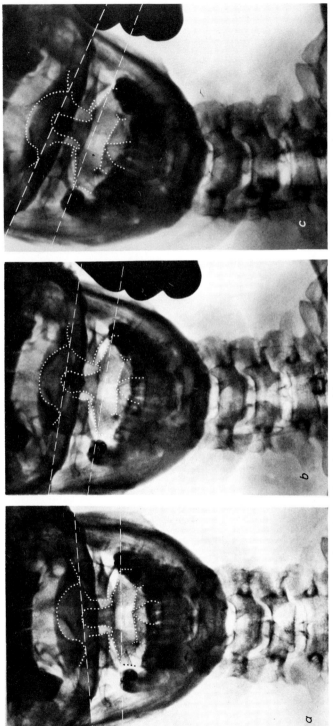

Figure 3.44 Blocked passive lateral flexion at the craniocervical junction. (*a*) In neutral position the atlas is slightly asymmetrical, to the right of the condyles and the axis. (*b*) Attempted passive left lateral flexion of the upper cervical spine has failed; there is no axis rotation, yet the atlas has moved to the left(!). (*c*) After treatment normal lateral flexion of the upper cervical spine is restored, with normal (slight) left rotation of the axis and shift of the atlas to the left

ante- and retroflexion, being the easiest movements, are usually the last to be blocked, and therefore movement restriction will show only in severe cases of blockage. On the other hand, ante- and retroflexion will easily reveal any hypermobility: increased shifting movements between C2 and C7, increased lordosis or kyphosis even in a single segment. At the craniocervical junction there may be the following signs of hypermobility:

1. Laxity of the transverse ligament between atlas and axis, with an increased distance between the anterior arch of the atlas and the odontoid, in particular at the tip of the odontoid. As a consequence the basion also shifts forward (*Figure 3.45*). At the same time the angle between the clivus and the odontoid decreases not only when the chin is held in, but also during anteflexion of the whole of the cervical spine.
2. There is hypermobility betwen occiput and atlas with increased shift of the basion and opisthion in relation to the atlas, without laxity of the transverse ligament (*Figure 3.46*).

Some morphological aspects

It is of course impossible to do justice to the vast field of morphology in this book; fortunately, it is adequately dealt with in the traditional literature, and only some aspects which are particularly important for us will be touched on here.

Anomalies

Anomalies may be important because they frequently imply some degree of change in function. This is particularly obvious in block vertebrae with coalescence of vertebral bodies and/or arches. These may be only partial, and in such cases we see a hypoplastic intervertebral disc, the vertebral bodies adjacent to that disc being narrower (*Figure 3.47*). This anomaly implies reduced or no mobility in a segment and produces compensatory hypermobility in the neighbouring segment (usually cranial) resulting ultimately in degenerative changes. A frequent anomaly is a transitional cervicothoracic vertebra C7 with large transverse processes and/or cervical ribs and without uniform processes; it is often asymmetrical.

Clinically the most important anomaly is a narrow spinal canal, because it may cause cervical myelopathy. A more useful method than measuring the width of the anterior–posterior diameter is to observe the altered proportion visible at first glance. Normally the spinal canal is wider than the vertebral body in the cervical spine. In the narrow spinal canal it is narrower and the shadow of the articular processes covers most of the breadth of the spinal canal (*Figure 3.48*).

The craniocervical junction, as a region of transition, is the site of frequent anomalies. The most important of these is basilar impression due to hypoplasia of the base of the occipital bone. In this condition the occipital part of the clivus is shortened and therefore the odontoid process is drawn up into the foramen magnum and is then situated considerably above the palato-occipital line in the lateral view; in the AP view it can reach the upper border of the foramen magnum between the condyles, and be high above the bimastoidal and bidigastric lines (*Figure 3.49*). At the same time the foramen magnum may be narrower than usual, unless there is also an Arnold–Chiari deformity. The changes may cause compression of nervous tissue not unlike that which occurs in a narrow spinal canal further down.

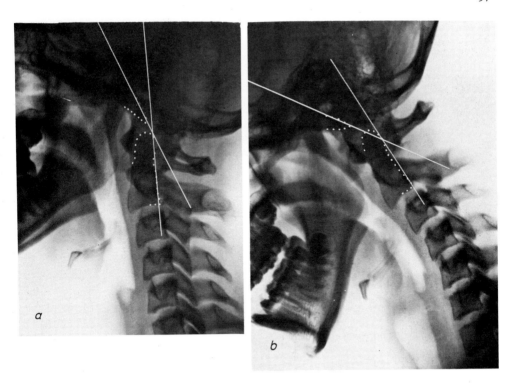

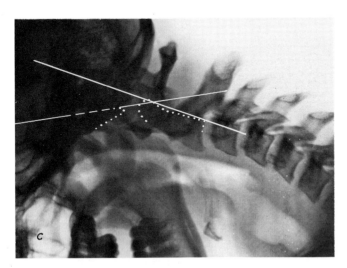

Figure 3.45 Hypermobility at head anteflexion with laxity of the transverse ligament of the atlas. (*a*) In the neutral position the articular facet of the anterior arch of the atlas is parallel to the odontoid process. (*b*) Slight and (*c*) maximum anteflexion: there is increasing angulation between the articular facets of the anterior arch of the atlas and the odontoid; note the change in the angle between the clivus and the axis and the anterior shift of the basion

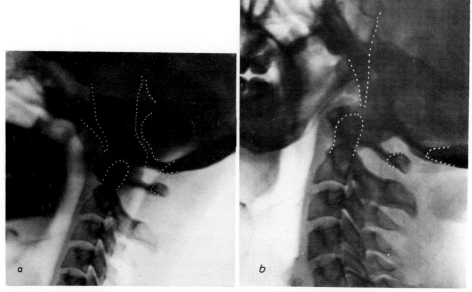

Figure 3.46 Hypermobility at head ante- and retroflexion between occiput and atlas. (*a*) At anteflexion (autotomogram during pneumography) the basion lies above the anterior arch of the atlas and the opisthion above the posterior arch; the arched course of the foramen Magendi has been drawn in. (*b*) At retroflexion the occiput has shifted 2.5 cm back (compare the relative positions of the basion and odontoid process and the opisthion and posterior arch of the atlas). For easier comparison, (*a*) has been turned 90 degrees clockwise

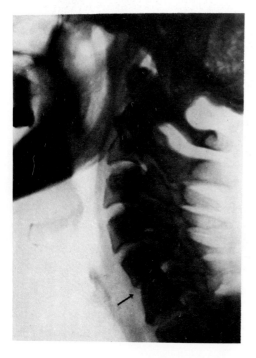

Figure 3.47 Incomplete congenital coalescence of C5 and C6 with a hypoplastic intervertebral disc and a short anteroposterior diameter of both adjacent vertebral bodies

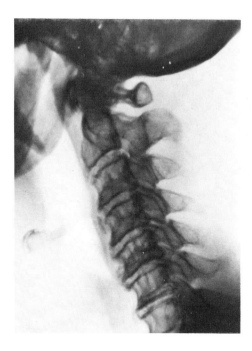

Figure 3.48 The narrow cervical spinal canal

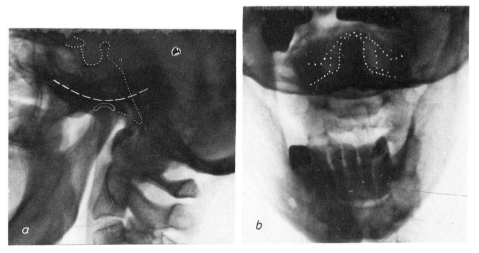

Figure 3.49 Basilar impression. (a) Lateral view with short clivus. (b) Position of the odontoid high above the condyles

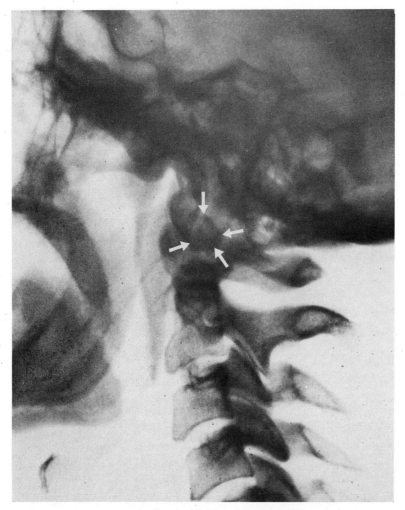

Figure 3.50 Os odontoides, side view (arrows) (Reproduced by kind permission of Dr G. Metz.)

In addition there is often hypoplasia or assimilation of the atlas to the occipital condyles. Less common is coalescence of the massa lateralis (usually one sided) with the axis. All the anomalies are more often than not asymmetrical, and this asymmetry concerns the whole of the craniocervical junction and may produce side shift of the atlas and even marked rotation of the axis in neutral position, which necessarily produces asymmetrical mechanisms of side-bending and rotation.

One important anomaly (malformation) is hypoplasia of the odontoid; another is the os odontoides, which implies pathological hypermobility (*Figure 3.50*). Another significant anomaly of the odontoid is increased reclination (Gutmann, 1981), which forces the atlas into a position of retroflexion and therefore places increased strain on the transverse ligament of the atlas during head anteflexion, and may cause laxity of that ligament.

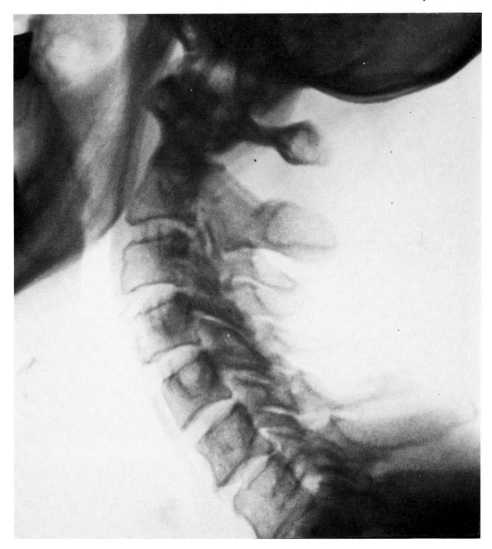

Figure 3.51 Spondylarthrosis with a horizontal course of the intervertebral apophyseal joints

Degenerative changes

Degenerative changes in the cervical spine are of special clinical interest when they impinge on the intervertebral foramina and may therefore interfere with both the spinal root and the vertebral artery. For this reason oblique views are useful (*see Figure 3.23*). These changes mainly concern the unciform processes (neurocentral joints), in particular their posterior parts. They are closely correlated to disc degeneration, as narrowing of the disc brings the unciform process of the lower vertebra into close contact with the lower lateral margin of the vertebra above.

Similarly, deformity of the articular processes may impinge on the intervertebral foramen. This is found in arthrosis of the apophyseal joints, which usually goes

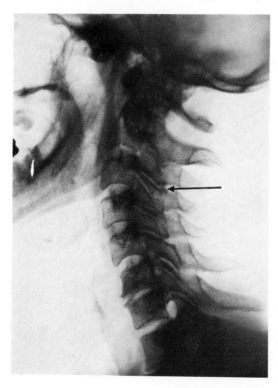

Figure 3.52 Difference in the oblique course of the apophyseal joints between C3 and C4 in the lateral view (arrow)

hand in hand with a horizontal position; in such cases the apophyseal joints become the *weight-bearing structures* (*Figure 3.51*). They are therefore very well seen in the AP view.

Finally I must point out the great significance of a change in the parallel course of both apophyseal joints in one segment, seen in an undistorted lateral view. This implies forced rotation of the cervical spine during retroflexion, producing narrowing of the intervertebral foramen on one side only (*Figure 3.52*).

4
Examination of locomotor function and its disturbance

Case history

As in other fields of medicine, examination starts with the anamnesis. Since vertebrogenic disorders represent the most important group, they will serve as the principal example. It is important to stress from the outset that diagnosis of disturbed function due to disease should not be made *per exclusionem* – i.e. only if all other (organic) causes are ruled out – but principally on positive evidence, of which a characteristic history is significant. We owe the main criteria to Gutzeit (1957).

Chronic intermittent course

Unless we see an acute condition in a young patient, we can usually ascertain by questioning that there have been previous attacks, perhaps going as far back as adolescence (e.g. low-back pain during menstruation in young girls). There are periods of complete recovery in between, and we should try to ascertain the frequency and duration of the attacks (and the free intervals), and the time of onset of the latest attack.

Involvement of the locomotor system

The function of the locomotor system and its disturbance can never be limited only to one structure, and therefore symptoms occur in various more distant parts of the system in the course of time, the variously located complaints having, perhaps, a common denominator – the vertebral column. This, too, has to be elicited by careful questioning; the patient will probably be unaware of the possible connection between, for example, headache, shoulder pain, pain in the region of the heart, or in the hip or knee, experienced at different times and perhaps after considerable intervals.

Susceptibility to strain and sustained posture

Function and its disturbances in the locomotor system are obviously influenced by strain imposed by enforced movement or sustained posture. One of the most important points in recording the case history is to determine *under what conditions* the attacks occur; this is not only of diagnostic value, but also important for therapy and prevention. This is the most crucial, but also the most difficult information to extract from the patient. It does little good to ask him *after what* his symptoms started, for he is likely to provide all the theories he has heard or formed for himself. What we need to know are the *immediate* circumstances in which pain was felt. This patients are often reluctant to tell, either because they cannot remember or because they find it irrelevant or unimportant; such statements as 'I was sitting, and when I got up from my chair . . .', 'I was shaving and when I looked into the mirror . . .', 'When I stooped to pick up this bit of paper from the floor . . .' are significant details. It is also important to learn which position or movement gives relief. It is important to know whether pain is provoked by a single brusque movement, by strenuous effort of some duration, or by enforcedly rigid position. Slight details may be important: the underlying cause of pain may be very different if it occurs during forward bending, while stooping (e.g. over a work bench), in maximum flexion (e.g. stooping to wipe a floor), or while straightening up from a stooping position.

Trauma

Trauma is one of the commonest causes of disturbed function and provides significant corroboration, even if structural damage is also present. We must insist on the fact that any excessive force applied to the body affects the locomotor system and the spinal column. This is particularly the case in head injury. Unfortunately the patient often forgets a minor trauma (such as an awkwardly performed somersault) and it is therefore advisable to ask what sports he indulges in. To give a typical example: a patient who 'never suffered any trauma' said that his hobbies were boxing and Rugby football!

Factors primarily influencing the autonomic nervous system

In vertebrogenic disturbances the mechanical factor is not the only one, and the reactions of the nervous system must also be taken into account. These include undue susceptibility to changes in the weather, particularly to cold and to high humidity; infectious diseases causing high temperatures; hormonal disturbances (more apparent in women because of the menstrual cycle); pain of locomotor origin which is heightened during menstruation; even allergy may be involved.

The psychological factor

Since the locomotor system is the instrument of our will, and pain is the most frequent symptom of disturbed function of that system, it is only to be expected that a psychological factor is frequently present in vertebrogenic lesions. Psychological involvement thus in no way excludes, but rather corroborates the diagnosis of vertebrogenic disturbance. It must be stressed that adequate treatment of the locomotor disturbance usually deals most effectively with the pain, giving the physician a much better chance to deal with the psychological problems, having understood the patient's main trouble. The course of treatment reveals the importance of the psychological factor as such and finally shows whether the patient recovers psychologically when relieved of pain, or whether the psychological conditions may not even cause relapse through muscular tension, as may happen, for example, in masked depression. Purely psychological pain is not common, particularly if the patient is capable of localizing the pain and describing it without frequent changes in the description.

Paroxysmal character

Those complaints in which autonomic nervous symptoms are prominent follow a typical paroxysmal course, e.g. vertebrogenic headache, vertigo, cardiac or other (pseudo-) visceral pain. Even if the patient describes the pain as constant, further questioning reveals that its intensity changes paroxysmally.

Asymmetrical localization

Vertebrogenic pain is rarely symmetrical, and is often one sided. This holds for radicular and pseudoradicular syndromes of the extremities as well as for headache, shoulder pain and pain in the chest.

The role of age

For differential diagnosis it is important to bear in mind that the most frequent pathological conditions should be evaluated according to the age of the patient.

We may expect juvenile osteochondrosis in adolescents, ankylosing spondylitis in young men and disc prolapse in young and middle-aged adults; after the age of 50 osteopenia (osteoporosis) may occur especially in women; progressive (destructive) osteoarthrosis especially of the hip and knee joint can be found in older men and women and so, too, can malignant disease. For this reason a history of pain in the locomotor system that begins after the age of about 50 and takes a progressive course must be treated with great circumspection.

Examination

The anamnesis is followed by clinical examination. There is perhaps no field of medicine in which clinical examination plays so decisive a role, and is so exacting, as in examination of locomotor function. Examination begins the moment the patient enters the doctor's office: the way he or she moves, sits down, undresses, etc. The patient must always undress for the first examination (to bra and briefs); natural movement is essential. Whatever the site of the trouble, important if not vital information may be missed if the patient remains fully dressed.

Examination of posture

Examination usually starts with the rear view; the plumb-line is placed between the heels. This is followed by the side view, observing the patient from the feet upwards. Any asymmetry should be noted: position and shape of the feet, the knees, the height of the gluteal folds, the position of the intergluteal line, the position of the hips, the (hanging) arms and the waist forming triangles which may or may not be symmetrical. This asymmetry is just as significant as a shift of the pelvis to one side in relation to the plumb-line. We should note any deformity due to scoliosis, such as asymmetrical height of the shoulder-blades, their prominence, the deviation of the spinous processes and the position of the head and neck. (Owing to rotation combined with scoliosis, deviation of the spinous processes is often masked in the erect position, but becomes very marked on forward bending.)

It is not usual to place equal weight on both feet, and shifting weight brings with it a shift in posture; this is important when patients are being photographed.

Asymmetry also concerns the musculature: the weight-bearing leg is usually slightly more strongly built than the other; one-sided hypotonia of the glutei is evident; the same applies to hypertonus of the erector spinae on one side. Asymmetrical fixation of the shoulder-blades can produce slight alar scapula on the side on which the shoulder-blade is higher. There can be marked asymmetry of the muscles of the upper extremity, of the face and of the eyes. On the ventral aspect the navel may deviate slightly to the side of the stronger muscles. The upper part of the trapezius muscle should have a slightly concave course, but if there is increased tension it is convex.

Symmetrical stance is usually examined with the patient on two scales (*Figure 4.1*), with the patient trying to put equal weight on each foot. This is also a way to test the patient's assessment of equilibrium. The scales used need not be very

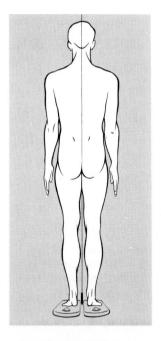

Figure 4.1 Examination of symmetrical stance on two scales in front of a plumb-line

sensitive, about 1 kg error either way being inherent to the method. In my experience a difference of up to 4 kg is within the norm for a patient of average weight (*see* Examination of equilibrium).

Examination of the side view begins at the feet, following the curvature of the knees (e.g. genua recurvata), then that of the spinal column and of the walls of the abdomen, and finally the chest wall. Lumbosacral hyperlordosis is due to increased pelvic tilt, for instance, if the gluteal musculature is weak; lumbar hyperlordosis is more characteristic of weakness of the abdominal muscles, which may be recognized by a protruding abdomen without signs of obesity, the navel being on the surface. A shortened pectoralis muscle produces increased thoracic kyphosis, but if its subclavicular part is shortened the shoulders are drawn forward. If the head position is normal a plumb-line from the outer auditory meatus passes through the collar-bone. If the head position is drawn forward there is hypertonus of the upper trapezius muscles with hyperlordosis of the upper cervical spine.

Examination of the patient standing should be followed by examination in the sitting position. This may show many differences, in particular where there is lumbar hypermobility with marked lordosis standing and marked lumbar kyphosis sitting. Even the position of the head may be greatly changed.

It is sometimes worth examining the patient from above, to detect possible relative rotation of the shoulder and pelvic girdle.

Examination of mobility

Only certain general principles will be dealt with here. We should examine active mobility, passive mobility and movement against resistance. Active mobility shows both muscular activity and joint mobility uninfluenced by the examiner. Any force applied by the examiner may be smaller, the same or greater than that used by the patient; we then have concentric (resisted) movement, isometric resistance, or eccentric movement. Each technique examines muscular function (the strength of muscle reaction and pain provoked in the muscles).

Passive movement shows the degree of mobility of joints and may at the same time reveal muscular tension or spasm. Examination of a particular joint may disclose mobility normal, increased, or restricted mobility. This may affect functional movement as well as joint play (*see* Chapter 2). The following changes should be looked for during examination:

1. Limited range of movement compared with the symmetrical joint or a neighbouring spinal motor segment, the 'pathological barrier' of American osteopaths; this has recently been registered remarkably successfully by a device constructed by Berger (1982) which is likely to prove very important for accurate analysis of impaired mobility (*see Figure 4.23,* page 128).
2. Resistance during motion, particularly during the examination of joint play.
3. Resistance or springing in the end-position. The pathological barrier, if engaged, does not spring. Here it is essential to take up the slack of both functional movement and joint play. This resistance in end-position has been registered by Figar and Krausová (1975) using a resistance transducer, in a blocked cervical segment before treatment, during a high-velocity thrust and after treatment (*Figure 4.2*).

A diagnosis of movement restriction (blockage) usually leads to interest in the direction of restriction, and therapeutic techniques are concerned mainly with mobilization in a specific direction. With movement restriction in the spinal column, however, it is sometimes of interest to note not only the direction of restriction but also which of the two intervertebral apophyseal joints is involved. However, this is not easy to determine, and in fact most techniques are effective if applied in the correct direction, whichever joint is affected.

The question of which side is affected is most readily solved in the lumbar region by simple clinical examination, because here axial rotation is not possible and

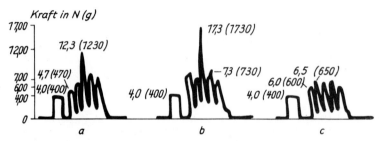

Figure 4.2 Recording resistance in end-position by the method of Figar and Krausova (1975). (*a*) Increased resistance in the blocked segment. (*b*) The force required for thrust manipulation in the blocked segment. (*c*) Equal resistance in all segments after manipulation. A weight of 400 g was used as a gauge

therefore a combination of restriction in the sagittal and coronal planes shows clearly which side is involved. It can be easily understood that on anteflexion the articular surfaces are in end-to-end position, whereas in retroflexion they are in full contact. During side-bending, however, the articulation on the convex side is in an end-to-end position as during anteflexion, while that on the concave side is in full contact as during retroflexion (*Figure 4.3*).

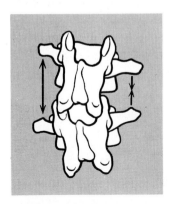

Figure 4.3 The mechanism of lateral flexion in the lumbar spine

Therefore, restricted retroflexion and side-bending to one side shows that the joint on the side of restricted lateroflexion is at fault, whereas restricted anteflexion and side-bending indicates that the joint on the side opposite to restricted lateroflexion is lesioned.

In the rest of the spinal column direct palpation of the transverse processes during ante- and retroflexion can be useful, but it is not easy to perform: during anteflexion the end-to-end position is reached only on the side of normal mobility, and therefore if anteflexion is restricted on one side the transverse process bulges slightly on the other side; during retroflexion, on the other hand, the joints reach full overlap only on the normal side, and therefore it is the side of restricted retroflexion that bulges slightly.

Palpation

A short paragraph dealing with palpation would be appropriate here, since this is the basis of our diagnostic techniques and is also essential for manipulation. Yet it is extremely difficult to describe exactly, in words, the information palpation provides; this is one of the reasons why manipulation cannot be learned from books alone.

Palpation of tissue structures seeks to determine the texture, resilience, warmth, humidity and the possibility of moving, stretching or compressing these structures. Concentrating on the tissues palpated, and pushing aside one layer after another, we distinguish skin, subcutaneous tissue, muscle and bone. Following a muscle we recognize the transition to the tendon, and finally the insertion. Palpating bone, we recognize tuberosities (and possible changes) and locate joints. Reflex changes due to pain affect all these tissues, and can be assessed by palpation; one of the most significant factors is increased tension.

We also palpate joint mobility, to assess resistance (binding) during movement, as well as the range of movement; approaching the extreme position, we sense increased resistance which may be gradual and elastic, or abrupt (without springing), i.e., we may engage a physiological or a pathological barrier. We also examine the relative mobility of tissues (skin, muscle and bone) in order to find possible adherence.

It is essential here to distinguish carefully between what we actually sense with our receptors, and the interpretation we give of our sensations; this is not always an easy thing to do, bearing in mind that palpation also implies subtle interaction with the patient's tissues.

Examination of the lower extremities and the pelvis

There is no need to repeat here what I have already said about the general examination of posture. It is important to assess the arch of the foot in both planes. To compare the feet it is useful to place one finger under the arch of each, from the medial aspect: where there is flat foot, the finger meets resistance. It may be even more revealing to examine the arch as it functions (in walking): from the medial aspect we can see whether the arch sags (decompensation of flat foot). For the function of the whole limb it is very important to note valgosity of the heel and the degree of external rotation of the foot (i.e. of the hip).

Examining the knee, we are interested both in varosity and in valgosity, and in the genu recurvatum.

Flexion in the hip joint while standing is characteristic of hip joint involvement in increased lordosis (unlike lumbago).

Examination of the pelvis, too, starts with the assessment of posture: the rhomboid of Michaelis is important here, the upper end corresponding to the end of the spinal column, the lower end to the coccyx, the lateral grooves to the posterior superior iliac spines.

For more detailed examination of the pelvis palpation is needed. First the iliac crests should be palpated. This is more difficult than is usually thought: it must be done from above, from the ribs down – the crests can be much higher than one would expect from the shape of the buttocks, i.e. close below the lowest rib. If the hips deviate to one side the iliac crests also deviate, and therefore it is not difficult to palpate the crest on the side to which the pelvis deviates, but greater pressure is needed to get on top of the iliac crest on the other side. The iliac crest thus appears higher on the side to which the pelvis shifts, unless great care is exercised.

To be sure that the iliac crests are at the same height it is wise to check with a spirit level (*Figure 4.4*).

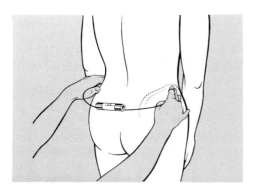

Figure 4.4 Comparison of the level of the iliac crests or other symmetrical structures, using a spirit level

The iliac crests should be palpated laterally (at the highest point) and followed towards both posterior superior iliac spines, and note taken whether the two palpating hands converge. Both the posterior and the anterior iliac spines point downwards and sidewards and have therefore to be palpated from below and from the side in order to find the corresponding points.

If both iliac crests are at the same height – and this is also true of the anterior and posterior iliac spines – the pelvis is horizontal and the legs are probably of equal length; if the iliac crest is higher on one side and the same is true of both anterior and posterior superior iliac spines, and if the fingers palpating the crests towards the posterior spines meet, there is pelvic obliquity and the most probable conclusion is difference in leg length.

Pelvic obliquity

Measurement of leg length is more difficult than might be thought, because the femoral heads and necks are hidden. Pelvic obliquity is thus the most reliable clinical sign of difference in leg length, unless this is caused by a difference in the length of the legs *below the knee*, a condition which can be readily assessed, e.g. with the patient supine, with knees flexed. The examination of a patient standing, with both legs straight, usually detects deviation of the pelvis towards the higher side; in typical cases the shoulder is lower on the side where the pelvis is higher. The (clinical) effect of a heel-pad should then be tested: if the pelvis is level after the heel has been raised on the lower side, there should be no side shift and the shoulders should have levelled out. However, this test is useful only if there is no major movement restriction.

At the same time weight distribution can be examined on two scales, with and without a heel-pad on the lower side, to see whether the patient is better able to assess equilibrium with or without the pad. The subjective reaction is tested by asking the patient whether she feels happier with a heel-pad, or whether it makes no difference. (In view of static correction an X-ray check is necessary. *See* pages 49–54.)

If we conclude that there is a difference in leg length we again check whether this is due to asymmetrical deformity at the knee (valgosity or varosity) or to a one-sided flat foot, in which case an arch support is more effective than a heel-pad.

Pelvic distortion

This is a curious phenomenon which must be distinguished from pelvic obliquity and is always secondary to some other lesion which must be found and treated. In the rear view the pelvis deviates slightly to one side (usually to the right) and is slightly rotated (usually to the left). Palpating of the iliac crests shows that they are more or less on the same level laterally, but as the fingers palpate towards the posterior superior spines they do not meet; one superior posterior spine (usually the right) lies higher than the other. This can be confirmed by direct palpation of the spines. In the front view the contrary is found: here the right anterior superior iliac spine is usually lower and the left higher. The two ilia seem to be distorted one against the other. Thus there is always a discrepancy if the iliac crests, and the anterior and posterior superior iliac spines, are compared, but relations vary so much here that the difference at the anterior or posterior spines may be greater or smaller, and the crests accordingly level or not; confusion with pelvic obliquity can easily occur.

For this reason, if examination shows signs of pelvic obliquity with some discrepancy on palpation of the most important points on the pelvis, the best approach is to get rid of the pelvic distortion first, and then to re-examine for pelvic obliquity.

Another feature of pelvic distortion is important because it points to disturbance of function: the 'overtake' phenomenon, in which on standing or sitting the left superior posterior iliac spine is usually the lower, but overtakes the right on stooping, becoming the more cranial of the two for a short time, about 20 s, after which the two spines are level and return to a symmetrical position.

Figure 3.12 (*see* page 62) shows that the sacrum must lie asymmetrically between the ilia in such a way as to create more tension on the side of the lower posterior superior iliac spine; as a result it follows the sacrum more promptly in stooping, causing the 'overtake'. The figure shows clearly that in the supine position there is greater external rotation of the leg on the side of the lower posterior spine, and there may be what Derbolowski (1956) has called a 'variable difference' in leg length – i.e. one leg may be apparently shorter in the supine position, while on sitting this is reversed.

More significantly, in this condition there is usually muscular imbalance in the pelvic region: spasm of the iliacus is frequent on the side of the lower posterior spine and the function of the gluteal musculature is frequently asymmetrical, but much depends on the cause of the pelvic distortion, which, as I have stressed, is always secondary.

Sacroiliac blockage

Although there is no active movement between the sacrum and the ilium, passive mobility can be examined, as well as springing. (Gynaecologists are familiar with the nutation movement of the sacrum during labour.)

In addition to the overtake phenomenon, the simplest screening method of diagnosing sacroiliac blockage is to examine restricted adduction of the thigh, with the hip flexed to about 90 degrees. The patient is supine. The examiner stands by the table and grasps the patient's furthermost knee, which is bent, and flexes the hip; with his other hand he fixes the anterior superior iliac spine to the table, from above. He then adducts the patient's thigh across the pelvis and compares the angle of adduction on the two sides. If there is normal mobility of the hip joint, adduction restriction is due to a blocked sacroiliac joint. At the same time the examiner can sense the absence of springing when he reaches end-position.

The sacroiliac joint can be sprung similarly: the patient is again supine, the examiner again grasps the knee and adducts the thigh across the patient's pelvis, but without fixing it with the other hand. Instead he continues adduction until the pelvis begins to rotate, i.e. the posterior spine begins to lift from the table. At this point the slack is taken up at the sacroiliac joint and the examiner places a finger of his free hand between the posterior superior spine and the sacrum, so as to palpate movement (springing). Without increasing adduction he now exerts slight pressure against the patient's knee in the direction of the axis of the thigh (taking up the slack) and from this position springs the joint by a gentle push in the same direction (*Figure 4.5*).

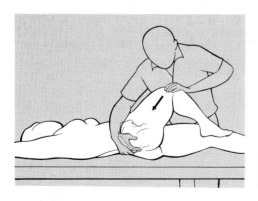

Figure 4.5 Springing the sacroiliac joint: with the patient supine, one leg flexed at the hip and knee and adducted across the pelvis, the therapist exerts pressure on the patient's knee

The force with which the sacroiliac joint is sprung in this technique produces a dorsal shift of the ilium against the sacrum, i.e. a movement mainly in the sagittal plane.

Mobility of the sacrum in relation to the ilium can be directly palpated with the thumbs below and medial to the posterior superior iliac spines while the patient marks time. In Chapter 6 another method will be described, which is used mainly for mobilization (page 222).

There is another very useful method for springing the sacroiliac joint. The patient lies on her side, and to stabilize the pelvis it is best if the lower leg is extended and the upper flexed, with the knee on the table. The operator puts his forearm (soft muscles) obliquely over the patient's iliac crest, so as to produce gapping between the posterior superior iliac spine and the sacrum. This is achieved by slight pressure in a ventromediocranial direction, but great care must be taken not to rotate the pelvis. Gapping is felt with the thumb of the other hand, between the posterior superior iliac spine and the sacrum (*Figure 4.6*). This technique thus

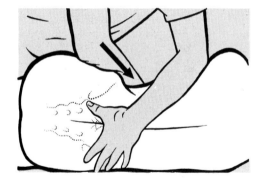

Figure 4.6 With the patient lying on her side the therapist springs the ilium in an oblique ventromediocranial direction, with his forearm, to produce gapping between the posterior sacroiliac spine and the sacrum, which he palpates with the thumb of the other hand

produces a movement of the ilium against the sacrum in the horizontal plane, and it is important to point out that it can reveal blockage even if the techniques described above show normal mobility. Rhythmic repetition of this manoeuvre evokes excellent mobilization, and it can be used as a high-velocity thrust by thrusting after taking up the slack (*see* page 222).

There are typical pain points at the upper and lower edge of the sacroiliac joint on the sacrum where increased resistance to springing may be felt, and a tender attachment point of the adductors at the symphysis. We find a slightly positive Patrick's sign and straight leg raising test, but no pain is felt if the patient is sitting up with his legs outstretched! There is some back bending and/or stooping restriction, and pain radiates in the S_1 dermatome.

A tender coccyx

A tender coccyx should never be missed at examination of the pelvis; it is far more frequently a sign of low-back pain than of coccygodynia (a much less common condition).

Correct palpation is crucial for diagnosis, but not as simple as it might seem. The point of tenderness is at the ventral aspect of the curved tip of the coccyx, and it is usually a very curved coccyx that presents this tenderness. Palpation is made even more difficult by the hypertonus of the glutei present in this condition. It may not be possible to reach the tip of the coccyx, and then no painful reaction can be registered.

In addition to this most important sign there is usually a visible hyperalgesic zone on the sacrum, looking like a cushion of fat covered by very smooth (taut) skin; Patrick's sign may be slightly positive on both sides, and the same is true of the straight leg raising test, as well as of spasm of the iliacus.

Ligament pain

Closely related to both sacroiliac lesions and to the tender coccyx there is the condition known as 'ligament pain' (Hackett, 1956; Barbor, 1964). It is examined and elicited by techniques that are thought to produce tension in the ligaments. According to Hackett (1956) and Barbor (1964) three ligaments are concerned: the sacroiliac, the iliolumbar and the sacrotuberous ligaments. The first two appear to be of considerable clinical importance. The following technique is used to provoke the pain. The patient lies supine on the table, and the examiner (standing by the table) grasps the further knee, flexes the patient's hip and adducts the knee; at about 90 degrees of hip flexion and adduction the iliolumbar ligament is tested; if flexion goes further (70–60 degrees) the sacroiliac ligaments are tested. If the operator feels resistance to further adduction he exerts pressure against the knee in the direction of the axis of the thigh, thus producing a gapping effect at the site of the ligaments, and maintains this pressure for several seconds. If the iliolumbar ligament is tender, the patient feels pain in the groin; if the sacroiliac ligament is tender, the pain radiates down the leg in the S1 dermatome (*Figure 4.7*). Before testing the ligaments the examiner must be sure the sacroiliac joints are not blocked in either the sagittal or the horizontal planes.

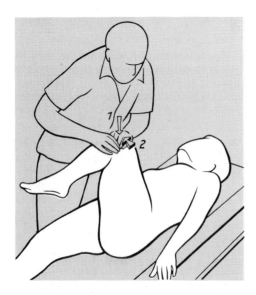

Figure 4.7 Testing ligament pain: the leg is flexed at the hip and knee; taking up the slack into adduction (arrow 2) and maintaining pressure along the long axis of the thigh (arrow 1), the therapist produces a gapping effect between the ilium and the sacrum (L5), producing tension in the sacroiliac (iliolumbar) ligament

On closer scrutiny, however, in the large majority of cases with a positive ligament test, resistance to adduction is increased on the painful side, so that the distance between the adducted knee and the table is considerably greater on the painful side. Obviously, ligaments cannot be the source of this increased resistance. This type of pain is found particularly in hypermobile patients suffering from static pain.

Testing the sacrotuberous ligaments seems less rewarding; it is simpler and more reliable to seek a tender ischial tuberosity.

Examination of the lumbar spine

Some criteria of pelvic examination, particularly with the patient standing, are also valid for the lumbar spine. Examination of mobility should start with active movement, and I recommend back bending. Here we are not only concerned with the total range of movement, but can follow it from the thoracolumbar region to the sacrum, noting regularity or local hypo- or hypermobility. Normally it should be possible to follow the movement down to the sacrum, as there is considerable mobility between L5 and S1 in retroflexion. If mobility ceases above S1, there is movement restriction in the segments above. In hypermobility, on the other hand, there may be a sharp bend in the thoracolumbar or in the lumbosacral junction. This is a frequent finding, and of importance; if back bending is not restricted but is painful, this may be a sign of tender spinous processes.

When examining side-bending care should be taken to see that the patient is in neither a forward nor a backward bent position, that the hands and arms slide sideways down the legs, and that the legs are straight and close together. The patient bends as far sideways as she can, and we note (1) how far down the fingertips reach; (2) whether the spinous processes arch symmetrically and regularly to both sides; and (3) whether there is rotation synkinesis. On side-bending it is normal for the pelvis to rotate towards the convexity of the curvature, i.e. to the right when bending to the left. Loss of this synkinesis is often the first sign of movement restriction in the lumbar spine and/or in the sacroiliac joints.

On anteflexion with the knees held straight, we note how close to the floor the fingertips reach, and at the same time the arch of the lumbar spine and the position of the pelvis, for it is important to distinguish whether the pelvis is much bent forward while the lumbar spine remains almost straight, or whether on the contrary the lumbar spine arches forward while the pelvis is only slightly flexed with regard to the legs. We then follow the arch of the spine, noting where it is exaggerated and where it is flattened. There is frequently a flattening at the thoracolumbar junction which should be regarded as physiological, and little or no kyphosis at the lumbosacral junction, with exaggerated kyphosis of the thoracic spine (which is not considered normal). Observing the patient from the rear we note whether the transverse processes and the erector spinae muscles are not more prominent on one side than on the other, in anteflexion. This is a sign of rotation usually found in scoliosis. In the thoracic region the corresponding phenomenon is prominence of the arch formed by the ribs. We should note not only how far the fingertips are from the floor, but also the contrary case – a patient who can lay her hands flat on the floor while bending forward with knees straight; hypermobility is as significant as restricted movement. The proportions of the patient – arm, leg and trunk length – must of course be taken into account.

Forward bending while standing may be painful and yet not restricted; one reason is the 'painful arc' described by Cyriax (1977). Almost at the beginning of forward bending the patient feels a sharp pain, and a slight evasive reaction can often be seen in the spinal column; forward bending may then proceed without difficulty, but on straightening up pain is again felt just before the erect position is reached. This phenomenon is never seen in anteflexion from the supine position, and is due to contraction of the erector spinae muscle on stooping; it is an important sign of true disc lesion. If, however, the patient feels pain only as she straightens up, this is a sign of articular blockage; in such cases back bending is also restricted.

If anteflexion is restricted while standing with knees straight, it should always be examined with the patient sitting on a chair; this localizes the movement restriction into the lumbar spine. If there is no such restriction the straight leg raising test is used, which will show restriction due to tension in the hamstrings.

Before examining movement restriction in individual segments of the lumbar spine it is advisable to examine tension (trigger points) in certain muscles corresponding to those segments. This will be dealt with in detail later.

Examination of individual segments in the lumbar spine

Tenderness is first examined by palpating the spinous processes with the fingertips; tenderness is usually not quite symmetrical, but more pronounced on one or the other side. Then the springing test is applied; this examines both resistance and tenderness of deep structures (mainly the discs and apophyseal joints) and avoids irritation of the spinous processes. The thenar eminence of one hand is placed on one transverse process and the hypothenar on the other; very slight pressure is exerted by the extended arm to take up the slack, and then spring the vertebra by a slight extra push (*Figure 4.8*).

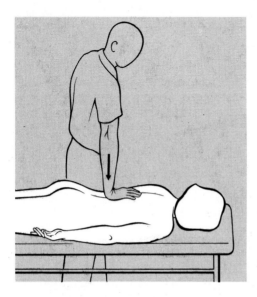

Figure 4.8 Examination of springing of the lumbar and thoracic spine, using thenar contact with the arm outstretched

Another method is to place two fingertips of one hand, one on either side of the spinous process, i.e. on the transverse processes of one vertebra; the hypothenar of the extended other arm is then placed across these fingertips, springing the vertebra after taking up the slack in the same way as before, again taking care to avoid irritating the spinous processes (*Figure 4.9*).

If increased resistance can be felt and the patient feels pain, this is probably due to articular blockage. If, however, there is no increased resistance and yet the patient feels pain, there is likely to be a disc lesion.

The springing test, however, cannot localize movement restriction or hypermobility in a single motor segment precisely. To achieve this specific mobility tests must be used.

TO TEST RETROFLEXION (EXTENSION)

The patient lies on her side with both hips and knees flexed. The examiner leans against the patient's knees with his thighs, fixing the spinous process of the upper vertebra of the examined segment with one finger, reinforced by the fingers of the other hand placed over it. He now exerts slight pressure against the patient's knees in the presumed direction of the intervertebral disc of that segment (the hip flexed

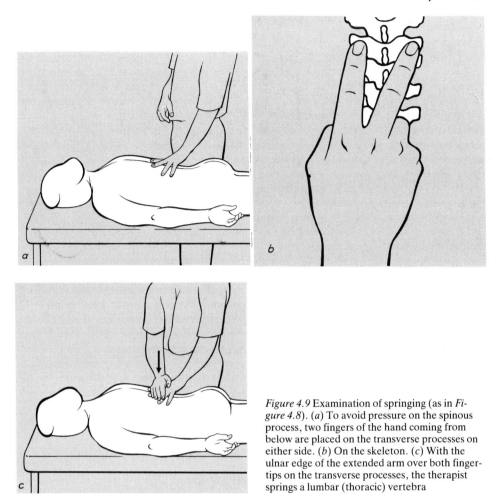

Figure 4.9 Examination of springing (as in *Figure 4.8*). (*a*) To avoid pressure on the spinous process, two fingers of the hand coming from below are placed on the transverse processes on either side. (*b*) On the skeleton. (*c*) With the ulnar edge of the extended arm over both fingertips on the transverse processes, the therapist springs a lumbar (thoracic) vertebra

at an angle of over 90 degrees) so as to take up the slack, and then springs the segment by a slight additional push with his thighs; he feels a slight shift of the pelvis and the lower vertebra against the one that is fixed. In cases of blockage no movement is felt if the slack has been properly taken up. If normal springing is felt dorsiflexion takes place between two adjacent vertebrae, as can be seen in an image intensifier. If there is hypermobility there may be some additional shift (*Figure 4.10*).

EXAMINATION OF ANTEFLEXION

The patient again lies on her side with flexed hips and knees. With one elbow the examiner fixes the upper thoracic region while pushing both flexed knees against the patient's abdomen, using his belly and thighs; this produces maximum anteflexion. With the index finger of the hand fixing the upper thoracic spine he palpates between the two spinous processes of the motor segment, sensing

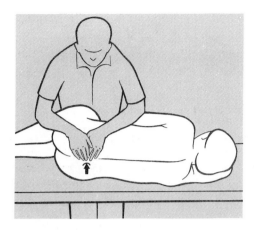

Figure 4.10 Testing retroflexion in one lumbar segment: the patient lies on her side, the therapist exerting springing pressure on both knees and fixing the upper spinous process with both hands

movement (separation of the processes) and tension (at maximum flexion). With his other hand over the patient's buttocks he reinforces flexion of the hips (this hand may also be used for palpation if the patient is very tall and the operator cannot reach the relevant segment with the upper hand). The most important technical detail in this manoeuvre is the fixation of the upper thoracic spine with the elbow while the knee is pushed towards the abdomen, i.e. in the direction of the elbow (*Figure 4.11*).

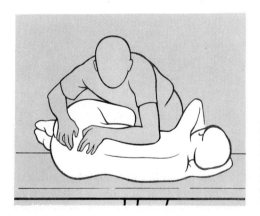

Figure 4.11 Testing anteflexion in one lumbar segment: the patient lies on her side, the therapist pushing the patient's knees against the chest, exerting counter-pressure with his elbow. The hand on the patient's buttock increases anteflexion of the pelvis, while the forefinger of the other hand palpates movement (tension) between the spinous processes

EXAMINATION OF SIDE-BENDING

The patient is in the same position as in the last section but care must be taken to see that both hips and knees are bent at right angles, the knees protruding slightly over the edge of the table; the legs below the knee are parallel to the trunk. The operator stands by the table, facing towards the patient's feet, and grasps both heels in one hand; with the knee closer to the table the examiner supports the patient's knees, thus creating a lever to side-bend the trunk. With the other hand he fixes the patient's flank, the heel of the hand creating a fulcrum at the level of the motor segment being examined, while he palpates between the spinous processes with one finger, from above, sensing movement and, finally, resistance. It is most important to keep the patient's hips and knees at right angles and to keep the knees propped up so that they do not lie lower than the buttocks.

Examination of the thoracic spine and the ribs

Active mobility is first examined, with the patient seated astride the table and performing ante- and retroflexion, side-bending and rotation. In rotation symmetrical movement can be assessed at sight by tracing the line formed by the spinous processes, especially in a slightly kyphotic position, and by noting the angle formed between the patient's shoulders and the table.

As in the lumbar spine, the spinous processes are palpated for tenderness; this is best done in a kyphotic position (*Figure 4.12*). Springing is performed by the same technique as that described for the lumbar spine.

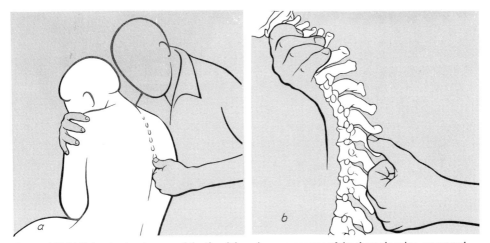

Figure 4.12 (a) Palpating tenderness of the tip of the spinous processes of the thoracic spine, separated by anteflexion. (*b*) Diagram

For the examination of passive movement the patient sits on the table with hands clasped behind her head and the elbows brought together in front of the face. To test back bending the examiner stands by the side of the patient, grasping both elbows from below, so as to extend her trunk and palpate with one finger of the other hand between the spinous processes of the segment being examined, sensing movement and then resistance in the end-position (*Figure 4.13*).

To examine forward bending the operator grasps the patient's elbows from above in order to anteflex the trunk, again palpating between the spinous processes with one finger of the other hand, for movement and for tension in the end-position. In both these examinations it is important to move the patient so as to provide maximum ante- or retroflexion at the site of palpation (*Figure 4.14*). It is also possible to examine ante- and retroflexion in a similar way with the patient lying on her side; this position is used for mobilization into retroflexion (*see Figure 6.35, page 225*).

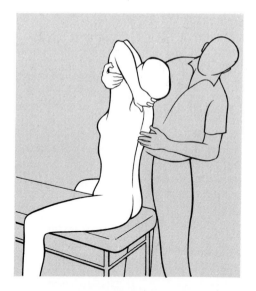

Figure 4.13 Examination of retroflexion of the thoracic spine

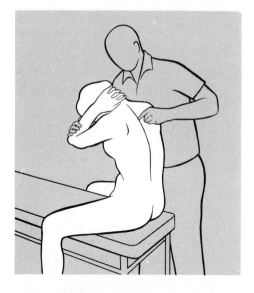

Figure 4.14 Examination of anteflexion of the thoracic spine

To examine side-bending the operator stands behind the patient with one hand round the patient's ribs at the level of the segment being examined, the thumb against the interspace between the spinous processes of the segment and the other hand against the patient's shoulder. He side-bends the patient with the latter hand while his other forms a fulcrum against the ribs, the thumb palpating the movement of the spinous processes and resistance in end-position. The bending movement may be performed at the level of the patient's shoulder; if the upper thoracic spine is being examined, this hand may be against the patient's neck; during examination of the thoracolumbar spine it may be below the shoulder. The other hand must always stabilize the chest from the side, creating a solid fulcrum, even if the palpating thumb appears to be far from the spinous processes when the patient is erect. During side-bending the thumb always reaches the spinous processes, owing to rotation (*Figure 4.15*).

To examine rotation the operator sits the patient astride the table and grasps one shoulder, passing his forearm under her axilla on the other side. He first carries out maximum rotation to one side, repeating the manoeuvre on the other side to compare the two. For examination of individual segments a slightly kyphotic

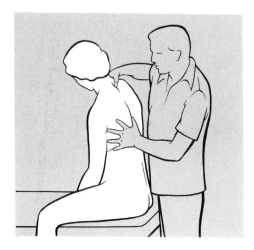

Figure 4.15 Examination of lateral flexion of the thoracic spine

position is recommended, making the spinous processes more accessible both to inspection and to palpation. If there is movement restriction the blocked segment is often visible: there is very little rotation if we follow from the lumbar spine into the thoracic up to the blocked segment, while there is hypermobility above it, so that the line of the spinous processes angulates. On the side where rotation is free we see the unbroken line of the spinous processes from the lumbar up to the thoracic region. Palpating the spinous processes of the blocked segment with two fingers, we feel no relative mobility, whereas on the normal side rotation will be felt first at the upper and a little later at the lower spinous process (*Figure 4.16*). It is most important for the examiner to rotate the patient exactly round her body axis, and to palpate with relaxed fingers which can follow the movement of the spinous processes. This is not easy, and it is therefore a great advantage to form a diagnosis by inspection; this is usually possible in kyphosis unless the patient is too obese. Rotation restriction is most significant in the lowest thoracic spine and at the thoracolumbar junction, less so in the middle or upper thoracic regions.

Mobility of the thoracic spine can be examined with the patient prone, breathing slowly in and out: not only can we see how the whole of the thorax lifts but the spinous processes can be seen spreading like a fan. This fan-like movement can be followed from the lumbar spine up to the cervicothoracic junction. As a rule, at the point where it is interrupted there is blockage; after treatment we see the normal mobility restored during breathing. The exception to this rule are patients with a faulty respiration technique who are unable to breathe into the posterior wall of the thorax even when prone.

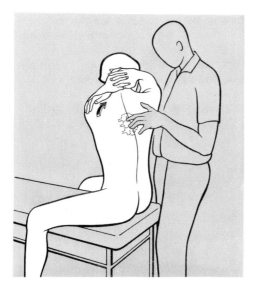

Figure 4.16 Examination of rotation of the thoracic spine

We now proceed to examine the thorax, particularly the ribs. Just as we palpate the spinous process for tenderness, so we palpate the most prominent part of the rib, the costal angle; in the region of the upper ribs we have first to abduct the shoulder-blade, by moving the elbow towards the shoulder of the opposite side.

In theory, a rib can be blocked both in the expiratory and the inspiratory position; from this it would follow that it ought to be more prominent if blocked in inspiration, and less so if blocked in expiration. Again it is wiser to rely on examination and comparison of mobility rather than on position; this means that we examine rib movement on both sides during breathing in and out, examining both by inspection and palpation. A particularly striking phenomenon is the 'overtake' phenomenon, found characteristically in the region of the upper ribs: palpation approximately in the nipple line, or even closer to the sternum, often

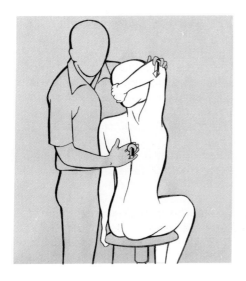

Figure 4.17 Palpation of resistance at the (upper) ribs at retroflexion of the thorax, according to Kubis (Personal communication)

shows that the ribs are not quite on the same level on the two sides. If the patient is asked to take a deep breath, the rib that stood lower will usually be higher than that on the other side, i.e. it has 'overtaken' the other rib. The side of lesser mobility is usually the side of mobility restriction.

Kubis (unpublished observations) has described the best method of diagnosing blockage by increased resistance to (passive) mobility during back bending: the patient sits on the edge of the table with the hand of the side to be examined behind her head, so that the elbow points upwards. The examiner stands on the other side, grasping the elbow from in front and provoking back bending. With the fingers of the other hand at the costal angle of the rib under examination he creates a fulcrum and senses resistance to back bending, resistance that increases if there is blockage (*Figure 4.17*).

It is important that the fingers fixing the rib should be level on the costal angle; curiously enough, the shoulder-blade is no obstacle to effective palpation. Resistance is felt through the shoulder-blade in blockage of the second to fifth ribs, i.e. the region where rib blockage occurs most frequently.

Examination of the first rib

In derangement of this rib pain is felt mainly in the shoulder and in the cervical region; there is a typical tender spot which can be palpated beneath the clavicle towards the manubrium sterni. The typical restriction of movement is impaired anteflexion of the rotated head: the examiner stands behind the seated patient and rotates her head away from the affected rib. With the radial aspect of the forefinger

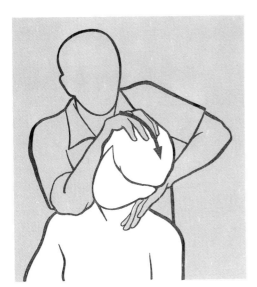

Figure 4.18 Examination of a blocked first rib by forward bending of the head rotated to the opposite side

of the other hand he creates a fulcrum parallel to and above the clavicle, over which the rotated head and neck are bent forward (*Figure 4.18*). The result of this manoeuvre is compared for both sides. Finally, increased resistance may be felt on springing the first rib from above (*see Figure 6.50*, page 236).

Examination of the cervical spine

After general inspection of the head and neck position we test active mobility –
ante- and retroflexion, side-bending and rotation. When dealing with the cervical
spine it is important not to omit examination of resisted isometric mobility, which
reliably reveals pain due to muscular lesions; this is frequently significant in acute
trauma.

The best position for the patient during palpation is supine, the head resting
against the examiner's thigh or belly, and slightly raised. In this position the
muscles are relaxed and we can palpate not only the spinous processes but also the
transverse and articular processes, while if the head is slightly raised we can palpate
the posterior arch of the atlas. In order to palpate the lateral aspect of the spinous
process of C2, which is one of the principal pain points, the head must be bent to
the opposite side. The transverse processes of the atlas are felt between the mastoid
processes and the ramus of the mandible, but they should be palpated from below,
with the patient seated, because they are more prominent than the transverse
processes of the lower cervical vertebrae (*Figure 4.19*).

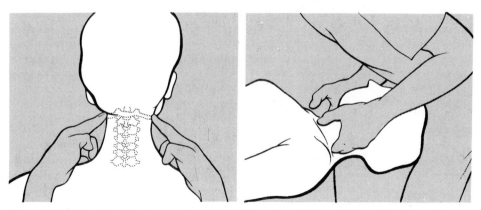

Figure 4.19 (*a*) Palpation of the transverse processes of the atlas with the patient seated; (*b*) cervical
spine supine

For exact orientation it is important to localize correctly the spinous processes of
C7; this is done in retroflexion of the cervical spine. Placing one finger on C7 and
the next on C6, we will note that while C7 remains in place, C6 moves forward and
is difficult to palpate in retroflexion. (NB: One should not rely on the vertebra
prominens being inevitably C7!)

Examination of passive mobility must begin with the mobility of the whole of the
cervical spine. The patient is seated and the examiner must fix (immobilize) the
shoulder girdle. He begins with passive retroflexion: standing by the side of the
patient he moves her head into retroflexion with one hand while the other fixes the
cervicothoracic junction. In passive anteflexion the patient's chin is drawn to the
sternum; this is a movement that is often restricted because of shortened neck
muscles. If maximum anteflexion is immediately painful, and there is no meningitis
or acute radicular pain, the pain felt by the patient is usually due to restricted
anteflexion of the occiput against the atlas; if, however, pain is felt after 15–20 s,

this is most probably ligament pain (*see* page 324, anteflexion headache). In order to examine side-bending of the cervical spine, the operator must fix the shoulder of the side *towards* which the head is bent and compare mobility in both directions. (If he fixed the shoulder *away from which* the head is bent he would then be examining the stretching of the trapezius muscle.)

Rotation

With the patient's head and neck erect – The examiner fixes the shoulder away from which the head is turned, with one elbow, observing how close he can bring the chin to the shoulder on one side or the other. Care must be taken to perform rotation of the head and neck round a vertical axis (*Figure 4.20*).

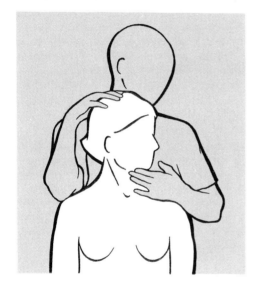

Figure 4.20 Examination of rotation of the entire cervical spine

   With the head in maximum anteflexion – The examiner stands behind the patient; with one hand on the occiput he moves the head and neck into maximum anteflexion, while his other hand holds the patient's chin. The rotation he now effects is mainly between the occiput and C2, i.e. between atlas and axis. Again, care must be taken to rotate round the axis of the head and the cervical spine, i.e. the operator moves the occiput from one side to the other, while the chin remains almost fixed. A word of caution: because the examiner is standing behind the patient, it is the occiput he sees, and he is therefore tempted to move the chin!
   With the patient's chin drawn towards the neck – As Jirout (1979) has shown, movement restriction of the C2/3 segment can be selectively shown by this movement. Again the examiner stands behind the patient, rotating the head with one hand on the occiput and one on the chin. The latter is necessary mainly to fix the chin against the neck, while it is the hand on the occiput that rotates the head, the axis of rotation being close behind the forehead.
   In retroflexion – This reveals blockage below C3; the greater the retroflexion, the more caudal the segment causing it. Here, too, the chin should be almost fixed while the hand on the occiput produces rotation. To fix the patient's shoulders, the

examiner should cross his arms, i.e. rotating the patient's head to the right he grasps the chin with his left hand (pushing the chin slightly to the right) and the occiput with his right, pushing towards the left and resisting rotation of the shoulder with his right forearm.

After these more or less screening techniques we must proceed to the most important specific techniques.

Side-bending

This can be performed with the patient seated or supine; in each case the examiner bends the patient's head sideways with one hand while the other creates a fulcrum with the aid of the medial aspect of the forefinger against the transverse process of the lower vertebra of the segment under examination. Both the range of movement and the resistance in end-position must be noted. In the supine position the patient's head is projected over the edge of the table and cradled in the examiner's hand. It is advisable to rotate the head slightly in the opposite direction to that of side-bending, and to lift it. To examine side-bending at C1/2, the cervical spine should be kept straight up to C2 while the operator rotates the head round an axis through the bridge of the nose (*Figure 4.21*). This technique is applicable from C1/2

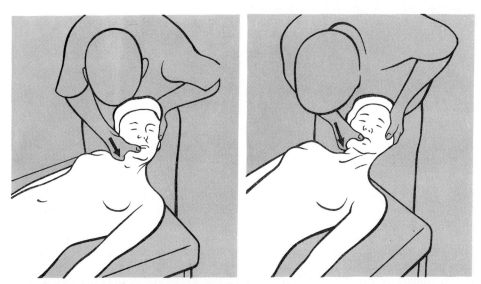

Figure 4.21 Palpation of passive lateral flexion of individual segments of the cervical spine with the patient supine: (*a*) in the lower cervical spine; (*b*) between atlas and axis

to C5/6 and even C6/7. Dealing with the cervicothoracic junction, if the patient is seated the examiner must take care to maintain the whole of the cervicothoracic spine erect, and the neck even in slight retroflexion, while the head must be slightly rotated in the direction opposite to that of the side-bending. With the thumb of the other hand he creates a fulcrum against the spinous processes of the lower vertebra of the examined segment (*Figure 4.22*). The same effect can be achieved with the patient lying on her side: the examiner stands in front of the patient, cradling her

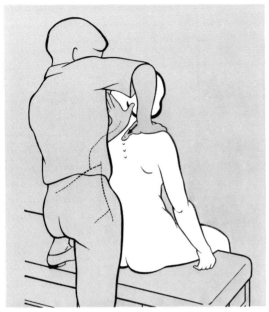

Figure 4.22 Examination of lateral springing at the cervicothoracic junction, by a push with the thumb against the lateral aspect of the lower spinous process of the examined segment

head and neck in his forearm and thus producing a side-bending movement, while the thumb of his other hand fixes the spinous processes from above (from the side – *see Figure 4.25*). In both cases the hand that side-bends the cervical spine also fixes (pushes) the spinous process of the upper vertebra, with the thenar.

Rotation

The patient is seated while the examiner stands behind her and fixes between thumb and forefinger of one hand the vertebral arch of the lower vertebra of the relevant segment, from one transverse process to the other. The examiner now rotates the patient's head (usually with his other hand on the chin) until he feels that the transverse process is engaged against his thumb or forefinger. He begins with the axis, establishing the range of movement between atlas and axis, proceeding from one vertebral arch to the next. The range of movement should increase step-wise from one segment to the next. If there is blockage in a mobile segment, the absence of this increase in one or both directions should be noted (*Figure 4.23(a)*).

This technique is particularly suitable for the demonstration of movement restriction of single mobile segments in the lecture hall, and equally suitable for optical registration. Berger (1983) has constructed a device (cervicomotograph): a helmet fixed to the ceiling by joints and rods. The patient is seated, looking at a fixed point in order to determine the neutral position of the head. Using the technique described here the operator first examines the segment C1/2 by fixation of C2, then C2/3 by fixation of C3, and on down to C5/6; capacity transducers in the rod joints make electronic recording of the range of movement possible. The resulting graph is a 'cervicomotogram' (*Figure 4.23(b)* and *(c)*).

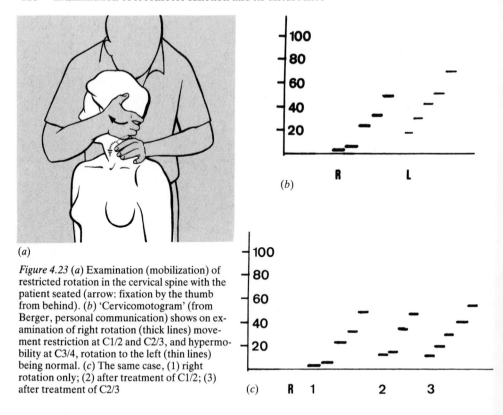

Figure 4.23 (*a*) Examination (mobilization) of restricted rotation in the cervical spine with the patient seated (arrow: fixation by the thumb from behind). (*b*) 'Cervicomotogram' (from Berger, personal communication) shows on examination of right rotation (thick lines) movement restriction at C1/2 and C2/3, and hypermobility at C3/4, rotation to the left (thin lines) being normal. (*c*) The same case, (1) right rotation only; (2) after treatment of C1/2; (3) after treatment of C2/3

There are two important technical details to be noted in this rotation technique: (1) if the examiner fixes the arch of a vertebra he must do so exactly in the neutral position, i.e. he must sense the correct position; (2) he must not use force to fix the vertebral arch; he simply stops turning the head at the moment when he feels the transverse process against his finger, i.e. resistance in the end-position.

Shifting techniques

These are used to examine joint play in the cervical spine and can be carried out in an anteroposterior and in a laterolateral direction. The examiner stands at the side of the seated patient and puts his arm round her head in such a way that his elbow is in front of her face or forehead, while his little finger grasps the vertebral arch of the upper vertebra of the segment to be tested. With the other hand he fixes the vertebral arch of the lower vertebra between thumb and forefinger. With his arm on the patient's head he now (1) pushes the head and the upper vertebra backwards, taking up the slack and finally springing the end-position against the thumb and finger of the fixing hand; or (2) he side-shifts the patient's head and upper vertebra against either the thumb or the forefinger of the fixing hand, first taking up the slack and springing the end-position (*Figure 4.24*). In this way he can examine the cervical segments from C2/3 down to C5/6 and also, in the anteroposterior direction, the occiput against the atlas – here I recommend slight anteflexion of the head. The fixing hand stabilizes the arch of the axis, but shifting occurs exclusively between occiput and atlas since no shifting movement can occur between the anterior arch of the atlas and the odontoid process.

From C6/7 to T1/2 or even T2/3 it is again only possible to carry out anteroposterior shifts, with the patient seated. The examiner applies his hand to the mass of the patient's upper trapezius muscle, from above, producing a backward shift, while he fixes the spinous process of the lower vertebra of the segment with one finger or the thumb of the other hand.

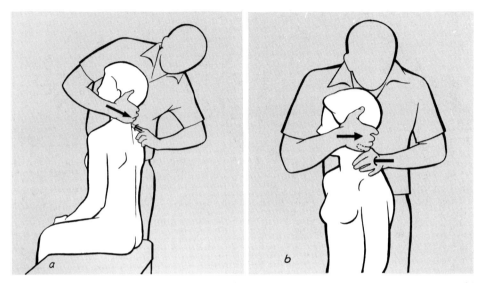

Figure 4.24 Examination of dorsal shift (springing) of the cranial against the caudal adjacent vertebra (*a*) in the cervicothoracic junction and (*b*) in the cervical spine: the head and cranial vertebra of the examined segment are shifted (backwards) while mobility (resistance) is felt at the spinous process or vertebral arch of the lower vertebra

Shift can also be examined with the patient lying on her side; the examiner stands in front of her, grasping her head in his arm and stabilizing it against his chest, while his little finger clasps the vertebral arch of the upper vertebra of the segment being examined. Again, the other hand fixes the arch of the lower vertebra between thumb and forefinger. The examiner may now push the patient's head backwards or upwards, i.e. laterally in the direction of the fixing thumb; downwards the movement is less effective. In the cervicothoracic region the hand coming from above again pushes against the mass of the upper trapezius muscle to produce a backward shift; it may also push upwards, producing a lateral shift against the spinous process of the upper vertebra, in the direction of the thumb of the other hand fixing the spinous process of the lower vertebra from above (*Figure 4.25*). It is important that the push from below should always be delivered at the level of the upper vertebra of the segment, so that there are no segments separating the examining hands! Both taking up the slack and springing should be carried out with minimum force. These techniques for examining shift (joint play) are among the most sensitive, revealing blockage in the cervical spine that is as yet unexposed by any other technique.

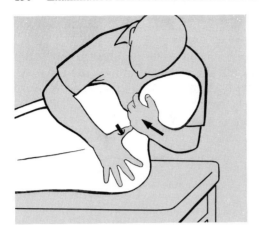

Figure 4.25 Examination of the cervicothoracic junction with the patient lying on her side

Movement between atlas and occiput

1. Without using any force, the examiner stands behind the seated patient with his fingers on her face and chin and brings the head into maximum rotation, stabilizing it against his chest and taking care to see that the head is erect, rotating correctly round a vertical axis. After taking up the slack he springs maximum rotation with the minimum of force. With a fingertip of the other hand he senses springing at the transverse process of the atlas. An alternative method is to fix the atlas with the thumb and forefinger, against the transverse process on each side, and to grasp the patient's head with the other arm (*see Figure 4.19,* page 124) so as to produce a very small rotatory movement while slightly side-bending the head in the opposite direction.

2. *Side-bending* – The patient lies supine with her head over the edge of the table; the examiner rotates the head so as to lock C1/2. He now side bends the head against the cervical spine (which is erect). Head rotation need not exceed 45 degrees, an important point to remember with elderly patients (*Figure 4.26*).

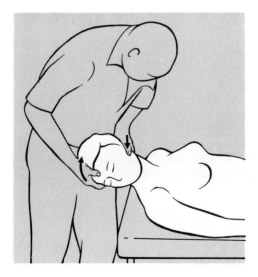

Figure 4.26 Examination of lateral flexion between occiput and atlas with the head rotated to the opposite side

3. *Retroflexion* – The patient is supine with her head over the edge of the table; the examiner places one hand on the chin and the other on the occiput, rotating it so as to lock the atlas/axis, and bending it back against the cervical spine. Care must be taken not to grasp the occiput too close to the atlas, so that the fingers meet no obstruction before full back bending is achieved (*Figure 4.27*).

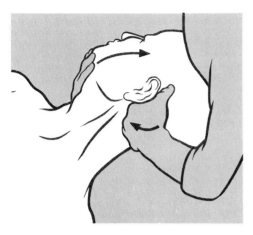

Figure 4.27 Examination of retroflexion between atlas and occiput with the head rotated

4. *Anteflexion* – The patient is supine on the table; the examiner places his hand under her occiput so that his thumb is resting against one transverse process of the atlas and his index finger against the other, producing fixation of the arch of the atlas. With his other hand on the patient's forehead he induces anteflexion (*Figure 4.28*). Anteroposterior shift of the occiput against the atlas has already been described under shift techniques (*see Figure 4.24*, page 129).

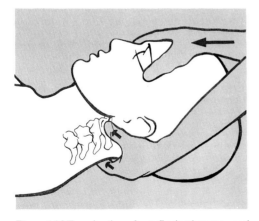

Figure 4.28 Examination of anteflexion between occiput and atlas with fixation of the transverse processes of the atlas

Examination of the extremity joints

Before going into detail I must stress once again that correct or disturbed function of the locomotor system concerns both the spinal column and the extremities, and that if pain is due to such a disturbance, function must be normalized, whatever its localization.

The examination of individual joints follows the pattern already established: active movement, resisted or isometric movement to show whether muscles are at fault, and passive mobility including joint play.

If passive mobility in a joint is impaired, there is a 'capsular pattern' (Cyriax, 1977) for each joint, i.e. if there is movement restriction in several directions it shows characteristic proportions, or pattern. If impairment does not follow this pattern we may conclude that the lesion is not in the joint but affecting it from without. The significance of joint play lies in the fact that its disturbance is the first sign of a lesion. The technique of examination of joint play is described in chapter 6, as it is identical with that of joint mobilization.

The shoulder

Active mobility includes abduction and elevation of the arm, rotation, anteflexion and retroflexion. The most striking disturbance is the 'painful arc' of Cyriax (1977) during abduction: the patient may feel sharp pain during abduction to even less than 90 degrees, but when she passes this point she can then raise her arm to a full 180 degrees. This phenomenon is due to disturbance of the subacromial bursa which facilitates the gliding motion of the head of the humerus, with the rotator cuff under the coracoacromial ligament.

Isometric resistance may show tenderness of some muscle insertions: against abduction, the supraspinatus tendon; against external rotation, the infraspinatus; and against raising the semi-flexed arm (like a waiter carrying a tray, *Figure 4.29(a–c)*), the long biceps tendon. Tenderness in the subscapularis must be diagnosed by direct palpation, as described in Chapter 6, page 270.

If passive mobility is impaired and the characteristic capsular pattern of the shoulder joint is present, the lesion is in the capsule of the glenohumeral joint, as is the case in 'frozen shoulder'. If we examine from the neutral position – i.e. with the arm in adduction, the elbow in right-angle flexion and the forearm facing forward – we find maximum restriction of external rotation followed by abduction and internal rotation. It is therefore important to examine external rotation very carefully: the examiner stands behind the seated patient and grasps the forearms close to the elbow, keeping the elbows closely adducted against the patient's trunk and using the forearm as a lever to produce external rotation (*Figure 4.30*). By drawing the patient's thumbs up her back, on both sides, we examine mainly internal rotation coupled with extension and adduction.

If it is only abduction that is restricted, and rotation is free, the lesion is in the subacromial bursa, whether there is a painful arc or not. In this case there is often impaired joint play. The examiner stands behind the seated patient and abducts her arm to 90 degrees, telling her to relax. With his other hand on the head of the humerus he exerts very slight pressure from above in order to take up the slack, and then springs the joint in the same direction. Interestingly, if there is a true capsular pattern and yet it is possible to abduct the arm to about 90 degrees, we find *normal* joint play, which again shows that the 'frozen shoulder' is *not* due to blockage. Joint

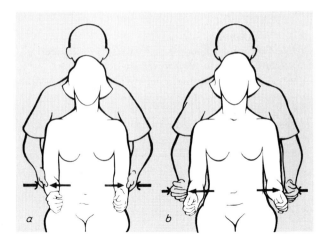

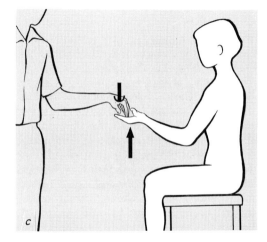

Figure 4.29 Examination against isometric resistance of the muscles of the rotator cuff at the shoulder: (*a*) against abduction of the adducted upper arm (supraspinatus); (*b*) against external rotation (infraspinatus); (*c*) against raising of the semi-flexed arm (long biceps tendon)

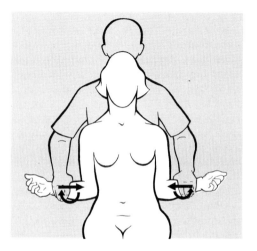

Figure 4.30 Examination of passive external rotation of the shoulder with the arms in adduction and elbows flexed at right angles

play, however, is certainly impaired if only abduction is involved, i.e. in what might be called 'periarthritis' if it were not preferable to drop this somewhat useless term and call it 'abduction lesion' (*Figure 4.31*). Care must be taken to place the hand on the head of the humerus and not on the labrum glenoidale of the scapula.

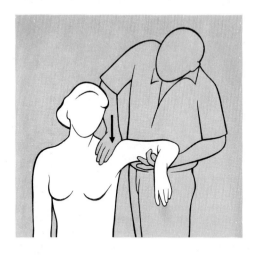

Figure 4.31 Examination of joint play (caudal shift) with the patient seated, her arm in 90 degree abduction; springing pressure is applied from above, on the head of the humerus

Two more joints may cause shoulder pain: the acromioclavicular and the sternoclavicular. Involvement of the former is a very frequent but rarely diagnosed condition, yet diagnosis is not difficult: if we push the elbow of the affected side against the opposite shoulder, the patient feels pain and the movement is restricted compared with the healthy side. Direct palpation of the joint is also painful. Pain due to blockage of the sternoclavicular joint is a rather rare condition: the patient experiences pain when moving the shoulder-blades and direct palpation reveals tenderness. There is one diagnostic pitfall to be avoided, however: tenderness of the medial end of the clavicle is far more often due to tension in the sternocleidomastoid muscle.

The elbow joint

Impairment here concerns mainly flexion and extension, the former suffering more (capsular pattern). As there are three bones articulating at the elbow, however, joint play is complex, and includes movement between radius and ulna. The most important clinical condition is pain in the epicondyles, where we find impaired lateral springing and typical muscle spasms which will be dealt with elsewhere.

The wrist joint

This is a complex joint consisting of the radius and ulna, the carpal bones and the joints of the distal carpal bones and the metacarpals. For clinical localization it is useful to know that the proximal skin fold on the dorsal aspect of the wrist in dorsiflexion corresponds to the radiocarpal joint, while the fold on the palmar aspect in palmar flexion corresponds to the carpometacarpal joints. Active movement consists in dorsal and palmar flexion and in radial and ulnar flexion. For correct treatment each of the movements must be fully understood.

Dorsal flexion takes place more in the mid-carpal joint, the distal row of the carpal bones gliding in a palmar direction. If this movement is impaired palmar gliding (joint play) must be restored.

Palmar flexion takes place more in the radiocarpal joints, the proximal row of the carpal bones gliding in a dorsal direction (joint play). If palmar flexion is impaired dorsal gliding must be restored.

Ulnar flexion consists in a radial gliding movement of the ovoid of the wrist in relation to the radius (and ulna), by which the hand rotates into ulnar flexion. This gliding movement of the proximal row against the radius must be restored if ulnar flexion is impaired.

The most complex of these movements is radial flexion. This movement is achieved by approaching the base of the first metacarpal to the styloid process of the radius. This is made possible by a localized dorsiflexion between the scaphoid and the trapezium, which can be palpated as a palmar protuberance in the proximity of the styloid process during radial flexion. Thus radial flexion cannot be carried out if the hand is in palmar flexion, while it is facilitated by dorsiflexion.

To restore this movement we must therefore restore joint play between the trapezium and the scaphoid, moving the former in a palmar direction. Even more frequently, however, radial flexion is restricted by yet another mechanism: impaired pronation of the radius against the ulna. On moving the hand into radial and ulnar flexion on a horizontal board we can easily see that the forearm makes a pronatory synkinesis during radial flexion and a supinatory synkinesis during ulnar flexion. Hindering this synkinesis by placing a thumb under the styloid process of the radius will prevent radial flexion. The same holds – in the opposite direction – for ulnar flexion. We must therefore examine and restore joint play in the elbow joint as well: for impaired radial flexion, lateral springing of the elbow joint should be used; and for ulnar flexion, medial springing. This is also the mechanism underlying styloiditis.

In addition to movement that can be carried out actively, there is of course joint play between each of the carpal bones and between the carpal bones and the forearm, and also between the carpal and the metacarpal bones, and even between the bases of the metacarpals. This has been shown to be of considerable clinical importance in view of the frequent occurrence of the carpal-tunnel syndrome. Whereas the gliding movements of joint play can normally be brought about with the minimum of force, indeed it is difficult to exert so little force as *not* to move these bones, in the carpal-tunnel syndrome there is increased resistance to joint play. It can only be diagnosed, however, by examining with the *minimum* of force. The clinical consequence is clear: we treat the carpal-tunnel syndrome by removing its main cause, disturbed joint play of the bones that form the walls of the carpal tunnel, bearing in mind that this function, too, is influenced by movement patterns controlling the upper extremity.

The finger joints will be dealt with in Chapter 6 (page 197).

The hip joint

Although the hip is an extremity joint, clinically it is part of the pelvis, and frequently the first symptom in lesions of the hip joint is low-back pain. The most constant signs to be looked for are Patrick's sign, a tender femoral head in the groin, restriction and tenderness on internal rotation, and pain on maximum abduction with the patient lying on her side. There is tenderness of the greater trochanter and, if the patient also complains of pain in the knees, tenderness of the pes anserinus on the tibia. The typical capsular pattern is maximum disturbance of internal rotation followed by extension, flexion and external rotation. The articular surfaces being largely congruous there is hardly any joint play in the sense of parallel shifting movement; there is only considerable distraction. In severe cases full extension of the hip is impossible and the typical posture develops: the buttock on the affected side becomes prominent and there is compensatory hyperlordosis of the lumbar spine.

The knee joint and the tibiofibular joint

The principal function of the knee is flexion and extension, but with the knee flexed there is considerable rotation. In disturbed function the capsular pattern shows maximum impairment of flexion followed by extension. Therefore, maximum flexion is examined first; since the surfaces of the tibia, fibula and patella are incongruous there is much joint play: proximodistal gliding of the tibia on the femur, lateral springing, and (clinically very important) shifting movements of the patella.

Although not directly connected, the tibiofibular joint plays a part in rotation of the leg if the knee is flexed, allowing some additional adduction and abduction of the foot. It can therefore be examined by comparing foot rotation with the patient prone and the knees flexed at right angles. The joint play consists in anteroposterior gliding with some rotation of the fibular head on the surface of the tibia. In lesions of this joint the fibular head is tender on palpation.

The foot

The function of the foot joints is best tested first by rotation around the long axis; the patient is supine, the examined leg flexed with the heel touching the table. The examiner grasps the foot with one hand at the first metacarpal head and the other at the fifth, and rotates it around the long axis, the centre of rotation being the talar head. If there is disturbed function of the foot joints, including the ankle, this rotation is impaired: either it deviates from the axis or, if an attempt is made to keep it on the axis, it is restricted and there is increased resistance. This is an invaluable screening test.

The ankle joint

This is a hinge joint in which dorsal and plantar flexion can be carried out. If there is disturbed function, dorsal flexion suffers more than plantar flexion (capsular pattern). When dorsal flexion is being examined it is important that the patient's knees be flexed, or else a short gastrocnemius muscle may impair dorsiflexion. Joint play consists in a dorsal shift of the tibia and fibula against the talus (*see* Chapter 6). It is important to realize that in this joint we find very frequently indeed that joint play is impaired without restriction of active mobility.

Examination of the joints of the foot

The complex of joints of the foot consists of the subtalar joint, Chopart's joint and the tarsometatarsal joint. They make possible pronation and supination (inversion and eversion), abduction and adduction of the foot. The techniques of joint play are invaluable for the examination of individual joints between the tarsal and the metatarsal bones.

The temporomandibular joint

This joint is of considerable clinical importance because it can cause pain in the face that may be mistaken for trigeminal neuralgia. Coupled with vertigo, this pain constitutes the Costen syndrome. This may point to a close connection with the craniocervical junction. At examination there is characteristic tenderness of the joint in front of the tragus; palpation is easier if the patient opens and shuts her mouth. No less important are trigger points in the masticatory muscles, which have to be palpated through the open mouth, including the temporalis muscle in the temple.

Muscular imbalance of masticatory muscles includes also increased tension of the digastric muscle palpated on both sides of the hyoid bone with tender attachment points at the hyoid and even a possible lateral shift of this bone, and increased resistance against a shift to the opposite direction. If there is free mobility is should be possible to place three knuckles between the upper and lower incisors. It is important to look for signs of malocclusion (missing teeth) or evidence of muscle dysfunction including buxism as possible causes of temporomandibular joint lesions.

Examination of reflex changes

Hyperalgesic skin zones (HSZ)

Examining segmental mobility and its disturbance, we naturally palpate the tissues where increased tension is sensed. Head (1893, 1894) discovered zones of increased sensitivity to pinpricks, but this method, however significant, has the disadvantage of relying solely on the patient's response. Methods of palpation may elicit pain, but even if they do not they always produce findings that the examiner can assess.

For the experienced examiner it may suffice to apply some pressure on the skin (and the underlying tissues). A very popular method is to form a fold of skin and roll it between the fingers (Kibler, 1958; Maigne, 1968); as it causes pain, this method provokes a reaction in the patient, while the examiner feels increased resistance to his folding of the skin and can see (and measure) the fold, which is thicker where a HSZ is found.

There are other methods of 'connective-tissue massage' (Leube and Dicke, 1951) which produce a similar reaction.

Recently I have developed a method that is proving diagnostically more reliable, is completely painless, and therapeutically very effective; this is the method of skin stretching. Any area of skin, large or small, can be stretched by the operator either with his fingertips or with his hands placed flat on the skin. The technique is simple: I first stretch the skin with the minimum of force, so as to take up the slack, and then feel springing in the end-position. This is compared in several directions over the tested area, which is also compared with the corresponding area on the healthy side. In a HSZ there is very stiff resistance after taking up the slack; after stretching in the end-position has been held for about 10 s this resistance can be felt to weaken, and normal springing is then restored. This can be measured if we mark the area with a pencil before taking up the slack, after doing so, and then after about 10 s stretching (*see Figure 6.128,* page 303). By this method it is possible to diagnose (and treat) even such small HSZ as can form between toes, over painful bone areas (spinous processes, xiphoid processes), and over and around scars.

Reflex changes in muscles – 'trigger points'

Muscles react to nociceptive stimulation by changes in tension; one of the most characteristic and clinically important reactions is the 'trigger point'. To quote Travell (1976): 'A trigger point in a skeletal muscle is identified by localized deep tenderness in a palpably firm band of muscle (muscle hardening); and at the point of maximum deep hyperalgesia by a positive "jump sign", a visible shortening of that part of the muscle which contains the band. To elicit the jump sign most effectively, one must place the relaxed muscle under moderate passive tension and snap the band briskly with the palpating finger'.

Not only local pain but also referred pain may be elicited from a trigger point. *Table 4.1* lists some important muscle trigger points.

TABLE 4.1. Important muscular trigger points

Muscle	*Clinical significance*
Quadriceps femoris, tensor fasciae latae	Pain at the upper edge of the patella
Thigh adductors	Lesion of the hip joint
Iliacus	Lesion of segment L5/S1 (coccyx)
Piriformis	Lesion of segment L4/5 (coccyx)
Rectus femoris	Lesion of segment L3/4 (hip)
Hamstrings	Lesion of segments L5–S1, pain at the tuberosity of the ischium and fibular head
Levator ani (per rectum)	Coccyx
Psoas and quadratus lumborum	Lesion of thoracolumbar junction (T10–L1)
Erectors spinae	Segment at the corresponding level
Rectus abdominis	Tenderness of xiphoid, symphysis, low back pain at back bending, abdominal viscera
Pectoralis	Thoracic viscera, upper ribs
Middle part of trapezius	Cervicobrachial and radicular syndromes of upper extremity
Subscapularis	Frozen shoulder, scapular pain
Supinator, finger extensors, biceps, brachioradialis	Radial epicondylalgia
Finger flexors	Ulnar epicondylalgia
Upper part of trapezius	Any cervical lesion
Sternocleidomastoid	Lesion of segment C0/1 and C2/3, pain referred to skull and face
Short extensors of the occiput (overlying the posterior arch of the atlas)	Lesion of the atlanto-occipital segment
Masticatory muscles	Temporomandibular joint, headache, facial pain
Digastricus	Pain at the hyoid, dysphagia

Reflex changes on the periosteum – pain points

There are numerous pain points on the periosteum in patients with disturbed function of the locomotor system. Frequently, like trigger points in muscles, pain points are highly characteristic of certain lesions and therefore have high diagnostic value (*Table 4.2*). Their disappearance (improvement) also serves as a valuable test for the efficacy of treatment. Frequently the tender periosteum is somewhat

TABLE 4.2. Important periostal points

Periostal point	Clinical significance
Calcaneal spur	Tension in plantar aponeurosis
Pes anserinus (tubercle of tibia)	Tension in long adductors, hip lesion
Fibular head	Tension in biceps femoris, blockage
Upper margin of patella	Tension in quadriceps or tensor fasciae latae
Posterior superior iliac spine	Frequent but not specific
Tuberosity of the ischium	Tension in hamstrings
Lateral aspect of the pubic symphysis	Tension in the adductors, sacroiliac blockage, hip lesion
Upper margin of the symphysis	Tension in the rectus abdominis
Coccyx	Tension in the gluteus maximus, levator ani, piriformis
Iliac crest	Lesion of thoracolumbar junction, tension in quadratus and gluteus medius
Greater trochanter	Tension in abductors, hip lesion
Spinous process (most frequently L5)	Tension in deep paraspinal muscles
Spinous process Th5,6 (Maigne's 'dorsalgie')	Low cervical lesion, thoracolumbar lesion
Spinous process of C2	Lesion of segments C1/2, C2/3, tension in levator scapulae
Xiphoid process	Tension in rectus abdominis
On ribs in the mammary and axillary line	Tension in pectoralis attached here, visceral pain
At sternocostal junction of upper ribs	Tension in the scalenus
Sternum just below clavicle	Lesion of first rib
Medial end of clavicle	Tension in sternocleidomastoid
Erb's point	Upper limb root syndromes, tension in the scalenes
Transverse process of atlas	Lesion of atlas/occiput segment, tension in sternocleidomastoid and recti capitis laterales
On the occiput	Referred from the posterior arch of the atlas and lateral aspect of spinous process C2
Styloid process of radius	Lesion at the elbow joint
Epiconyles	Lesion of the elbow joints, tension of muscles attached at epicondyles
Attachment of deltoid	Lesion of scapulohumeral joint
Condyle of mandible	Lesion of temporomandibular joint, tension in masticatory muscles
Cornua of hyoid bone	Tension of the digastricus, dysphagia

changed on palpation, as though it formed a soft bump. Many periosteal pain points are sites of attachment of tendons or ligaments (enthesopathy), and the tenderness is apparently related to increased muscular tension, e.g. the greater trochanter, fibular head, Achilles' tendon and attachments. If spinous processes are tender on one side, this correlates with the side of muscle spasm and with restricted rotation to that side.

Where joints can be palpated directly they are tender on palpation if there is any lesion. This is true for the intervertebral joints, which can be particularly well palpated in the cervical region with the patient supine; for the rest of the spinal column deep paraspinous palpation is required, with the patient prone. All extremity joints are accessible to palpation, and this is very important in affections of the hip joint which is palpated in the groin, of the acromioclavicular and sternoclavicular joints palpated at the lateral and medial end of the clavicle, and of the temporomandibular joint palpated before the tragus.

Root syndromes

I have repeatedly stressed that mere reflex changes in a single segment, including radiating pain, hyperalgesia and even dysaesthesia, do not constitute sufficient grounds for a diagnosis of root syndrome. Conclusive evidence of a root lesion is provided by neurological deficit: hypoaesthesia, hypoalgesia, muscular weakness with hypotonia and/or atrophy, increased idiomuscular excitability and decreased tendon reflexes. Unless these signs are present we may suspect root lesion but require further proof. There are two signs, however, which strongly suggest a root syndrome: pain and/or dysaesthesia radiating as far as to the toes or fingers; and the straight leg raising test below 45 degrees.

The individual root syndromes will be dealt with in Chapter 7. The dermatome chart of Hansen and Schliack (1962) is reproduced here (*Figure 4.32(a–e) and (g)*) together with that of Keegan (1944) (*Figure 4.32(f)*) for the leg. It should be pointed out that to this day there is no generally accepted dermatome chart, which may perhaps be explained by the fact that dermatomes vary from one subject to the next. An important point in the Hansen and Schliack (1962) chart is their 'cervicothoracic and lumbosacral hiatus': segments C5–T1 and L2–S2 do not appear on the trunk, but only on the extremities. On the scapular line on the back there is a 'step' which these authors consider to be the region where the dorsal and ventral rami meet.

In conclusion, it can be said that there is a wealth of detectable signs of reflex changes due to painful (nociceptive) stimulation in the skin and underlying tissues, in muscles, periosteum, tendons and ligaments, all of which can be diagnosed clinically and some of which can be registered (skin temperature, electric resistance, etc.). These signs enable us to make a clinical diagnosis and to locate those changes which can be the object of specific and adequate therapy.

Examination of disturbed equilibrium

I have already shown that the spinal column plays an important role in maintaining or disturbing equilibrium, and it is therefore necessary to assess this factor in cases of disturbance, if possible by direct clinical examination.

Hautant's test is very suitable for this purpose: the patient is seated in a chair which supports her back, with both arms stretched forward. The examiner stands facing her, with his thumbs pointing at the patient's hands. The patient closes her eyes while the examiner watches for a few seconds, to see whether the patient's hands deviate to one side in relation to his own thumbs (*Figure 4.33*). After examination in the neutral position, it is repeated in different head positions: turned to the left, to the right, bent forward, bent back. While the patient changes the position of her head the examiner holds her hands in neutral position to prevent deviation due to synkinesis of the arms.

This test has two great advantages: being seated and propped up, the patient feels safe even if dizzy and deviation is not caused by nervousness, as is often the case in Romberg's test (with the patient standing). The second advantage is that with the patient's back leaning against a chair, only side deviation of the arms is possible. In Romberg's test, on the other hand, in which the swaying of the body with eyes shut is tested, the change in the direction of swaying that occurs in head rotation (forwards or backwards) is interpreted as the result of labyrinth imbalance,

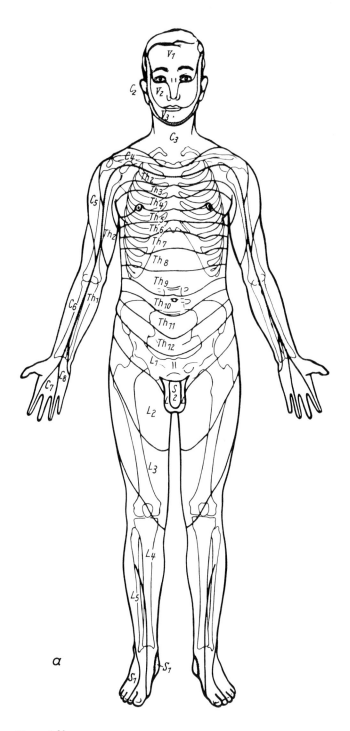

Figure 4.32

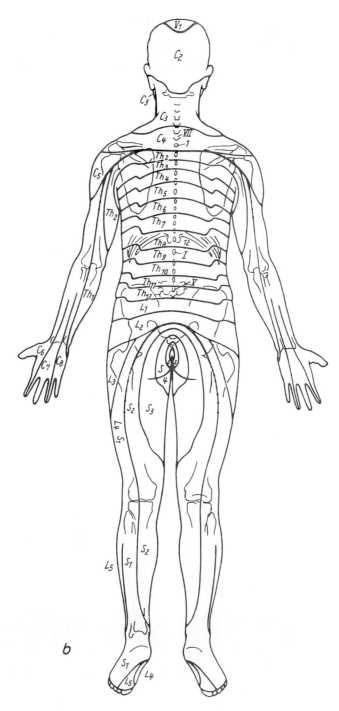

Figure 4.32

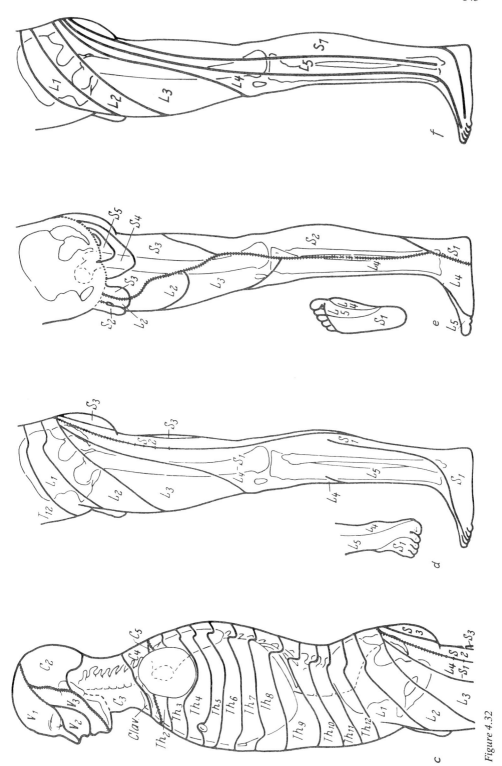

Figure 4.32

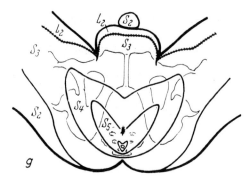

Figure 4.32 The dermatome chart given by Hansen and Schliack (1962) (*a–e* and *g*) and by Keegan (1944) (*f*): dermatomes on the (*a*) ventral, (*b*) dorsal, (*c*) lateral aspects of the trunk; (*d*) on the inner and (*e*) outer aspect of the leg and foot; (*f*) on the outer aspect of the leg; (*g*) at the perineum

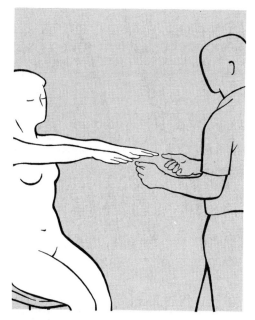

Figure 4.33 Hautant's test: the patient is seated with the back supported and the eyes closed; the examiner watches deviation of the outstretched arms by comparing the position of the patient's arms with his own thumbs

the patient swaying in the direction of the affected labyrinth. In Hautant's test, any deviation that takes place when the patient turns her head is the result of the head position relative to the trunk, i.e. the position of the cervical spine. We can thus distinguish pathogenic and relief positions of the head, i.e. positions that cause or increase deviation, and those that abolish deviation if it has been found in the neutral position. In fact, the reaction to changed head position in cases of imbalance due to cervical lesion is so characteristic that we can speak of a 'cervical pattern' (*see* page 327).

This very simple examination is carried out if the patient complains of disturbed balance and if the test standing on two scales shows a difference greater than 4 kg.

Berger (1983) has constructed a simple apparatus to register this deviation: the patient is seated as before, with eyes closed; in one outstretched hand he holds a pencil and moves it from right to left and back for about 1 cm on paper that is moving at a constant speed. In this way deviation can be registered for various head positions (*Figure 4.34*).

Diagnosis is corroborated (or reversed) if deviation disappears (or persists) after treatment.

It is necessary to distinguish between disturbance of balance caused by the position of the neck, and disturbance due to the position of the head with the rest of the body, in space, i.e. to labyrinthine lesions. To make this distinction we must

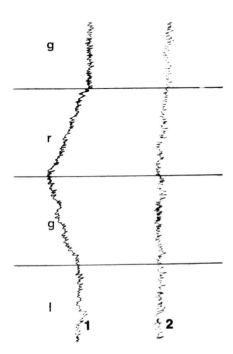

Figure 4.34 Cervicovertigogram (by courtesy of Berger): the patient holds the head in various positions, with eyes closed, and makes oscillatory movements with the outstretched arms; these movements are recorded by pencil on a moving strip of paper. (1) During head rotation to the right (r) there is deviation to the left; with the head straight (g) the arm returns to mid-position; and during head rotation to the left (l) there is no deviation. (2) After treatment of restricted rotation of the occiput/atlas to the right, there is no longer any deviation

change the position of the patient's head *and* trunk simultaneously (sitting up, lying down, turning from one side to the other) to determine which position causes vertigo. This type of vertigo is usually very intense but of short duration, so that it is enough to watch the patient's reaction. We should, however, insist on the patient keeping her eyes open while changing position; we can then observe spontaneous nystagmus, which usually lasts only a few seconds. (The patient will always tend to close her eyes in this type of vertigo.)

To determine the role of the vertebral artery in vertigo De Kleyn's tests are useful; here, too, it is the position of the head relative to the trunk that is decisive, i.e. neck position. If the head is bent back and rotated to one side, blood flow is impaired in the vertebral artery on the side *away from* which the head is turned. Hence, if the vertebral artery on the side *towards* which the head is turned is insufficient due to disease, symptoms will occur. The test is carried out with the patient supine, her head in retroflexion over the end of the table. Turning the head first to one side and then to the other, we examine nystagmus in end position and watch the patient for symptoms of dizziness, nausea, etc. This test is particularly conclusive if there is no movement restriction in the position that causes symptoms, thus ruling out blockage as their possible cause. For diagnostic purposes it may therefore be necessary to treat movement restriction (e.g. if left rotation in retroflexion is restricted and causes symptoms) and repeat the test after mobility has been restored. If the symptoms do not recur then they were due to the movement restriction; if they persist, then they are due to vertebral artery insufficiency (in this case, on the left).

Examination of disturbed muscle function

The great difficulty here is that there is no exact delimitation of what is to be considered normal, and diagnosis must be based almost exclusively on clinical examination. Polymyoelectrography using surface electrodes is so cumbersome that its use is very limited.

Clinical kinesiological examination should comprise:

1. Neurological screening.
2. Examination of muscle strength (muscle tests).
3. Examination of short muscles, fasciae, etc.
4. Examination of hypermobility.
5. Examination of posture standing and sitting.
6. Examination of simple movement.
7. Examination of gait with variations such as walking on tip-toe, on the heels, with arms raised, etc.

In the neurological examination those signs are of special interest that are characteristic of minimal brain dysfunction: marked asymmetry in particular of the face and the extremities, restlessness, clumsiness, etc.

Muscle testing was originally introduced to examine paresis of individual muscles or of muscle groups in such diseases as poliomyelitis. Essentially, muscle strength is examined in the course of simple co-ordinated movements which make it possible to examine only one specific muscle or muscle group. Standard conditions must be maintained, so that results are comparable. Results are graded as follows:

0. No muscle activity at all.
1. Muscle twitch without locomotor effect.
2. Movement with exclusion of gravity (i.e. only in the horizontal plane).
3. Movement against gravity but not against additional resistance.
4 and 5. The ability to perform movement against resistance: (4) against little resistance; (5) normal muscle activity.

Since in our patients true paresis is found only in root syndromes, changes are usually found between grades 4 and 5, although the abdominal muscles and deep neck flexors may exhibit grade 3. Thus the distinction between grades 4 and 5 is not fine enough for our purpose.

Without going into details about muscle testing, it is essential to stress the following principles: the *position* of the patient must be constant; *fixation,* because this determines which muscles the patient brings into play; *direction, speed* and *resistance* must be constant throughout the movement. Isometric examination can reveal the degree of force in the muscle but not important faults of co-ordination.

For the type of disturbance to be expected in our patients it is necessary to modify the original muscle test in some particulars; the most important techniques will be described here. In the section on disturbed movement patterns I have distinguished those muscles with a tendency to weaken ('predominantly phasic muscles') and those muscles with a tendency to hyperactivity (tautness – 'predominantly postural muscles') after Janda (1972).

Examination of muscles tending to weakness

Gluteus maximus (*Figure 4.35*)

Before performing the 'classic' muscle test we examine (hyper)extension of the hip, with the patient prone, in order to diagnose the pattern. Electromyography has established that the prime movers in hip extension are the hamstrings, followed almost immediately by the gluteus maximus and the erector spinae. It is advisable to palpate the hamstrings and gluteus with one hand and the two lumbar erectores spinae with the other. If the gluteus maximus is weak, contraction is retarded, weaker than on the healthy side, and may even be absent – yet the strength of hip extension need not be noticeably reduced. In very marked overactivity of the lumbar erector spinae with marked hypertonus, even with the patient prone, this muscle may contract first, before the hamstrings.

The muscle test proper is performed with the patient prone, her knee flexed so as to inhibit the hamstrings. Resistance is applied against the thigh, above the knee, throughout the movement. If we wish to facilitate the gluteus maximus to the greatest extent, we examine hyperextension of the hip with the leg in external rotation.

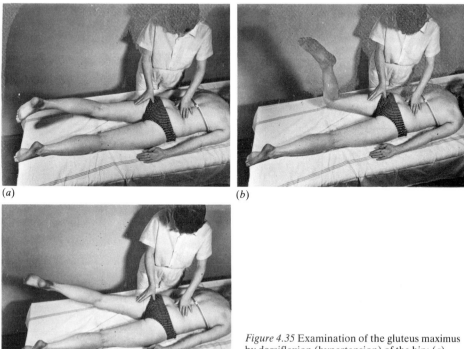

(a)

(b)

(c)

Figure 4.35 Examination of the gluteus maximus by dorsiflexion (hypertension) of the hip: (*a*) with the leg straight; (*b*) with the leg flexed; (*c*) with the leg in external rotation

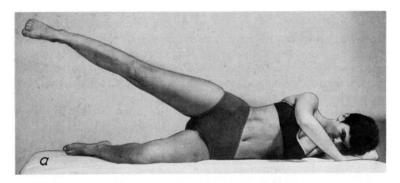

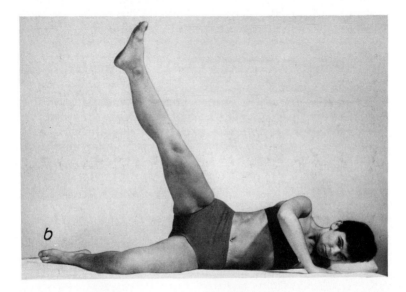

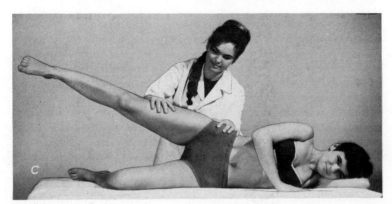

Figure 4.36 Examination of hip abduction with the patient on her side (gluteus medius and minimus): (*a*) pure abduction correctly carried out; (*b*) false abduction by substitution by the hip flexors, particularly by the tensor fasciae latae; (*c*) the 'classic' test for the abductors (the examiner palpating the tensor fasciae latae with the fingers and the gluteus medius with the thumb)

Gluteus medius (*Figure 4.36*)

We first examine spontaneous abduction of the hip with the patient lying on her side, the under leg slightly bent at the knee and hip. First we observe the patient to see whether she makes a true abduction, or a combined movement rotating the leg outwards while flexing the hip. True abduction employs both the tensor fasciae latae *and* the abductors (glutei medii and minimi); the combined movement is produced mainly by the tensor fasciae latae. It is therefore advisable to palpate the tensor fasciae latae with one finger and the gluteus medius with another, to see whether both contract during abduction. If there is outward rotation and hip flexion (incoordination) the gluteus medius is contracting too late, too little, or not at all. During the muscle test the requisite resistance is given against the lower third of the thigh from the side, and the pelvis is fixed in such a way that incoordination is prevented. Even then one should palpate the contraction of both the tensor fasciae latae and the gluteus medius.

Rectus abdominis

The usual test of the rectus abdominis is for the patient to sit up from the supine position, with flexed knees: to 'curl up', lifting first the head, then the shoulders, and then the rest of the trunk, with the operator fixing the feet and pelvis. For our purposes it is better if the patient flexes her legs and sits up unaided with arms stretched forward (*Figure 4.37*). This can *only* be done if the abdominal muscles are functioning well – if these muscles are very strong, the patient may be able to sit up with her hands held behind her head. Although bending the legs inhibits the hip flexors to some degree, sitting up is always the result of co-ordinated synergy of the abdominal muscles and the hip flexors. To examine the recti abdominis alone, the examiner puts his hands under the heels of the supine patient, telling her to press the heels downwards. She is then told to lift her head, shoulders and trunk, in

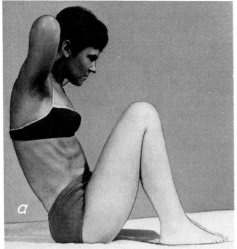
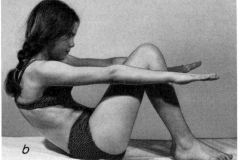

Figure 4.37 Examination of the rectus abdominis: the patient sits up with flexed knees, without fixation: (*a*) 'excellent'; (*b*) normal strength

succession; the moment the patient starts using the hip flexors, the pressure of her heels on the examiner's hands ceases. The stronger the abdominal muscles, the higher the patient can lift head and shoulders without relaxing the pressure of the heels.

Lower part of the trapezius (*Figure 4.38*)

To test this muscle the patient must be prone, with the arm on the tested side stretched forward; with one hand the examiner grasps the outstretched arm above the elbow, while the other grasps the inferior angle of the scapula, telling the patient to pull her arm and shoulder down; the examiner resists this movement with both hands, and if the lower trapezius is weak the resistance of the hand holding the inferior scapular angle is sufficient to prevent the scapula from moving down. For

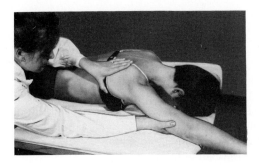

Figure 4.38 Examination of the lower part of the trapezius: the patient moves the shoulder-blade actively, in a caudal direction (against resistance)

our purposes, i.e. to diagnose incoordination, mere inspection is usually sufficient: we tell the prone patient to pull one shoulder down (in a caudal direction). If this movement is carried out correctly, the inferior scapular angle moves in a caudomedial direction (i.e. in the direction of the fibres of the lower trapezius muscle). If this muscle is weak, however, the inferior scapular angle moves medially like a hook and protrudes under the skin, not unlike an alar scapula. This is why the caudal movement, usually forceful, can be so easily prevented by the examiner's hand.

Serratus anterior

This muscle is tested with the patient on all fours; care must be taken to see that she puts her weight not on her knees but on her arms, and that the shoulders are abducted. The patient is watched to see whether an alar scapula appears. To make the test more difficult, the patient may be told to bend her elbows. Although this test concerns mainly the serratus anterior, it is also affected by a weak lower part of the trapezius.

Deep flexors of the neck (*Figure 4.39*)

To test these muscles the patient is supine and is told to pull her chin towards her chest in an arching movement. The examiner fixes the patient's chest with one hand while the other, on her forehead, resists flexion of the head and neck. This movement must be carefully distinguished from that of the patient pushing her

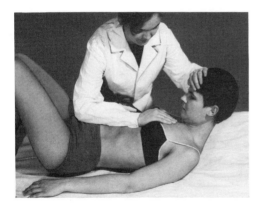

Figure 4.39 Examination of the deep neck flexors

head forward, which will usually happen if the deep flexors are weak (incoordination), bringing into play the sternocleidomastoids and even the scalenes. There is a useful quantitative test: we ask the patient to lie with her head raised as though intending to read (without lifting the thorax). Normally this position can be maintained for half a minute or even longer, but patients with weak deep neck flexors can only hold it for a few seconds.

Examination of short (tight) muscles

We have already seen which muscles tend to shorten – the 'predominantly postural muscles' of Janda (1972). In principle we observe how far a muscle can be stretched without the use of force; as this is done mainly by the same manoeuvres as post-isometric relaxation, only those techniques that differ will be described here.

Triceps surae (soleus)

If this muscle is shortened, dorsal flexion of the ankle joint is restricted. This can be tested by asking the patient to squat down: if the triceps surae (soleus) is normal, she should be able to place the whole foot on the floor, including the heel, but if the soleus is shortened, the heel will not touch the floor (*Figure 4.40*). If, however, it is only the gastrocnemius that is shortened, as is frequently the case, dorsiflexion of the ankle joint will be reduced if the knee is stretched and increased if she flexes the knee (*Figure 4.41*). For this reason it is a mistake to examine the mobility of the ankle joint with the knees extended.

Hamstrings

The hamstrings are tested the same way as in the straight leg raising test. The leg that is not being examined should be fixed to the table from above. The hamstrings are considered shortened if the stretched leg cannot be raised to an angle of 80 degrees from the horizontal. Unlike in the straight leg raising test for root syndromes, the patient feels only the stretch under the knee, but no real pain. This is the most frequent reason why a subject cannot touch the floor when bending forward with straight legs.

152

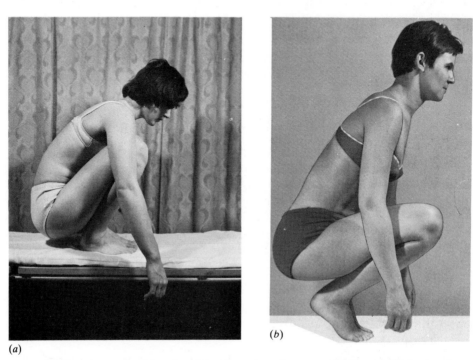

(a)

(b)

Figure 4.40 Screening test for shortening of the soleus: the patient squats. (*a*) Normal; (*b*) shortened (the heel does not touch the floor)

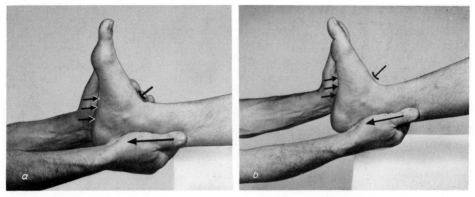

Figure 4.41 (*a*) Examination of dorsiflexion of the foot, with leg stretched; (*b*) with knee bent. Marked increase in dorsiflexion with the knee bent is characteristic of a short gastrocnemius

Hip flexors (*Figure 4.42*)

These comprise the iliopsoas, the rectus femoris and the tensor fasciae latae. They are examined in the position for Mennell's tests. The patient is supine with the buttock at the edge of the table, the leg of the examined side hanging over the edge. The patient grasps the flexed knee of the other leg and draws it towards her chest close enough to flatten lumbar lordosis. In this position it is possible to assess the relevant changes by inspection: if the iliopsoas is shortened the knee of the leg hanging over the edge of the table will be raised instead of being below or on the level of the patient's hip. If the rectus femoris is shortened, the knee will show too little flexion; if the tensor fasciae latae is shortened the leg will be slightly abducted and the patella deviated slightly outward.

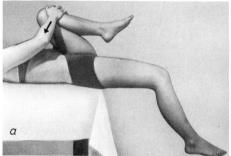

a

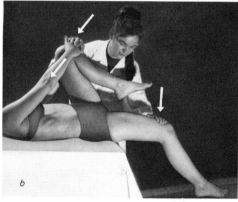

b

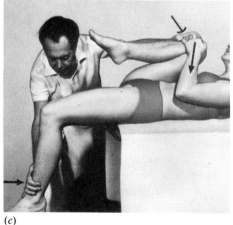

(c)

Figure 4.42 Examination of the hip flexors: the patient is supine with her buttocks at the end of the table; she pulls one bent knee to the abdomen, to flatten lumbar lordosis, while the leg to be tested hangs over the edge of the table. (*a*) The examiner notes whether the thigh is raised above the horizontal and whether there is extension of the knee; (*b*) pressure on the knee from above to test shortening of the iliopsoas; (*c*) bending the knee produces hip flexion if the rectus femoris is short

The examiner can now proceed to consider each muscle, with the patient in the same position. With one hand he reinforces the fixation of the knee (held in the patient's two hands) and then (1) exerts pressure on the other knee from above so as to determine the exact extent of shortening of the iliopsoas; (2) increases flexion of the knee of the free leg (over the edge of the table) or tells the patient to flex it actively. If the rectus femoris is short the knee will immediately rise above the horizontal; (3) the examiner will try to adduct the knee. If the tensor fasciae latae is shortened there is immediate resistance to adduction, and the iliotibial tract can be seen to form a groove on the lateral aspect of the thigh by tightening.

The (lumbar) erector spinae (*Figure 4.43*)

There is a simple test for orientation: the seated patient is told to draw her forehead to her knees. This is hindered by a shortened erector spinae, but there are many factors that may invalidate the test: if the patient has a short trunk and long thighs she will perform the movement easily even with a short erector spinae; conversely, if her trunk is long and thighs short, she will fail even with a normal erector spinae. I therefore prefer a modification of the test: the patient, seated, fixes her pelvis by placing the hands on the iliac crests, and simply humps her spine. If the lumbar part of the erector spinae is shortened, no lumbar kyphosis is obtained.

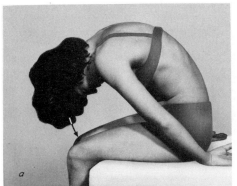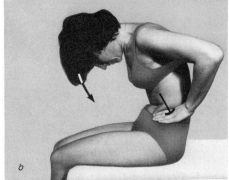

Figure 4.43 Examination of short erectores spinae, the patient sitting, with knees bent: (*a*) drawing the forehead to the knees; (*b*) humping her back while fixing the pelvis with her hands

Clinically no less important than a shortened erector spinae is hypertonus of this muscle, especially in the thoracolumbar region; it is most often found in patients with increased lumbar lordosis. It may be seen when the patient stands relaxed, and disappear on retroflexion (first degree); it may be found on retroflexion and disappear when the patient is prone (second degree); in the most severe cases it is found even when the patient is prone. These are the cases in which hip extension from the prone position is initiated by the erector spinae.

The quadratus lumborum (*Figure 4.44*)

The state of this muscle can be assessed while the patient bends sideways, but difference in leg length must of course be ruled out first. For exact assessment the patient lies on her side and lifts the upper part of her body by adducting the elbow and side-bending the trunk. Care must be taken to see that she does not lift her pelvis, which is best fixed from above by the examiner.

The technique of examination of the pectorales, upper trapezius and levator scapulae is identical with relaxation treatment, and will be described in the relevant chapter. At inspection a short pectoralis is shown by round or forward-drawn shoulders, while hypertonus of the upper part of the trapezius is revealed by the upward convex 'Gothic' shape of the shoulders (*Figure 4.45*). For rapid assessment

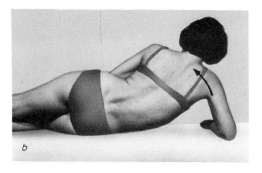

Figure 4.44 Examination of the quadratus lumborum: the patient lies on her side, lifting the upper part of her body by adducting the elbow (the pelvis must not be lifted and may be fixed by the examiner)

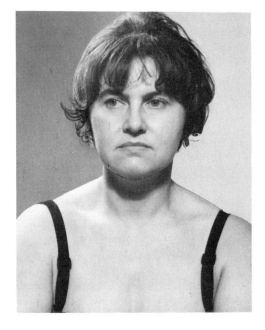

Figure 4.45 Typical appearance of a patient with hypertonus and hyperactivity of both upper trapezii, 'Gothic shoulders'

of both upper trapezii and the other neck extensors, the simplest test is to draw the patient's chin to her chest. If the neck extensors are short a gap of one or two (or even three) fingers' breadth remains. Short neck extensors are the most frequent cause of inability to bring the chin down on to the chest.

Examination of hypermobility (range of movement)

Not only weakness and tautness, but hypermobility, too, is mainly the consequence of muscular activity or is determined by the muscular system. The significance of hypermobility for pathogenesis has already been pointed out; here we are concerned only with examination and diagnosis.

To Sachse (1969) goes the credit for elaborating guidelines for the assessment of normal range of movement, and for attempting to determine the concepts of hypomobility, average mobility and hypermobility, all within the range of the normal. It is nevertheless important to bear in mind the great variability not only between individuals, but also according to age and sex. What may be considered hypermobile in an adult male may be perfectly normal in a female or an adolescent or child. With these limitations in mind, range A (in the diagrams) stands for hypomobile to normal, range B for slightly hypermobile and C for marked hypermobility. I shall give the criteria of Sachse with additional data from Kapandji (1974) and describe some examination techniques.

The spinal column

The total range of spinal mobility is given by Kapandji (1974), on the basis of X-ray examination, as 145 degrees for anteflexion, 135 degrees for retroflexion, 75 degrees for lateroflexion to one side, and 90–95 degrees for rotation to one side.

This is difficult to assess clinically; each of the principal sections of the spinal column must be examined separately.

LUMBAR SPINE

The average range of retroflexion is 35 degrees according to Kapandji (1974). Clinical examination shows a sharp bend either at the lumbosacral or at the thoracolumbar junction in cases of hypermobility. In order to determine the range within the normal, Sachse (1969) gives the following test: the patient lies prone with bent elbows pointing backwards and hands flat on the table by her shoulders. By extending her arms at the elbow she lifts the upper part of her body while the examiner fixes the pelvis from above; in this way the lumbar spine is forced into retroflexion. Range A is from up to 60 degrees at the elbow, range B between 60 and 90 degrees and range C above 90 degrees (*Figure 4.46*).

The average range of anteflexion is 60 degrees. Clinically this is tested by the patient bending to touch the floor, with knees and fingers stretched. Range A goes up to the point where the subject touches the floor with her fingertips, B from this performance to putting the knuckles on the floor, and C beyond this, the patient not only able to lay her hand flat on the floor, but sometimes even to bring the chest to the thighs (*Figure 4.47*). This most popular test, unfortunately, shows not only the degree of anteflexion of the trunk but also the extensibility of the hamstrings. For simple trunk anteflexion, therefore, it is better for the patient to sit and touch her knees with her forehead (*see Figure 4.43(a)*), range A covering the range of anteflexion up to where this is possible, and range B is where the patient can put her forehead between her knees.

The average range of lateral flexion is 20 degrees to each side; the clinical criterion according to Sachse (1969) is the shift of the axilla relative to the mid-line. In range A, the axilla of the convex side should come to rest above the intergluteal line; in B it should rest above the buttock of the other side, while in C the axilla shifts beyond the lateral aspect of the buttock of the other side (*Figure 4.48*). The range of axial rotation is given by Kapandji (1974) as 5 degrees but is not clinically tested. When testing stooping and side-bending the examiner must take into account the mobility of the hips and the proportions of the patient: there may be 'false' hypermobility due to a long trunk and short legs, or 'false' hypomobility due to long legs and a short trunk, while the length of the arms plays a role in stooping.

Because of its unfavourable consequences, however, the most important sign of lumbar hypermobility is hyperlordosis when standing relaxed and exaggerated lumbar kyphosis when sitting relaxed.

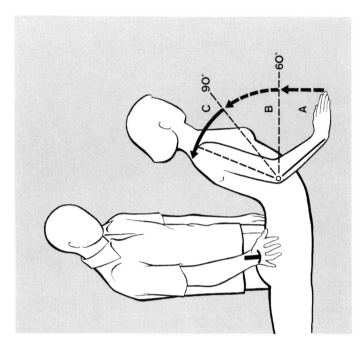

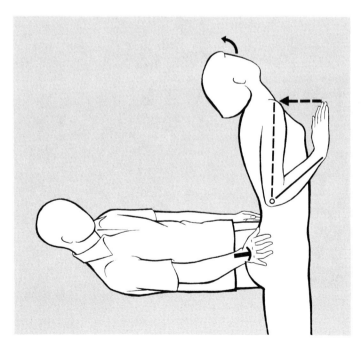

Figure 4.46 Testing the range of lumbar (trunk) retroflexion. Range (*a*) hypomobile to normal; (*b*) slight hypermobility; and (*c*) marked hypermobility (After Sachse, 1969.)

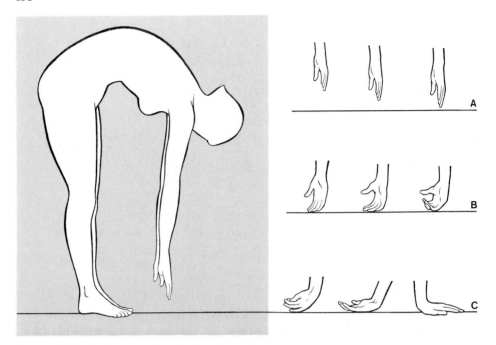

Figure 4.47 Testing the range of lumbar (trunk) anteflexion

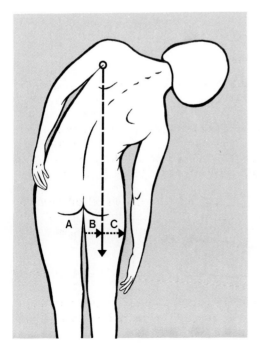

Figure 4.48 Testing the range of lumbar (trunk) lateral flexion

THORACIC SPINE

Trunk rotation is tested clinically. Kapandji (1974) gives 35 degrees to each side as the average. The patient sits astride the table, turning first to one side and then the other. According to Sachse (1969) range A is up to 50 degrees to each side, B from 50 to 70 degrees and C beyond 70 degrees (*Figure 4.49*).

Obviously the tests for stooping, retroflexion (extension) and side-bending show the mobility of the whole trunk, including the thoracic spine, but in clinical practice they are used (with the patient standing) for assessment of the lumbar spine.

Kapandji (1974) gives the range of movement for the thoracic spine as 45 degrees in anteflexion, 25 degrees in retroflexion and 20 degrees to each side in lateroflexion.

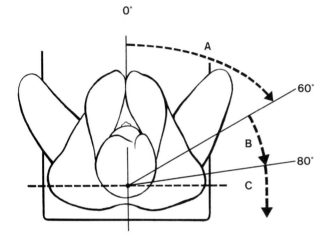

Figure 4.49 Testing the range of trunk rotation (thoracic spine)

CERVICAL SPINE

Here, too, it is mainly rotation that is clinically tested. According to Kapandji (1974) this is only 50 degrees to each side, while Sachse (1969) gives range A as up to 70 degrees to each side, B from 70 to 90 degrees and C over 90 degrees. Rotation is tested in the *erect* position by bringing the patient's chin above the shoulder. The discrepancy between the anatomical and the clinical data is due to the fact that rotation takes place in the erect position, and thus also involves the upper thoracic spine. On slight forward bending rotation stops at C7 and the range is reduced to about 50–60 degrees (*Figure 4.50*).

The range of anteflexion (Kapandji, 1974) is 40 degrees, that of retroflexion 75 degrees and of lateroflexion 35 degrees to each side. The range of mobility at the craniocervical junction has been given in the chapter on functional anatomy and X-ray examination.

Some extremity joints

Here again I give the figures as determined by Sachse (1969). The metacarpophalangeal joints: at passive dorsiflexion range A is up to 45 degrees, B between 45 and 60 degrees and C beyond 60 degrees (*Figure 4.51*).

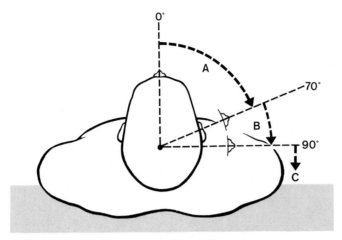

Figure 4.50 Testing the range of head (cervical) rotation

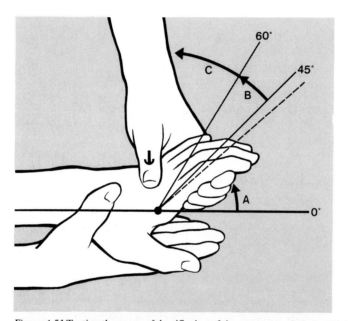

Figure 4.51 Testing the range of dorsiflexion of the metacarpophalangeal joints

Elbow joint: there is more valgosity in the hypermobile elbow, and the following test is therefore clinically valuable. The patient holds both arms before her chest, palms upwards, with her forearms held together from elbow to wrist; she is told to stretch her arms, keeping the elbows together. Range A mobility will enable the patient to keep the elbows touching up to an angle of 110 degrees, B to 110–135 degrees, while beyond this is range C (*Figure 4.52*).

Shoulder girdle: here the characteristic test is to bring the elbow towards the shoulder of the opposite side; range A mobility enables the patient to bring the elbow to mid-line, range B from there to a point halfway between the mid-line and

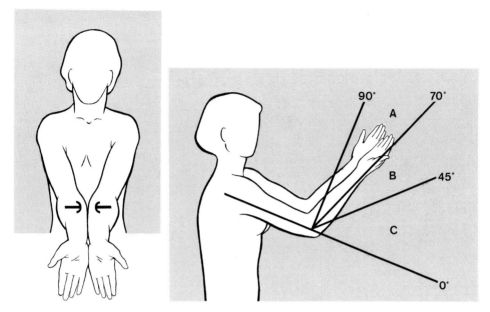

Figure 4.52 Testing the range of elbow extension, both elbows kept touching

the other shoulder, while in range C the elbow may touch the opposite shoulder (*Figure 4.53*). Another test is to try to make both hands meet behind the back, one from above and the other from below. With range A mobility the fingers may not touch, or may just come into contact; in range B the fingers may touch or overlap as far as to the first phalanx; in C the whole hand may overlap (*Figure 4.54*). In this test it is important not to allow for hyperlordosis.

If we intend to examine the scapulohumeral joint by itself, it is most convenient to test only pure abduction while one hand fixes the shoulder-blade with the clavicle, from above. Range A is up to 90 degrees, B from 90 to 110 degrees and C over 110 degrees (*Figure 4.55*).

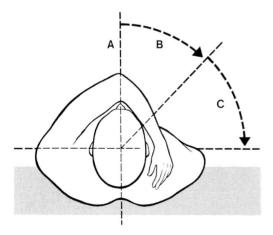

Figure 4.53 Bringing the elbow towards the shoulder of the opposite side

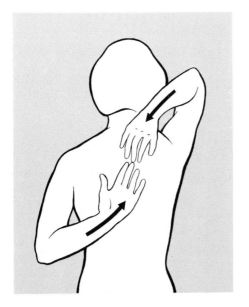

Figure 4.54 Making both hands meet behind the shoulder

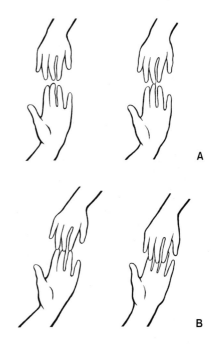

A

B

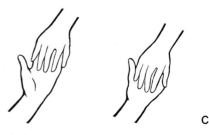

C

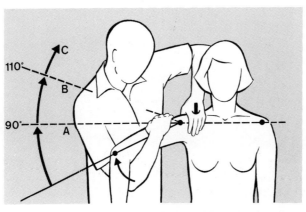

Figure 4.55 Testing the range of abduction of the scapulohumeral joint, with the shoulder-blade fixed from above

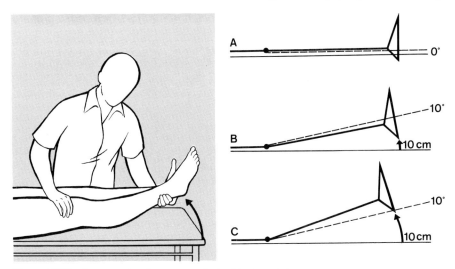

Figure 4.56 Testing extension (hyperextension) of the knee joint

The knee joint: here we test extension (or hyperextension), range A being up to full extension (180 degrees), range B up to 10 degrees hyperextension (190 degrees) and C beyond this figure (*Figure 4.56*).

The hip joint: here internal and external rotation are tested, range A being up to 90 degrees (external plus internal rotation), B between 90 and 120 degrees and C more than 120 degrees (*Figure 4.57*).

It is important to test the range of mobility in various regions of the body, because there may be hypermobility in one and average or even reduced mobility in another, without restriction of movement.

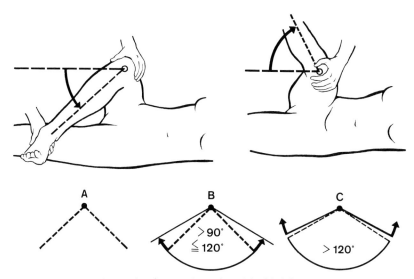

Figure 4.57 Testing internal *and* external rotation of the hip joint

Examination of co-ordinated movement (locomotor patterns)

The examination of individual muscles and the assessment of overall mobility are followed by the study of more complex movement patterns, or stereotypes. We begin with assessment of posture with the patient standing, as described at the beginning of this chapter (*see Figure 4.1,* page 106).

This is followed by examination in the sitting position, on an adjustable stool (*Figures 4.58* and *4.59*). The examiner notes the position of the feet and of the iliac crests, the course of the (lumbar) spine and the tonus of the abdominal and gluteal musculature. In correct posture, seated, the feet are flat on the floor, the thighs horizontal and the pelvis rotated (tilted) forward if possible; there should be slight lumbar lordosis (no kyphosis) and no flabbiness of the abdominal or gluteal muscles.

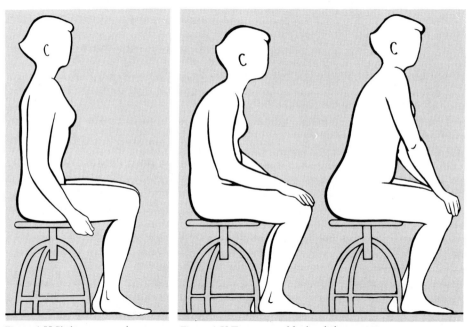

Figure 4.58 Sitting on a stool: correct posture

Figure 4.59 Two types of faulty sitting posture

Stooping and straightening up (*Figures 4.60* and *4.61*): for correct stooping one foot should be placed in front of the other and both knees should be slightly bent. The trunk bends forward, starting with the head, the body curling up from the head downwards as the gluteal and abdominal muscles contract. The erector spinae first contracts and then relaxes during maximum stooping. Conversely, at straightening up the knees stretch while the trunk uncurls, starting with the lumbar spine, followed by the thoracic spine, the neck and finally the head. This, too, is the result of co-ordinated contraction of the gluteal, abdominal and back musculature. The

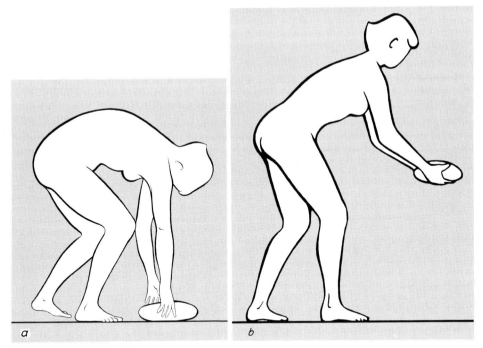

Figure 4.60 (*a*) Stooping and (*b*) lifting an object correctly

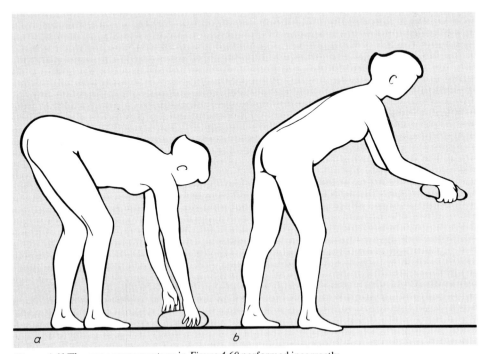

Figure 4.61 The same movements as in *Figure 4.60* performed incorrectly

trunk must never be lifted like a rod (lever!) nor must the abdomen be allowed to bulge.

Trunk rotation, sitting (*Figure 4.62*): this test is more closely concerned with the thoracic spine and shoulder girdle than were the previous tests. Again the pre-condition is correct sitting posture on a stool, with a test object (such as a book) in the hand resting on the lap. Special attention must be paid to relaxation of the arms and shoulders, which must not be drawn forward. The patient is now asked to place the book on a shelf behind her, at the level of her head; special attention must be paid to trunk rotation, the action of the back and abdominal muscles, fixation of the shoulder-blades and tension in the upper part of the trapezius.

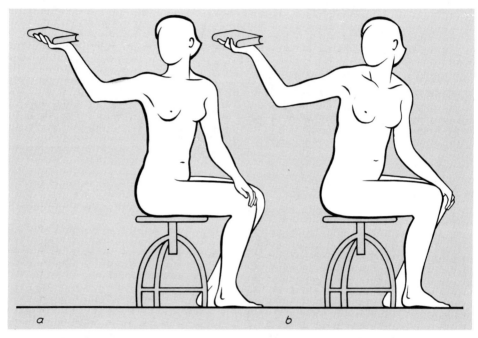

Figure 4.62 Trunk rotation, seated, holding an object in the hand: (*a*) correct; (*b*) faulty

If the test is performed properly we see harmonious rotation from the thoraco-lumbar junction upwards while the pelvis and legs remain in place; abdominal and back muscles are moderately active, the inferior angles of the scapula do not diverge and the neck musculature, in particular the upper part of the trapezius, remains relaxed.

Test movements for the head and neck (*Figure 4.63*): first we observe the head position with the patient standing and sitting; lordosis should not be too marked and if there is a flat thoracic spine the neck will also be straight. The angle between the mandible and neck should be about 90 degrees. During head turning the examiner observes neck rotation as well as muscular activity: the patient should be able to avoid lateroflexion, lordosis should not increase, the shoulders should not be lifted nor should one shoulder be drawn forward; the sternocleidomastoid should not be overstrained.

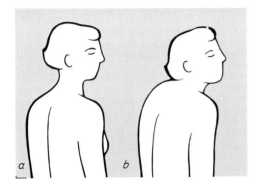

Figure 4.63 Head rotation, seated: (*a*) correct;
(*b*) faulty

Lifting the arms (*see Figure 6.123*, page 299): when lifting the arms the patient
also raises her shoulders, contracting the upper fixators of the shoulder girdle
(upper part of the trapezius and the levator scapulae), fixation of the shoulder-
blades from below (by the lower part of the trapezius) being insufficient.

Weight carrying (*Figure 4.64*): here the typical fault is a forward-drawn position
of the head and shoulders, causing tension in the upper fixators of the shoulder
girdle. If a weight is to be carried correctly the shoulders are behind the line of
gravity of the body and the head and neck remain erect.

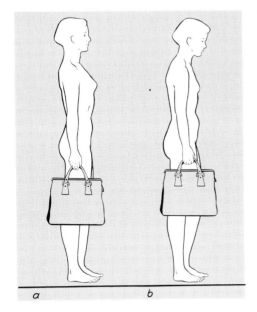

Figure 4.64 Carrying weights: (*a*) correct; (*b*)
faulty posture

Standing on one leg (*Figure 4.65*): special attention should be paid to the muscles
and joints of the supporting leg, the line of gravity of the body, the pelvis, in
particular the iliac crests, and the hip stabilizers, especially the gluteal musculature,
and the spinal curvature.

In correct posture on one leg, all joints of the supporting leg are in the line of
gravity; the centre of gravity, compared with stance on two legs, moves forward to
the second and third metacarpal head. The pelvis should remain horizontal and

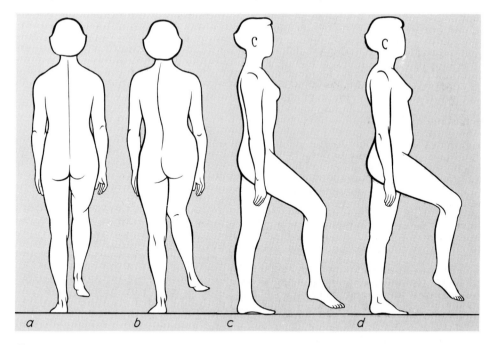

Figure 4.65 Standing on one leg, back view: (*a*) correct; (*b*) faulty. Side view: (*c*) correct; (*d*) faulty

spinal curvature should therefore be almost unchanged. The stabilizers of the hip, in particular the gluteus medius, should contract. Both flexors and extensors of the hip as well as the abdominal and back muscles, and the quadrati lumborum, should contract in a co-ordinated fashion to stabilize the hip and trunk. If the hip abductors are weak, the most frequent fault, the patient will lift the iliac crest of the side *opposite* to the supporting leg (Déjérine, 1901), bringing the centre of gravity above the supporting leg and thus relieving the abductors. (Trendelenburg's sign, the lowering of the iliac crest on the unsupported side, is rare; it is seen in severe cases of congenital hip luxation but not even in myopathy with extremely weak muscles.)

Walking: the examiner takes particular note of how the heels touch the ground, how weight is shifted from one leg to the other, how the pelvis moves with the spinal column, the position of the head and the movements of the arms.

In normal gait the steps are even and the weight is placed equally on each leg in turn. The pelvis should remain almost horizontal, but it does sway from side to side, more so in women than in men. The spinal column curves from one side to the other in a series of waves, the greatest excursion being in the mid-lumbar region; there is some counter-excursion in the thoracic spine, the thoracolumbar junction remaining above the sacrum. The head should move very little and the arms should swing symmetrically or slightly more pronouncedly on the left, the movement coming from the shoulder. The shoulder-blades are fixed from below, the upper fixators of the shoulder girdle relaxed. The centre of gravity of the body and that of the head should shift as little as possible, either from one side to the other or up and down, i.e. the patient should neither waddle nor rock.

Asymmetrical gait and stiffness can also be detected aurally, and the examiner must listen carefully. Certain faults become more marked if the patient closes her eyes, walks on tiptoe or on the heels; these should be examined as required.

Finally patients should be examined, if possible, in their typical working position (e.g. typing, lifting weights, reading, at a machine, etc.).

Examination of respiration

We have already seen in Chapter 2 that respiration is first examined at rest in the supine position and then with the patient seated or standing. In the supine position abdominal respiration should predominate. Under postural conditions the trunk broadens from the waist; the examiner therefore places his hands on the patient's lower ribs, from both sides. If breathing is correct, the hands are moved apart, but if the patient lifts her thorax as she breathes, the examiner's hands move upwards. If this faulty breathing pattern (with raised thorax) is very pronounced, the thorax may remain in the inspiration position even while at rest, the upper clavicular grooves are deep and the sternocleidomastoids, scalenes and upper fixators of the shoulder girdle are taut. During inspiration the collar bones are lifted, too. In less severe cases this fault is noticeable only when the patient takes a deep breath while sitting; but in more severe cases it can be seen even during breathing at rest and in the most severe cases it is evident even at rest in the supine position (*Figure 4.66*). Respiration can be so badly co-ordinated that a patient may draw the abdomen in during inspiration and push it out while breathing out.

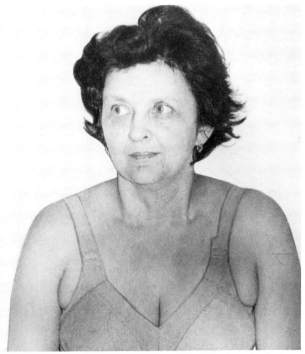

Figure 4.66 Lifting the thorax during inspiration: marked tension in the sternocleidomastoidei, scaleni and the upper part of the trapezii; very deep supraclavicular fossae on both sides

Inspiration and expiration should be about the same duration; the patient should be able to breathe in for 7–10 s or longer, breathing out for the same length of time (except for professional singers, who breathe out for much longer). There are, however, patients who cannot breathe in (or out) for more than 4 s, although they suffer from no respiratory disease! Both inspiration and expiration are audible; the nostrils expand during the former and narrow during the latter. It is important that the facial musculature should be relaxed, particularly the lips, the muscles of the jaw and the tongue.

The examiner should watch carefully for asymmetry, particularly in a patient who lifts her shoulders during inspiration.

In the prone position the respiratory wave of the thoracic spine should be observed during deep breathing. The absence of a wave, and no restriction of the thoracic spine, implies a faulty breathing pattern.

Syndromes

The lower crossed syndrome (after Janda, 1979)

There is imbalance in the following pairs of muscles: (1) weak glutei maximi and short hip flexors; (2) weak abdominals (recti abdominis) and short lumbar erectores spinae; (3) weak glutei medii and short tensors of the fasciae latae and quadrati lumborum.

There is not only antagonism but also 'competition' or substitution: for weak glutei medii by the tensors and quadrati lumborum, for weak abdominals by the

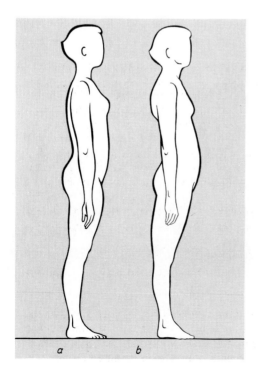

Figure 4.67 (*a*) Increased pelvic tilt and (*b*) lumbar hyperlordosis

iliopsoas in hip flexion, for weak glutei maximi by the erector spinae (and the hamstrings). Obviously, in this syndrome the correct mechanism of curling up in sitting up from the supine position and in stooping is interfered with; the result is increased forward tilt of the pelvis as well as increased lumbar lordosis (*Figure 4.67*). The hamstrings are usually short in this syndrome, but this is frequently a compensatory mechanism that lessens pelvic tilt.

The upper crossed syndrome

There is imbalance in the following muscle groups:

1. Between the upper and lower fixators of the shoulder girdle (i.e. the upper trapezius, levator scapulae and frequently the scalenes on the one hand, and the lower trapezius and the serratus anterior on the other).
2. Between the pectorales and the interscapular muscles.
3. Between the deep neck flexors (longus cervicis, longus capitis and omo- and thyrohyoideus) on the one hand, and the neck extensors (cervical section of the erector spinae and upper part of the trapezius) on the other.

In addition there may be shortening of the uppermost part of the ligamentum nuchae with fixed lordosis in the upper cervical region.

Obviously, if the lower fixators of the shoulder girdle are weak, the upper fixators must become hyperactive and tense. Hyperactivity of the pectorales produces round shoulders, forward-drawn shoulders, neck and head; weak deep neck flexors with short extensors produce hyperlordosis of the upper cervical spine. In addition to the relevant movement patterns, the respiration stereotype is also usually affected.

Stratification syndrome

In this syndrome strata of hypertrophic and weak muscle groups alternate: in a caudocranial direction there are hypertrophic ischiocrural muscle groups, hypo-trophic weak gluteals and under-developed lumbar erectores spinae, and above these the bulging hypertrophic thoracolumbar section of the erectores spinae; these are followed by flabby interscapular muscles with hypertrophic taut upper fixators of the shoulder girdle above them.

On the ventral aspect the lower section of the recti abdominis bulges, but more laterally there is a groove corresponding to the taut oblique abdominal muscles; lateral from this the abdominal wall may bulge again in the region of the waist ('pseudohernia').

This syndrome implies imbalance in the stratum of hypermobility (laxity) that alternates with strata of increased tension, hypermobility being most pronounced in the low back region.

Testing

Clinical examination provides a wealth of data concerning the functioning of the locomotor system and reflex changes in the tissues. This enables us not only to establish diagnosis, but to compare *before* and *after* therapy using the techniques to be described below, which produce an immediate reflex effect. Immediate testing, i.e. comparison of the state before and after treatment, thus constitutes a feedback which enables us to assess not only treatment but diagnosis on the spot, an aspect that is indispensable for the critical therapist. This becomes clear if we compare our procedure with that of the pharmacotherapist, whose clinical results are always difficult to assess in view of the ever-changing and frequently unpredictable course of the disease. It is all the more important, therefore, that we can see immediately clear effects, or complete failures. However, a positive test is *not* tantamount to therapeutic success, because if we have treated an irrelevant lesion the effect may be but short lived. If the immediate effect is incomplete, this leads us to look carefully for yet another lesion.

In principle, every deviation from the norm found at clinical examination can be made the object of testing; obviously the most rewarding are findings that can be measured: range of movement of joints, parts or mobile sections of the spinal column, and the straight leg raising test. However, improvement in the straight leg raising test should be considered reliable only if there is a marked difference in performance before and after treatment (20 degrees or more) and if the test has become much less painful. Side deviation in Hautant's test is also significant, as is asymmetrical distribution of weight on two scales before and after treatment. Systematic testing can easily show that even slightly paretic muscles in radicular syndromes acquire strength immediately after successful manipulation or even after traction, and that even the tendon reflex may improve.

It is also possible to test reflex changes: muscle spasm, trigger points, hyperalgesic zones, the skin fold or skin stretching may all be influenced immediately by manipulation, local anaesthesia or needling, or simply by skin stretching or post-isometric muscle relaxation. Instrumental methods such as the measurement of skin temperature, conductivity, plethysmography etc. may also show reflex changes affected by any type of therapy.

Although one should not rely solely on subjective assessment, it is of course most significant if the patient herself (as is frequently the case) feels and appreciates immediate relief after the appropriate treatment. It is in fact good policy to let the patient herself palpate pain points and trigger points before and after treatment, so as to assess the effect herself. If the therapist palpates after treatment, the patient sometimes doubts whether the same amount of force has been applied as before treatment, since she feels less.

In addition to its diagnostic value, testing is useful for indication of further therapy; e.g. if traction has brought relief, further traction treatment is probably indicated.

The course of examination with special regard to chain-reaction patterns

There is an important question: what should the case sheet of a patient with disturbed function of the locomotor system look like? A 'manipulative case sheet'?

Once the examination techniques are known the question of how to obtain useful results in practice and avoid errors as far as is humanly possible must be addressed.

The answer is not simple, since the object of examination, disturbed function of the locomotor system and its reflex changes, concerns many different fields of medicine. Some patients present themselves with problems belonging to the field of general medicine, others with neurological, rheumatological, orthopaedic, gynaecological, otiatric and other symptoms; in some cases the trouble lies in disturbed joint mobility, in others in disturbed muscle function, while in other cases pain with its specific reflex reactions dominates. To examine each patient from all of these aspects would demand far more time than the clinician has at his disposal.

We must therefore approach each case from the point of view of the patient's complaint, and proceed from one finding to the next. Experience has shown that the findings follow certain patterns (chains) so that if we find (a) we expect (b) and must then look for (c).

If the patient is absolutely unknown to the examiner, he must first look at gait and posture, see how the musculature is developed, make screening tests of cervical, thoracic and lumbar mobility, palpate the pelvis with the patient standing, examine Patrick's sign and adduction of the flexed thigh with the patient supine, and examine rotation of the foot.

Since, however, the patient can be expected to provide information about his complaints, we may proceed accordingly. For instance, if a patient comes with headache troubles (and negative neurological findings) we must thoroughly examine mobility of the craniocervical junction and the typical pain points on the posterior arch of the atlas and the lateral aspect of the spinous process of C2. If the head is held in the forward-drawn position, we look for a stiff thoracic kyphosis, for taut pectoralis muscles, for hypertonus of the upper trapezius and levator scapulae and for weak lower parts of the trapezius. If the patient adopts this forward-drawn position when seated, we look for increased lumbar kyphosis in the sitting position. We should never fail to note a raised thorax during respiration, and consequently examine the scalenus muscles. If there is restriction in the craniocervical junction we examine the upper ribs, the temporomandibular joint and masticatory muscles.

In shoulder pain or a painful upper arm we pay attention not only to the whole cervical spine including the craniocervical junction, but also to the cervicothoracic junction, the upper ribs and the humeroscapular joint; we have to expect a painful arc during abduction, examine joint play with the arm horizontal and examine the clavicular joints. Painful muscle insertions should be sought; we must palpate the epicondyles and examine joint play of the carpal bones. Here, too, disturbance of muscle function in the region of the shoulder girdle is important, and again a forward-drawn position of the shoulders, in view of pain during weight carrying.

Even for low-back pain we must give a screening examination to the upper cervical spine and then examine the position of the pelvis and some characteristic muscles (psoas, iliacus, erector trunci, piriformis, rectus femoris); we must perform the springing test with the patient prone, and lying on her side; we must examine the sacroiliac joints and the coccyx. If stooping is restricted on standing, we examine anteflexion sitting and then perform the straight leg raising test. Then we look for typical pain points and test the ligaments. If posture is affected, the muscles that govern pelvic inclination should be systematically tested, and if low-back pain is provoked by weight lifting, the patient's stooping stereotype should be examined.

These examples may suffice. I will now point out typical chain reactions making orientation easier. These chains or patterns correspond to basic functions of the locomotor system and their disturbance.

1. Gait concerning mainly the lower extremity with (a) a supporting phase (extension) and (b) a swinging phase (flexion).

(a) Impaired extension: increased tension in foot and toe extensors, all hip flexors and adductors with tender attachment points, overstrain of knee and hip joints, inhibition of the glutei, lesion of the sacroiliac joint, thoracolumbar junction and L3/4.

(b) Impaired flexion: increased tension in foot flexors and blockage of the articulations, painful calcaneal spur, tension in triceps surae with painful Achilles tendon, a blocked fibular head and sacroiliac joint, tension in gluteus maximus and levator ani with a painful coccyx, and in the gluteus medius with a painful trochanter major; blockage of segments L4/5 and L5/S1.

2. (a) Body statics (upright posture) and (b) respiration, concerning trunk and neck (spinal column).

(a) (i) There is increased tension in the following muscle pairs with the corresponding attachment points: sternocleidomastoid and short extensors of the craniocervical junction; of the scaleni and deep neck flexors on the one and the trapezius and levator scapulae on the other hand; the pectoralis and the interscapular muscles; the iliopsoas and the recti abdominis on the one and the erector trunci and the quadrati on the other hand.

(ii) Most important blockages: in all key regions, i.e. the craniocervical junction, the cervico-thoracic junction, the thoracolumbar junction and the lumbo-sacro-iliac junction; there is frequently a stiff thoracic kyphosis.

(b) (i) There is increased tension in the scaleni, the upper shoulder girdle fixators, the sternocleidomastoids, the short extensors of the craniocervical junction and the pectorales with the corresponding tender attachment points.

(ii) There is blockage at the craniocervical junction, the cervicothoracic junction, the upper ribs and the midthoracic spine.

3. Prehension concerning mainly the upper extremity having two phases: (a) extension and (b) flexion.

(a) Impaired extension: tension in finger and wrist extensors, supinators, the biceps with pain at the lateral epicondyle and styloid process with blockage at the elbow; tension in the infraspinatus, deltoideus, upper shoulder girdle fixators with blockage of the mid-cervical spine.

(b) Impaired flexion: blockage of carpal bones (carpa tunnel syndrome), tension of finger and wrist flexors, of the pronator with pain at the medial epicondyle, tension in subscapularis, pectoralis, latissimus with lesion of the glenohumeral joint, tension in the scaleni, the sternocleidomastoids with lesion of the 1st rib and cervicothoracic junction (thoracic outlet syndrome), and craniocervical junction.

4. (a) Keeping the visual field constant – viz under (2).

(b) Food intake, respiration and speech, concerning head and neck. Disturbance causes tension in the masticatory muscles with pain at the temporomandibular joint, tension of the digastricus with pain points at the hyoid, movement restriction of the craniocervical junction with tension in the short extensors and the sternocleidomastoid, increased tension of the scaleni and pectorales with typical pain points and lesion of the cervicothoracic junction and upper ribs.

There is marked tendency to one-sidedness in all chain reactions. Visceral pain usually causes flexion (impaired extension).

Note: By treating one link of a chain, we usually obtain relief of other affected parts.

Problems of differential diagnosis

There are two main categories: the first concerns headache, visceral pain etc., which may be due either to disturbed function of the vertebral column or to some other lesion of the locomotor system such as muscle spasm, or to visceral disease. This category covers the whole field of medicine, and the problem will frequently have to be solved with the collaboration of specialists in the relevant branches of medicine.

The second category concerns lesions in the locomotor system which may be due either to disturbed function or (mainly or partly) to structural changes (pathology). This involves differential diagnosis in the locomotor system itself, i.e. the main object of our therapy; errors in differential diagnosis in this category are most unfortunate and lie entirely within our responsibility.

In general terms, the pitfalls are inflammatory, metabolic or neoplastic diseases. Some screening tests should be performed as a routine procedure (erythrocyte sedimentation rate, uric acid level and X-ray pictures). However, particularly in the initial stage of the disease, it is usually impossible to recognize the true nature of the condition, and such patients may be just as well treated with reflex (physical) therapy, including manipulation, as with analgesics. The great advantage of the up-to-date techniques described in this book is that they cannot harm the patient.

If it is impossible to recognize pathology in the initial stages, the course of the disease should give sufficient warning; the most important signs are repeated relapses, the decreasing effect of all therapeutic measures and progressive deterioration. There is one important warning note to sound: however desirable it is to test immediately after treatment, a positive result, i.e. immediate improvement of objective findings, and subjective relief, *do not preclude* pathology, including tumours, because of concomitant blockage and other reflex changes that are susceptible to adequate therapy.

I will now list some typical pitfalls and suggest how they may be avoided. If relapses occur regularly at the same segment of the spine, despite preventive measures (including remedial exercise), the principal cause will be visceral disease affecting that segment, tumour, or some other pathology of corresponding localization. When sacroiliac blockage recurs in young patients we must consider the possibility of ankylosing spondylitis. In women after the climacteric, on the other hand, osteoporosis must be borne in mind.

Differential diagnosis is particularly difficult but important in the acute stage after injury. There are cases in which we can achieve immediate relief, but it is essential to rule out major trauma such as fracture, luxation, torn ligaments or muscles and muscle sheaths, and haematoma.

Abnormal function may be due to anomaly, in which case direct treatment is useless and futile – another reason why X-ray examination is desirable. Once the anomaly is recognized we must try to attain compensation or substitution of impaired function.

The most frequent diagnosis requiring differentiation is that of disc prolapse, with or without pathology. This problem will be dealt with in Chapter 7.

Since the most prominent symptom in our patients is pain, it is important to differentiate between physical, psychological and partly psychological pain. There is an unfortunate tendency in the medical profession – though an understandable one – to dismiss pain as psychological if no physical signs are present. However, since most doctors are not familiar with the examination of disturbed locomotor function and its reflex changes, it is my belief that they simply fail to recognize the most frequent cause of pain. If the patient is able to give a fairly precise description and localization of his pain, I feel one should be reluctant on that account to regard it as merely psychological. As we have already seen, in doubtful cases the physical and psychological components will be distinguished during the treatment, when repeated comparison of (changing) physical signs and the patient's own assessment of them will provide objective criteria.

There is a special problem, however, in cases of masked depression, which frequently take the outward form of vertebrogenic pain and may even cause lesions by exaggerated muscle tension and a cramped posture in particular in the cervical region, with headache as the principal complaint; low-back pain is also frequently presented.

The diagnosis cannot be established at the first examination, but here again, the course of treatment should alert the therapist to the possibility that there is something more than pain due to disturbed locomotor function. Once we take into consideration the possible existence of masked depression, we should enquire into any history of depression in the family and the patient's own past. The most important symptom is *disturbed sleep*: characteristically, the patient falls asleep normally but wakes within a few hours and cannot go back to sleep. Here the decisive criterion is the effect of anti-depressive drugs; if the underlying cause of the 'vertebrogenic' pain is masked depression, the symptoms will clear up.

A brief warning must be given here: *subarachnoid haemorrhage* and acute wry neck in a labile patient may be difficult to distinguish. In some cases of acute wry neck with nausea, vomiting, and a panic reaction, and when there is pain at head anteflexion – all symptoms provoked by the autonomic nervous system – lumbar puncture is mandatory. Conversely, the principal symptom in subarachnoid haemorrhage may be acute neck pain, and the main sign on examination may be restricted anteflexion of the head.

Another warning must be issued, concerning intracranial tumours particularly of the posterior fossa, with occipital headache and a forced head position which can easily be mistaken for wry neck.

Muscular pain as a constant symptom of disturbed function of the locomotor system must be distinguished from myosotis, particularly from a myosotis that is not yet severe; this is a difficult problem. The changing site of the pain, and the fatigue, suggest psychological pain. Laboratory findings are often ambiguous. The most significant feature is that only those muscles that show changed muscular tonus are tender, especially when painful *hypotonus* is present.

To conclude this chapter on differential diagnosis, and diagnosis altogether, I must stress that diagnosis of disturbed function of the locomotor system is a new field of clinical medicine, and as such is still a difficult one. Any pathological lesion is first made manifest by disturbed function. Moreover, patients referred for pain due to 'mere' disturbed function are mostly out-patients who cannot be examined as thoroughly as those in a hospital ward. The physician in charge of such cases must always be aware of the innumerable pitfalls around him; no danger is greater than that of over-assurance. This chapter on differential diagnosis cannot be more than a warning.

5

Indications for treatment

Indications for treatment should be the result not only of clinical diagnosis but also of pathogenic analysis, determining which lesion is most important at a given moment and is therefore likely to be the most effective object of therapy. Every measure we take should thus result from a fresh examination, to keep up to date with the course of the patient's condition. For if our therapy is determined by the principles set out here, it is *effective* and at control examination the condition of the patient should have changed, implying a change in further treatment. If the patient's condition is unchanged, treatment was not adequate and should not be repeated. A series of repetitive therapeutic measures of the same type is more often than not out of place. Critical assessment of the preceding treatment and constant correction of planned therapeutic measures are essential.

Methods of treatment

1. Manipulation.
2. Traction.
3. Reflex therapy:
    (a) massage;
    (b) post-isometric relaxation;
    (c) skin stretching;
    (d) anaesthesia – needling;
    (e) electrical stimulation;
    (f) acupuncture;
    (g) treatment of scars.
4. Remedial exercise.
5. Correction of faulty statics.
6. Immobilization (supports).
7. Pharmacotherapy.
8. Surgery.
9. Regimen.

Manipulation

Manipulative treatment is indicated if there is movement restriction (blockage) of a joint or a spinal mobile segment, and if this is considered *relevant* to the patient's symptoms. As stated in Chapter 1, no specific disease or complaint need be indicated for manipulation (headache, lumbago, etc.) but only a pathogenic lesion (i.e. blockage), which should, however, be relevant to the patient's problem.

Bearing this in mind, many of the questions frequently asked can be answered easily: what about spondylosis, disc prolapse, scoliosis, juvenile osteochondrosis, spondylolisthesis, osteoporosis, or ankylosing spondylitis? The answer is straightforward: these conditions do not form the objective for manipulative treatment. Nevertheless, if in such conditions movement restriction (blockage) is found and considered harmful, then it should be treated with *adequate* manipulative techniques.

To give some examples: as the pathogenic importance of spondylosis is questionable, if movement restriction is the main disturbance of function the patient's symptoms will probably resolve after manipulation. In disc prolapse concomitant blockage may cause the patient's condition to deteriorate considerably, so that after treatment of the blockage the clinical condition may be greatly improved. To what extent this will happen cannot be easily foretold, but it is *always* worth trying provided we use the right technique. Scoliosis is certainly not an objective for manipulation, since in itself the condition does not usually cause pain. If a patient with scoliosis feels pain, and blockage is present, it is probably the cause of that pain and should be treated. Manipulation is indicated if blockage interferes with remedial exercise. In both juvenile osteochondrosis and osteoporosis stiffness (immobility) is harmful, and normal mobility improves trophicity. Adequate gentle mobilization techniques are therefore indicated to restore mobility. Spondylolisthesis (and many other anomalies such as basilar impression) cannot be influenced by manipulation, but in their final stages are more often than not symptom free. Blockage can be and frequently is the true cause of symptoms. In ankylosing spondylitis movement therapy is indicated, and mobilization techniques are most appropriate – they have to be applied, however, to those segments that *still* show some degree of mobility.

The reason for these somewhat sweeping statements is that the basic techniques described in this book are very gentle and also very effective for mobilization, using muscular facilitation and inhibition, i.e. the inherent forces of the patient. It is most unfortunate that in the minds of most people, physicians and laymen alike, manipulation is tantamount to thrusting techniques – techniques that should rather be the exception.

It cannot be overemphasized that if movement restriction is severe, if there is much pain and muscle spasm, if several segments or an entire section of the spinal column is affected, then thrusting techniques are ruled out, for they are not only too violent, but more often than not ineffective as well, whereas mobilization techniques capable of dealing with muscle spasm overcome movement restriction gently. With a few exceptions we never begin treatment with a thrusting manoeuvre, and if manipulative treatment is required frequently, thrusting techniques would be definitely harmful.

After this eulogy of gentle mobilization let us turn to the real role of thrusting techniques. The most important occasion for their use is when after mobilization the experienced therapist has the impression that restriction has not entirely been overcome in (preferably) a single segment, because there is still some resistance to be felt, or a pain spot remains tender (this tenderness usually disappears when restriction has been removed). This remaining symptom is then treated by a high-velocity thrust, the segment or joint being well prepared for this manoeuvre by the preceding mobilization. The thrust should succeed with the minimum of force, and if it does not the therapist should desist. It is as if he asks the structure he is manipulating whether it is ready to accept a thrust or not; if it is ready, it will 'click' or 'pop' with the greatest ease, but if this does not happen the manipulator should desist and go back to gentle mobilization again. Another situation in which a thrust is useful is that of very slight and painless blockage, with minimum muscular spasm, which is nevertheless thought to be clinically relevant because, for example, it is in a key region. A thrust is by far the quickest way of dealing with this. It can be seen from *Figure 4.2* (page 108) what slight force is applied in an expertly performed high-velocity thrust.

In this connection it is worth quoting Stoddard's (1961) system of recording degrees of joint mobility (*Figure 5.1*).

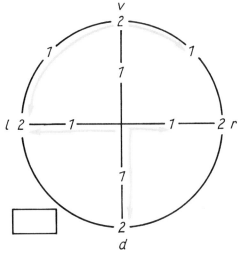

Figure 5.1 The degree of blockage: here the segment C7–T1 is blocked at rotation and side-bending to the right (primary block) and at side-bending to the left and back bending (secondary block). By drawing in an arrow extending beyond the circle it is possible to indicate hypermobility (After Stoddard, 1961.)

0 = No mobility – ankylosis; not suitable for manipulative treatment.
1 = Severe restriction; only mobilization techniques to be applied.
2 = Slight restriction; both mobilization and thrust techniques can be used.
3 = Normal mobility; best left alone, but if there is movement restriction in some directions while in others the joint is free, treatment in a free direction can be useful (Maigne, 1968), and is usually very gentle, the 'indirect method' of the American osteopaths.
4 = Hypermobility; all types of manipulative treatment, particularly thrust techniques, should be avoided.

From the technical point of view we distinguish between techniques which produce relative shift of articular facets and those which produce distraction (gapping). As a rule the latter are the most effective.

Contraindications

This problem is given much space in the medical literature, but in my opinion it is rather a pseudoproblem. With up-to-date techniques no harm should ever ensue from manipulation, and in fact the problem boils down to the need to avoid technical mistakes. To put it briefly, what is contraindicated is faulty technique.

What are the crucial faults? These are (1) the predominant use of thrust techniques; (2) applying a high-velocity thrust before the patient is properly relaxed and before taking up the slack (*see* Chapter 6); (3) trying to force manipulation of any type against painful muscle spasm or in a direction that causes pain; (4) thrust techniques should be avoided in cervical back-bending and rotation, because of possible impingement on the vertebral artery.

In this connection I must also stress that too insistent *examination* of mobility in a painful direction can be positively harmful, and at the craniocervical junction even dangerous.

The discussion of contraindications derives from the fact that serious complications have been described in the literature, even with a fatal outcome (Grossiord, 1966; Lorenz and Vogelsang, 1972; Krueger and Dazaki, 1980), the Memorandum of the German Association of Manual Medicine, 1979, and most recently Dvořák and Orelli, 1982). Basing their calculations on the results of a questionnaire sent to doctors of the Swiss Association of Manual Medicine, the last two authors compute the number of serious complications after manipulation (thrust techniques) at 1:400 000. By far the most important cause of serious complication is undoubtedly damage to the vertebral artery.

Unfortunately it is an almost constant feature of this literature that the technique responsible for the damage is not described – as if postoperative complications were described with no details of the operation technique used. There is one example quoted by Dvořák and Orelli (1982), however, which seems to me so characteristic that I shall comment on it here:

> A female patient of 35 collapsed while attending a funeral, and had suffered from wry neck for 3 weeks afterwards. 'She was manipulated three times within 1 week by a qualified chiropractor (the patient was supine and the manipulation consisted in rotation, reclination and extension of the head)'. This was followed by a short period of unconsciousness and later by tetraplegia; artificial respiration had to be applied and maintained for 36 hours. Recovery took several weeks and was complete 4 months later.

Thrust techniques in acute wry neck (torticollis) are questionable in themselves, but to use the dangerous combination of 'rotation, reclination and extension' is courting disaster (*see* De Kleijn's test, pages 145–146).

From this description of a possibly dangerous 'technical mistake' something like a contraindication can be deduced: if it is a mistake to perform manipulation in a painful direction, then manipulative therapy must be discarded altogether if we produce pain in *all* directions. In fact, in mere disturbance of function (i.e. the objective of manipulative therapy) pain is never found in all directions at once; distraction as a rule brings relief, and therefore pain in all directions at once is usually a sign of pathology and manipulation is out of place.

For obvious reasons manipulation of hypermobility is undesirable, but not manipulation of a blocked segment in an otherwise hypermobile patient.

This brings us to another category of 'contraindications' which is often strongly emphasized: tumours, in particular those with destructive changes; acute inflammatory conditions (such as tuberculosis); fracture, etc. It is clear that no one in his senses would try to treat this type of pathology by manipulation; on the other hand, we know that particularly in the initial stages of such conditions diagnostic error is often unavoidable. The specialist sees such patients in hospital, at a later stage, when the diagnosis is already easier. Yet, using adequate gentle techniques, the patient should come to no more harm than from the administration of analgesics – and suffer fewer side-effects. To make the point even clearer: if in a case of diagnosed pathology concomitant blockage is considered harmful to the patient's condition (as it frequently is), there is no reason why this blockage should not be treated if we know how. I have myself given manipulation in acute decompensation of (benign) posterior fossa tumour, with excellent temporary results. Blockage at the craniocervical junction can cause great deterioration in patients with insufficiency of the vertebral artery, and should be treated by expert manipulation. It is most unfortunate that this condition is considered by many to offer a contraindication, simply because technical errors in this situation are particularly disastrous.

The course of manipulative treatment

In a routine case which is neither very severe nor very acute we treat those restrictions of movement which we think clinically important, in particular those in key regions, even if painless (i.e. clinically latent). After treatment the patient is told she may expect some unpleasant reaction at the end of the day, or during the next day or two, and if possible is advised about what to correct (or avoid) in her daily regimen. About 2 weeks is a reasonable interval for control examination, the organism having had time to react and to adapt itself to restored mobility.

In a way the control examination is almost more important than the first examination; our diagnostic conclusions on first examination might be called a working hypothesis (except for very simple cases), a hypothesis on which we base the first therapeutic steps; it is at the second examination that we try to draw conclusions and decide on a plan of treatment.

If the patient feels clearly improved it is likely that the conclusions reached at first examination were well founded, and we proceed to treat what remains to be cleared up. We may invite the patient for re-examination after 3 or 4 weeks, and if all goes well, again after 6 weeks. However, even if improvement is steady, we should follow up the patient for several months, in view of the typical chronic and relapsing course of these disturbances.

If the patient feels no improvement at the second examination, the first question must be: did she feel better for a few days, or not at all? Treatment sometimes produces a very marked but short-lived effect. At re-examination two distinct conditions may be found: (1) the findings are the same, i.e. treatment has given no results or (which is not much better) the condition has relapsed; (2) our original findings have been corrected but new factors are now producing similar symptoms.

In the latter case, we can consider the patient improved even if her complaints (her pain) seems to be the same. There is even a highly characteristic pattern in the cervical region: the lesions tend to move in a caudal direction from one treatment to the next, until they disappear.

In the former case, however, we must ask ourselves whether the first diagnosis was correct, or complete; whether we did not overlook an underlying condition which may have produced relapse (blockage at a key point at the other end of the spinal column, an awkward position at work, etc.); or whether the case is not altogether more serious than it appeared at first.

If the case is very severe, i.e. if the blockage is hard and painful, and there is restriction of larger sections of the spinal column, then this type of treatment is insufficient and repeated mobilization is required, i.e. two or three times a week. In such cases we should always teach the patient self-treatment (mobilization) which she can perform several times a day.

If manipulation has brought no relief at all, nor any change, it may be given another chance, but only after careful re-examination and reassessment of the whole case, because the most likely reason is diagnostic error. If the effect is always good but short lived, followed by relapse, we must seek the underlying cause. This then becomes our main concern (e.g. cardiac ischaemia in recurrent lesions in the upper thoracic spine), for to go on treating movement restriction in such cases would be more than useless.

Obviously, as a rule more serious cases will not be treated by manipulation alone and can be expected to have a chronic course. It is then important to follow up the patient for a considerable time, 6 months or more, at intervals.

The possibility of indicating manipulation for the purpose of prevention must also be considered. True, manipulation is indicated only if we think the movement restriction is clinically relevant. On the other hand, when administering manipulative treatment we should never overlook blockage in key regions, because this is most likely to cause relapse. In other words, we indicate manipulation for clinically latent blockage in key regions in order to *prevent* relapse. This is in effect introducing the preventive aspect into therapy, a regular feature of rehabilitation. Bearing this in mind, there is a strong case to be made for manipulative treatment, for example, in children, physically very exposed individuals, etc. (*see* Chapter 8).

Traction

Traction is essentially a form of manipulation, but unlike other methods it is generally accepted in traditional medicine. Within the framework of manipulative techniques, traction of the lumbar and cervical spinal column plays a specific role; it is particularly useful in true radicular syndromes and in the lumbar spine whenever the diagnosis of disc lesion is made. In fact if traction relieves symptoms in the lumbar region, then the diagnosis of disc lesion is corroborated. In both the cervical and the lumbar region traction can be very useful in such conditions as acute wry neck and acute lumbago. The essential technical details will be given in Chapter 6.

There is one important point to be made, however: whatever our opinion of the usefulness of traction, it is essential to test each case and apply traction only where it gives relief. If there is no relief, we must first modify the technique and then desist if it still fails. One of the reasons why traction is sometimes badly tolerated is blockage, which must first be treated by manipulation before traction can be applied (e.g. in radicular syndromes).

Reflex therapy

It would be a great mistake to think that when mobility is restored to the mobile segment by manipulation, all painful changes there will automatically disappear, even if we frequently find them reduced. They can also, of course, be found in cases where there is no segmental movement restriction. In these cases other methods of reflex therapy are indicated.

Massage

This term covers a great variety of techniques which have developed from time immemorial; they are applied to the soft tissues and even to the periosteum. It is not within the scope of this book to deal with massage in any detail. Rationally applied, i.e. from the clinical point of view, it should be used when and where changes are found in the tissue, changes that consist mainly in altered tension. The experienced masseur adapts his technique so as to give relief, i.e. to lessen tension in the muscles as well as in the skin and the connective tissues. Deep friction may be applied to pain points on the periosteum.

Bearing this in mind it would seem that massage is a universal method applicable in all reflex changes produced by pain (nociceptive stimulus); indeed it is widely used in this way. Some techniques are pleasurable, giving immediate relief and being very popular with patients. There are other massage techniques, which are painful. Unfortunately, the effect of massage is usually only short lived, while the procedure is very time consuming. It is moreover a purely passive form of treatment, demanding almost no co-operation from the patient.

We therefore prefer to indicate massage only as a preparation for other, more active and more effective methods of treatment, and not as the sole therapy.

Post-isometric muscle relaxation (PR)

This method, which will be described in detail in Chapter 6, has a similar effect to that of the spray and stretch method (Travell and Simons, 1983) and appears to be a specific method to obtain muscle relaxation. It is effective not only in the treatment of pain points (trigger points) in the muscle, but also of many if not most pain points on the periosteum if these are points of attachment of muscles with increased tension, or points of referred pain originating in the muscle. It is (with a few exceptions) completely painless and the patient can (and should) be taught self-treatment. It is clearly effective only if there is increased tension in the muscle; otherwise it is useless.

Skin stretching

This method is as specific in hyperalgesic skin zones as is PR where there is increased muscle tension. It has of course an effect similar to that of some massage techniques applied to the skin, like rolling a fold of skin (the 'pince roulé' described by Kibler (1958), or the technique of Leube and Dicke (1951)) but unlike these techniques it is completely painless, much less time consuming, and again can and should be used by the patient himself. Skin stretching should only be indicated for increased tension in the skin, or, more precisely, for increased resistance to stretching in a specific area of the skin. It can be applied even to a very small area of the skin, such as the hyperalgesic fold between the toes in a radicular syndrome, or the skin over a periosteal pain point, with very good effect. Being entirely painless, it can be used even in hyperalgesic skin in causalgia.

Local anaesthesia, needling

One of the most widely used methods of treating painful lesions is local anaesthesia, or needling. It may appear unorthodox to deal with these two methods together, yet one does not simply use local anaesthetics to relieve pain for the short period during which the anaesthetic has effect; the popularity of local anesthesia is due to the fact that its effect far outlasts the direct (pharmacological) effect of the anaesthetic, and seems not to be dependent on it; in fact, Kibler (1958) uses sodium bicarbonate, and even subcutaneous air or gas have been used. Direct proof has been provided by Frost, Jesse and Siggard-Andressen (1980) in their 'controlled double blind comparison of Mevipacain injections versus saline injections for myofascial pain', showing that if anything, the physiological saline solution was more effective. The common denominator of all these methods is, of course, the use of the needle. The effect, however, appears to depend very much on the needle touching the painful structure exactly, if possible so as to reproduce the pain the patient complains of, whether an anaesthetic is used or not. If we succeed in finding the exact spot, we produce analgaesia immediately, whether we use local anaesthetic, a saline solution, or simply a dry needle (Lewit, 1979).

Local anaesthetics are of course necessary if we want to induce anaesthesia of nervous structures, for example in nerve-root infiltration or epidural infiltration in radicular pain.

One special method using local anaesthesia is that of producing blobs on the skin by *intracutaneous* application within a hyperalgesic skin zone. Here again a similar or more intense effect can be obtained by using distilled water.

It is interesting that just as after manipulation, so after successful local anaesthesia or dry needling, the immediate relief we obtain is often succeeded the next day by a painful reaction, after which the therapeutic effect establishes itself. This treatment should therefore not be repeated before 6 or 7 days have elapsed. Repetition is indicated if the method has proved successful, yet some pain remains.

Electrical stimulation

Here we obviously face a variety of methods with similar effects, which are apparently interchangeable. To these must be added such new methods of physical therapy as transcutaneous electrical stimulation, and other forms of electrotherapy which produce a similar effect on skin receptors and in the subcutaneous tissue. They have to compete, too, with other traditional methods including not only massage, but poulticing, cupping, capsicum plasters etc. The clinician has therefore a wide range of choice, the 'ideal' method being painless, without risk, without side-effects and if possible applicable by the patient himself.

Acupuncture

It would be burying one's head in the sand not to mention the ancient method of acupuncture in this context, the more so as it is now widely used and discussed. There can be no doubt that acupuncture, too, achieves its results by evoking reflex mechanisms. Difficulties arise the moment we attempt closer analysis and classification of the mode of action. The orthodox acupuncturist indicates treatment according to disease, without reference to the pathogenesis, although the more 'enlightened' admit that acupuncture should be used in cases of disturbed function rather than in structural pathology. The choice of acupuncture points according to the viscera and of 'meridians' without clinical examination of these points is based purely on tradition and not on scientific verification. For scientific analysis, therefore, it will be necessary to examine not only the complex method as a whole, but its simpler elements, one by one.

One such element is the effect of the needle; dry needling was reintroduced to modern medicine by Travell and Rinzler (1952) and I myself proved the analgesic needle effect (1979) in 271 out of 312 applications of the needle to pain points, in 241 patients. There is sufficient clinical evidence of the efficacy of the treatment.

On the other hand, there appears to be a growing tendency even among modern Chinese doctors to choose their points not according to the traditional 'meridians', but on the basis of the segmental theory of innervation. Instead of needling, electrical stimulation is also being introduced (Chang Hsian Tung, 1979). Melzack (1975) on the other hand, has tried to establish a far-reaching analogy between the pain and trigger points of Travell and Rinzler (1952) and the traditional acupuncture points. Gunn *et al.* (1976) found that of 100 acupuncture points chosen at random, 70 were motor points in muscles. Many acupuncture points are attachment points of muscle tendons which can be treated by post-isometric relaxation if they are tender (e.g. the head of the fibula, the Che gu (4 equ L 14) point as the attachment point of the adductor brevis).

Gaymans (1982) was able to show that by pressure on acupuncture points he could facilitate or inhibit muscles. There seem to be interesting correlations between acupuncture points and the motor system.

On closer examination it seems that many acupuncture points can be tender at palpation, that increased tension can be palpated on the site and that the skin over them may show increased resistance to stretching. In other words, if clinical examination of acupuncture points were to become a routine, a more rational application of the treatment would ensue. This is borne out, too, by the results of electrical measurement of skin resistance at the sites of acupuncture points.

The importance of such a rational approach would be that it might enable us to indicate cases in which acupuncture is really the method of choice, and preferable to other methods acting through reflex mechanisms.

Treatment of scars

It is curious that as a rule acupuncturists seem to be unaware of perhaps the most rewarding effects of needling (local anaesthesia) in the treatment of scars. This is based on the Huneke phenomenon (*see* page 4). The problem is one of correct diagnosis; when and under what conditions is a scar (usually a quite irrelevant one) a focus which can become the cause of a lesion that would not normally be connected with it?

Under what conditions should we consider the possibility and look for such scars? (1) If the patient relapses and there is no other apparent reason either in the segment or elsewhere in the locomotor system; (2) our findings seem too insignificant to explain the case history; (3) if the cause of the scar (often an operation wound that did not heal properly, or suppuration) coincides with the time when the present symptoms started or became much worse.

Any scars found should be examined for tender spots on deep palpation, with increased resistance ('adhesions'); there may also be a hyperalgesic skin zone round the scar, best detected by skin stretching. To produce the Huneke phenomenon we may first stretch the skin, and if the result is not satisfactory we may then infiltrate or apply the needle to the pain spot within the scar. If treatment is successful both the resistance and the pain spot within the scar should disappear, and the lesion for which the patient is being treated (headache, radicular pain, etc.) should then *markedly* improve, and with lasting effect.

Remedial exercise

Having dealt with methods of treatment indicated mainly to combat pain in the motor system we may now turn to those concerned directly with locomotor function. Here remedial exercise plays a prominent role. There are two principal types that concern us here. In the first type the patient uses his muscles to restore joint mobility, i.e. self-mobilization techniques; these will be described under the heading of mobilization and manipulation techniques, to which they belong, as will techniques of post-isometric muscle relaxation carried out by the patient himself.

Here I am concerned only with the second type of remedial exercise, intended to correct locomotor patterns or stereotypes, or muscular imbalance, which is frequently the real cause of painful disorders in the 'periphery' of the locomotor system.

In disturbed function of the locomotor system the objective of remedial exercise is a faulty motor pattern or stereotype which has been *diagnosed* and is considered *relevant* to the patient's problem. Without this diagnosis and subsequent assessment of the importance of the faulty stereotype in the pathogenesis of the symptoms, remedial exercise is simply a waste of time. Herein lies the role of the physician, the technical aspect being left to the physiotherapist. The doctor, who is familiar with the diagnosis, will of course be able to evaluate the results achieved by the physiotherapist. This is very important because remedial exercise can be not only very time consuming but also extremely frustrating.

The emphasis is thus placed on diagnosis, but as a rule this can be established only after the acute pain has been treated by the physician, as otherwise the patient's movements are so distorted that it is impossible to say what is due to pain and what reveals faulty movement patterns.

The second criterion for indicating remedial exercise is the relevance of the faulty stereotype to the patient's problem. Here the decision is not as simple as the indication of manipulation for movement restriction or needling if a significant pain point is found. Remedial exercise is always time consuming, and time should not be wasted. Faulty movement patterns are extremely frequent, moreover, and to embark on a course of remedial exercise in every case would be most unrealistic. We therefore indicate remedial exercise where we think the faulty movement patterns are so important that without correction, relapse of the painful condition is inevitable. Indeed, it is frequently indicated precisely on account of relapses. Nevertheless there are cases where we can be sure, without waiting for the patient to relapse. One criterion is the degree of muscular imbalance; in other cases we must consider the conditions under which relapses occur: if a patient suffers from lumbago on stooping or lifting weights, and his movement pattern in stooping and weight lifting is bad, then obviously he has to be taught to correct this fault. The same is true of carrying weights, of sitting at the typewriter, or of standing for long periods. The most disastrous of all faulty patterns, however, is faulty respiration: severe incoordination of respiration may jeopardize the result of any treatment of the locomotor system.

To make remedial exercise as effective as possible, and to make it a routine procedure, it is essential to limit the goal as strictly as possible. We should not attempt to teach patients 'ideal locomotor patterns', but only to correct the fault that is causing the trouble. If we do this, it is possible in most cases to obtain results within a few weeks, even after a few sessions. If we try to achieve more at the outset, it may take months or years.

It is no less important to know how and when to indicate remedial exercise than to know the limits of its possibilities. Unlike manipulation or local anaesthesia, remedial exercise requires the *active* and intelligent co-operation of the patient, and this is by no means always easy to achieve. Locomotor patterns can be extremely firmly fixed and if the patient is no longer young, it is very difficult to change them. It is thus generally easier to train a younger patient than an elderly one. Even more important is the question of motivation. If the patient is not really interested in improving his condition, the physiotherapist is simply wasting her time. It cannot be sufficiently emphasized, however, that the art of the good physiotherapist consists almost as much in motivating her patient as in her technical competence.

In addition to motivation, intelligence plays a great role and its lack can be a seriously limiting factor. Here I must remind the reader of what was said in Chapter 2 about individuals incapable of forming good motor patterns. There are people of high intelligence who are almost handicapped the moment locomotor skills are called for – and here we may fail even with an intelligent and willing patient.

Finally, the physical condition of the patient may be a limiting factor: heart disease, a high degree of obesity, weak abdominal musculature after repeated operation for hernia, decompensating scoliosis and other conditions may all restrict the effectiveness of remedial exercise.

Despite these limitations, remedial exercise should constitute the most important task of the physiotherapist; we should therefore single out for remedial exercise those cases that are most significant and rewarding, so that she does not waste her time too much on the passive procedures such as massage, and the many forms of electrotherapy.

One might ask whether and under what conditions this type of remedial exercise should be prescribed for purely preventive reasons. This is a reasonable consideration in view of the unfavourable conditions under which the locomotor system develops in technically advanced countries, producing imbalance of muscle groups, frequently in children. This is almost an insoluble difficulty at present, mainly because group therapy is not easy to arrange. Certain Yoga techniques, in particular respiration exercises, can be taught in groups; the 'spinal' yoga exercises may also be considered.

Treatment of faulty statics

The diagnosis of faulty statics has been described in Chapters 3 and 4. In so far as the cause is muscular imbalance or external influences, faulty statics must be treated accordingly. Here we are concerned with obliquity, particularly in the pelvic region, and whether to correct it by a heel-pad or by raising one buttock in the sitting position. This is a more important decision than would appear at first sight; it is effective only if the aid is *constantly* used, i.e. if we are aiming at a permanent change in function.

Such a decision can be straightforward, for instance, if the difference in leg length is due to fairly recent trauma. In flat foot on one side only, we can see the effect of an arch support if the patient stands with her weight on the outer edge of the sole, and we observe that this straightens the pelvis.

In the majority of cases, however, obliquity develops slowly during growth, and as it increases compensation develops, and assessment is impossible without exact

X-ray analysis such as that described in Chapter 3. However, indication of static correction can never be a question of X-ray diagnosis alone, but must be decided on clinical grounds.

Clinically, static pain is characterized by a chronic course, as a rule deteriorating under conditions of static load, i.e. standing or sitting. On examination we expect signs of pelvic obliquity and deviation, and pelvic shift (*see* Chapter 3), and correction should bring about clinical improvement. As shown, however, spinal statics can be checked reliably only by X-ray under standard conditions; hence it would usually be incorrect to indicate static correction on clinical grounds alone. If clinical and X-ray findings are in agreement, we are justified in indicating correction.

There are some practical points that must be stressed here. The first is the immediate reaction to a heel-pad. If a thin sole of about 1 cm is put under the foot of a normal subject, and he is told to put his weight equally on both feet and keep his legs straight, he will object. A subject with pelvic obliquity may respond to this situation in three different ways: he may find it positively comfortable, he may feel no difference, or he may object. In the first two cases we can expect the patient to tolerate correction well from the outset, and he should be instructed to wear the pad in his house-slippers as well as in his outdoor shoes. In the last case, however, there may be an unfavourable reaction, and time is needed for the patient to adapt. He should be told to stop using the pad if the pain increases; he must try to adapt to the correction gradually, and must be checked up on at regular intervals of a few weeks.

It is not a matter of indifference which type of correction is used. A heel-pad fitted into the shoe is practical, but has the disadvantage that the shoe fits less well. If possible, it is better to lower (shorten) the heel of the other shoe. This is advisable only where the difference is from 1 to 2 cm. Where the difference is greater, the whole sole must be thicker on the side of the short leg so as not to make too much difference between the position of the two feet; another possible solution is to lower one heel and raise the other.

If the pelvis is level, and there is thus no apparent difference in leg length but obliquity at the base of the vertebral column has to be corrected, we shall find that obliquity is the same whether the patient is sitting or standing. Here it is advisable to prescribe correction (a thin board) under one ischial tuberosity when the patient is seated.

The most frequent and most serious fault in sitting, of course, is excessive lumbar kyphosis due to hypermobility of the lumbar spine. If we do not prescribe supports we should advise the patient to sit in the oriental manner, with feet crossed and knees apart, or on her heels in the Japanese way. Another position is that advocated by Brügger (*see* page 295), in which the pelvis is rolled forward and the thoracolumbar spine much better balanced, or simply to raise the back of the seat, like a saddle.

Immobilization and supports

In acute lesions of the locomotor system, muscle spasm clearly indicates that rest and immobilization is required. This can be particularly evident after acute trauma, when the healing of damaged tissue makes immobilization imperative. Immobilization itself becomes a problem, however, once the condition becomes chronic, and if we aim at full recovery, i.e. the restoration of normal function, immobilization presents an outright obstacle. Thus immobilization, for us, can never be more than a temporary measure in preparation for rehabilitation, i.e. improvement of function. Only in cases where there is no hope of functional recovery can permanent immobilization be indicated, as a necessary evil.

Unlike immobilization, however, supports need not greatly interfere with mobility while protecting the patient against static overstrain. Unfortunately, static overstrain is extremely frequent in working conditions in technically advanced countries, and hypermobile subjects with lax muscles and ligaments frequently find it difficult to adapt, in particular if, as in most modern means of public transport, jolting is added.

We therefore recommend car drivers to use an inflatable cushion for the small of the back; hypermobile subjects suffering from headache can wear a soft supporting collar while riding in bus or Underground; elderly or obese patients with weak abdominal musculature can wear a firm abdominal belt. For patients with ligament pain in the pelvic region a firm pelvic belt worn mainly at night (Cyriax, 1977) is very helpful (*see* page 301 for details). Most of these supports should only be worn under conditions of static performance, and not while moving (except for the abdominal belt).

Pharmacotherapy

As we are dealing with disturbances that mainly concern the function of the locomotor system it is easy to see that pharmacotherapy can only act within certain limits. It is difficult to conceive of a drug that could correct faulty functioning of a restricted spinal segment, or a faulty pattern of respiration or weight lifting. On the other hand, disturbed function in itself is not tantamount to disease and pain. It also causes reflex changes which are felt as painful, and therefore drugs that reduce reflex segmental reactions to nociceptive stimulation and can raise the threshold of pain can be most useful, particularly if we find the response to disturbed function excessive.

Therefore, it is sometimes useful in some cases to prescribe drugs that lower the response of the autonomic nervous system, and if pain is acute, analgesics of the non-steroidal anti-inflammatory type should be administered. Opiates should be avoided, but sedatives are often to be recommended.

It has recently become fashionable to combine analgesics with myorelaxants, and there are drugs available that combine the two approaches. These may be used advantageously in cases where muscle tension is a prominent feature, but they should not be prescribed indiscriminately. In patients with a tendency to hypermobility, and a flabby musculature, even if they have painful muscle spasm (trigger points) at the site of the lesion, these drugs can have an adverse effect, increasing the existing muscular imbalance and laxity. In such cases only specific treatment of the muscles showing increased tension is indicated.

Where there are signs of depression or a suspicion of masked depression, the administration of mild anti-depressives can be most rewarding, and we should not hesitate to give them a fair trial.

As a rule the intramuscular application of corticoids is *not* indicated in disturbances of function. The popular practice of local application of corticoids to pain points (on the periosteum, etc.) should never become a routine procedure.

Pain points usually react to local anaesthesia or dry needling; if they are the attachment points of muscles they react to PR or to other forms of reflex therapy. Corticoids should be tried only if these far more physiological methods (which produce no side-effects) have failed. If the corticoids do not show the desired effect they should never be repeatedly administered.

Surgery

If the clinical condition of the patient is due to disturbance of function *alone*, there should be no question of surgical intervention. However, disturbed function may be the consequence of an anatomical lesion requiring surgery; it will frequently be our task to decide whether this is not, in fact, the case. The most frequent condition in which the question arises is that of root compression and other sequelae of disc herniation, a condition in which we may often succeed by conservative measures aimed at restoring function, but where it is important to decide when surgery is likely to be more successful (*see* page 333–334). Another case is that of pathological hypermobility, e.g. in spondylolisthesis. This condition in itself can be clinically mute and compatible with perfect health; however, in the evolutive stage there may be considerable symptoms due to pathological hypermobility, which may constitute an indication for surgery. This is even more likely in hypermobility due to a free os odontoideum.

Regimen

This is probably the most important and most effective approach both to treatment and to prevention of disturbed function in the locomotor system. I have left it to the last because it is not a therapeutic measure in the true sense of the word, and there is a special chapter devoted to the question. However, as I have pointed out elsewhere, one of the important aspects of taking down a case history is to discover the possible source of the patient's trouble in his daily regimen and we should be able to advise him on how to avoid the most harmful habits. Indeed, if we succeed in detecting these important clues, we should be able to give him very useful advice after the first examination.

Conclusions

Indicating methods of therapy is the practical application of all that has been said in the theoretical parts of this book. Since symptoms are usually the result of several factors, we have to single out each time the factor or lesion that we think the most important at the moment, while we have the patient before us, and also which lesion we think is most accessible to treatment.

    If we succeed in our intentions, a different therapeutical approach will probably be needed when we next see the patient. Our aim is not to promote one type of therapy but to improve function and relieve symptoms by the most adequate and efficient method. This involves a very difficult problem, that of evaluation. It is hard to say whether the patient has improved because of manipulation, remedial exercise, or needling. On the other hand, to carry on with manipulation when movement restriction is no longer important, or to continue needling when there is no pain point to justify it, is out of place. However, in typical situations this need not be an obstacle, if statistics are not held to be the only criterion of success. If an acute appendicitis is cured after the removal of the inflamed organ no statistical evaluation is required. If after manipulation mobility is restored in a segment and remains good after several control examinations, then we have achieved what can be achieved by this method. If a pain point disappears after needling or post-isometric relaxation of the muscle and does not recur, or if a patient has learned how to normalize respiration and does not slip back into her old habits, then something has been achieved even if there remains another lesion which still causes symptoms and has yet to be treated.

This may seem an unusual and unorthodox approach, but it is also a demanding one, for it precludes routine procedures and knows few 'routine' patients. It is highly rewarding, however, both for patient and for physician.

6

Therapeutic techniques

In the preceding chapters the importance and the diagnosis of disturbed function of the locomotor system have been explained, and I have described the clinically significant reflex changes involved and indicated the most important therapeutic methods. It would be impossible to describe all these techniques in detail in this chapter; I shall confine myself principally to manipulative techniques and the specific forms of remedial exercise, with a few ancillary techniques.

MANIPULATION

The sole aim of manipulation is to restore normal joint mobility, including joint play. Two major types of manipulation can be distinguished: (1) mobilization techniques; and (2) thrusting techniques. I will start, however, with a few general principles.

The positioning of the patient

The patient should lie (or sit or stand) so that she can relax, so that the joint to be treated is accessible, and so that one of the articulating bones is either fixed by the patient's own weight or can easily be fixed by the therapist. The height of the manipulation table from the floor should be adjustable as required; in general it should correspond to the distance of the therapist's fingertips from the floor when he stands erect with arms hanging loosely down and fingers stretched.

The position of the therapist

This is in many ways decisive for the therapist's technique. He must be comfortable in order to be relaxed, and his relaxation is essential in order to procure relaxation of the patient. As a rule the direction in which the therapist's hand moves continues the line of his forearm, but whenever possible the movement should come from the whole body; it often comes from the feet, as in throwing the discus. The therapist's movement must never be forced, cramped or exhausting; if he is easily tired he must be making a technical error. For manipulation of the spinal column the body of the therapist and that of the patient must move in harmony, like a couple of dancers; this is the secret of gentle, flowing and elegant technique and is also valid for examination.

Fixation

One of the bones articulating in the joint being manipulated should be fixed while the other is mobilized. In extremity joints it is usually the proximal joint that is fixed, i.e. supported by the table or by the body of the therapist. For effective fixation it is advisable to move only one joint. In the spinal column fixation is achieved by correct positioning ('locking') and where possible by direct contact with the therapist's hands. Good fixation of the pelvis can be obtained if the patient sits astride the table.

The position of the joint and the direction of treatment

The joint to be treated must not be in a position in which the capsule and the ligaments are overstretched, i.e. it must not be locked. The direction of treatment (manipulation) may correspond to the impaired joint mobility or to joint play, i.e. to relative shift or distraction (*Figure 6.1*). According to Kaltenborn (1973) the

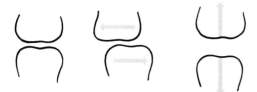

Figure 6.1 Possible directions of joint play

direction of joint play is not purely haphazard, and depends on whether the concavity of the joint is proximal or distal (*see Figure 2.4,* page 16). In the former case shift of the distal partner, which has to be restored, is in the opposite direction to the impaired movement, whereas in the latter case the shift of the distal partner is in the same direction as impaired mobility. For this reason the first phalanx should be shifted mainly in a palmar direction (if flexion is restricted) and the carpal bones against the radius in a dorsal direction if palmar flexion is restricted (*see Figure 6.3,* page 199).

Taking up the slack

This is a crucial step before treatment begins and is technically almost identical with the beginning of mobilization. We try to bring the joint into its extreme position either of normal function or, more frequently and particularly in extremity joints, of joint play. Distraction of the joint is helpful. In the spinal column it is not always possible to make the distinction between mobility and joint play, the movement of a single mobile segment (in itself impossible to achieve by active movement) playing to some extent the role of joint play. This end-position is never reached suddenly in normal movement; sudden resistance in the end-position is a sign of blockage. We know that we have taken up the slack the moment we sense the *first slight* increase of resistance. This must be carried out very *gently*, with the patient *relaxed*. The most important source of error is to mistake active resistance by the patient for the sign that we have taken up the slack. This invariably happens if we cause pain – something to be avoided at all costs.

Manipulation proper

After taking up the slack we have two main means of restoring restricted movement: (1) by gently springing the joint in end-position (mobilization); or (2) by making a thrust from end-position.

MOBILIZATION

At the first slight increase in resistance while we are taking up the slack we first make sure we have indeed reached the end-position, by slightly decreasing the range of movement and then increasing it again, to establish whether we meet resistance at the same point; in other words, we spring the joint in end-position, which is exactly what we do in passive mobilization. Repeating this procedure several times will show that even in a normal joint the range of movement increases, i.e. we reach end-position (take up the slack) after a longer interval. In a restricted joint this increase will be much more pronounced. There are two mistakes to be avoided in this type of springing (repetitive) mobilization: (1) we must be careful to remain in end-position and not return to the neutral position of the joint, i.e. the range of the springing movement must be small and very well controlled; (2) springing back is even more important for the restoration of mobility than is the pressure we exert; therefore even if the range of movement increases, we must never increase our pressure. The joint must be allowed to move back almost to the initial end-position. In this way the range of springing will increase but never the amount of pressure we exert.

This type of mainly passive mobilization is effective in joints that are not excessively fixed by muscle spasm when blocked, such as the sacroiliac and acromioclavicular joints, and many extremity joints. It is less effective in the spinal column, however, and here passive mobilization is used mainly as a preparation for thrusting techniques, and as after-treatment. To make mobilization of the spinal column fully effective we have learned, in recent years, to use techniques of muscular facilitation and inhibition.

Mobilization using muscular facilitation and inhibition

Some techniques aim at specific muscles or muscle groups, while others have a more general effect.

Isometric contraction of muscles in tension, followed by relaxation – Isometrics (Mitchell, 1979) or, as I prefer to call it, PR – post-isometric relaxation. Unlike the widely used technique developed by Kabat (1965), we use only *minimal* resistance during the isometric phase. After the slack has been taken up, the patient exerts only a minimum of pressure in the opposite direction from that of the movement restriction, holding it for about 10 s. She is then told to 'let go', and the operator *waits*, or even repeats the 'let go!', until he feels that the patient has truly relaxed. Only then does he carry out his movement in the direction of the restriction – but then only to the point where the slightest resistance is felt, i.e. only so far as the patient's relaxation will allow. It is important to profit from her relaxation as long as the range of movement increases spontaneously; this may be for 10 s or even longer. When the therapist feels no further relaxation the procedure is repeated from the newly gained position: the ground that has been won must not be lost again. If relaxation has been satisfactory, the time allowed for isometric resistance may be slightly reduced, but if relaxation is insufficient resistance may be prolonged for up to half a minute. This procedure can be repeated for as long as the therapist continues to observe increasing range of movement, but usually 3–5 repetitions suffice.

Active rhythmic repetitive movements by the patient in the direction of the restriction, producing reciprocal inhibition in the antagonist in spasm.

Direct repetitive rhythmic muscle pull, under certain conditions, to produce mobilization directly – e.g. the therapist causes rhythmical contractions of the scalenus in order to mobilize the first rib, or of the psoas to mobilize the thoracolumbar junction.

These techniques are applied to specific muscles or muscle groups, but the first is by far the most important. The following techniques have a far more generalized effect.

Respiration (*see* page 35ff.) – It is of great practical significance that as a rule inspiration has a facilitating and expiration an inhibiting effect on muscles. Therefore, it is usually appropriate to combine inspiration with isometric resistance and expiration with relaxation. However, there are important exceptions to this rule: during retroflexion of the thoracic spine, maximum expiration produces additional mobilization of the thoracic spine into retroflexion by contraction (facilitation) of the thoracic erector spinae, while in a kyphotic position of the thorax deep inspiration produces mobilization into flexion. Even more important is the mobilizing effect of respiration during side-bending (Gaymans, 1980), due to alternating facilitation and inhibition of individual segments of the spinal column (*see* page 35). As the even segments are facilitated during inspiration and inhibited during expiration, in these segments we combine the isometric phase with inspiration, and relaxation with expiration; in the odd segments this is reversed. To be effective, respiration must be sufficiently slow, and deep. The intense facilitatory (inhibitive) effect on muscles of respiratory synkinesis can be usefully applied.

Eye movements – These facilitate the movement of the head and trunk in the direction of the patient's gaze and inhibit movement in the opposite direction. This holds for lifting the head and trunk as well as for stooping and rotation; it is *not* true for side-bending, but looking up facilitates straightening up from side-bending. Eye movements should not be exaggerated, however; according to Gaymans (1980) maximum excursion has an inhibitory effect.

Combinations. It is obvious that these methods lend themselves to useful combination, in particular PR with respiration and eye movements. This has the enormous advantage of automation: instead of telling the patient to 'press with minimum force – only a few grams' we now tell her to look to the right and breathe in slowly (if rotation to the left is restricted), and then to look to the left and breathe out, thus automatically producing the correct resistance during the isometric phase, followed by relaxation. For the mobilization of side-bending in an even segment, after taking up the slack we ask the patient to look up and breathe in slowly, and then to look down and breathe out.

I shall draw attention here to some of the problems of correct combination, which is not always an easy matter. Since looking up facilitates inspiration and inhibits expiration, and looking down vice versa, looking up must not be combined with expiration nor looking down with breathing in. We must also bear in mind that looking up facilitates retroflexion and looking down facilitates anteflexion (stooping), which may or may not be useful in a given case. Thus in mobilizing side-bending in an even segment it will be useful to proceed in the manner described in the preceding paragraph. If, however, we wish to mobilize an *odd* segment, it would be wrong to tell the patient to look *up* and breathe *out* during the isometric phase, because looking up inhibits expiration. It would be equally wrong to tell the patient to look down, for that would inhibit the straightening-up reaction needed during the isometric phase, while the situation would be even worse if the patient looked up during relaxation. Therefore we do *not* combine respiration with eye movements in mobilization of side-bending in an *odd* segment. In the cervicothoracic junction it is essential for the neck to be held in retroflexion during the mobilization of side-bending. It is therefore very convenient to combine looking up with inspiration, but not looking down with expiration, because the patient will bend her neck forward if she looks down.

It is very important that the patient breathes slowly, so that both the isometric and the relaxation phase are long enough. It is therefore useful first to tell the patient, for example, to look to the right and only a moment later to tell her to breathe in slowly; similarly, to tell her to first look to the left and only then to breathe out slowly. If a patient finds it difficult to breathe slowly, they should be told to hold their breath for a few seconds at the end of inspiration. However, a patient with such bad co-ordination that slow breathing (no more than 4 seconds) cannot be attained, must be taught to breathe correctly, because such faulty respiration is incompatible with normal functioning of the motor system. If our combinations are well thought out, they not only improve the technique by what we may call automation but they also increase its effectiveness by the summation of stimuli; frequently two or three repetitions are sufficient to restore normal mobility.

THRUSTING

This technique consists in a fast but not forceful movement of small amplitude, starting from end-position (i.e. after taking up the slack). A barrier seems to give way, and as a rule we hear a 'click'. Immediately afterwards we sense hypotonia and observe increased mobility.

The thrust must be applied *only* after the slack has been taken up completely, and this is possible only if the patient is completely relaxed. There are three technical pre-conditions: (1) we must be able to sense the moment of complete relaxation; (2) the patient having relaxed properly, the end-position is reached (the slack is taken up) with a minimum of force; (3) the thrust must start from the end-position, i.e. we must never release tension before delivering the thrust, as when we lift the arm before delivering a blow – the typical beginner's error, because it corresponds to a type of movement we are used to. Here, however, it is a crucial mistake, because it enables the patient to contract his muscles and in this way to thwart our manoeuvre, which is effective only if the patient's musculature is taken by surprise.

With these conditions fulfilled, thrusting manipulation is never forceful; as can be seen from *Figure 4.2* (page 108), the thrust corresponds to a weight of not more than 1000 g. Although the high-velocity thrust is typical of thrusting techniques, there are situations in which a relatively slow increase in pressure ('low-velocity thrust') may suffice to obtain complete release and even the 'click'.

Testing

Immediately after treatment, whether this consists in mobilization or thrusting techniques, the effect must be checked by testing (*see* Chapter 5).

Records

Methods of documentation are legion: diagrammatic, typed, variously coloured, etc., and every practitioner will adopt the one he or she finds most suitable. The essential is that in every case the technique used and its precise location, side and direction are recorded. Without this documentation it is impossible to evaluate results, to learn from failure or to deal with possible complications as described in the literature.

After these general remarks, I will now deal with the individual joints.

Extremity joints

In the manipulation of extremity joints we use almost exclusively techniques aimed at restoring joint play. Since examination of joint play is technically identical with the mobilization of these joints, I shall describe both here.

Interphalangeal joints

For mobilization (and examination) dorsopalmar and laterolateral shifts and distraction can be used. The therapist fixes the proximal phalanx between the thumb and forefinger of one hand, either against the table or his own body, while with the thumb and forefinger of his other hand he mobilizes the distal phalanx in the required direction. It is advisable to keep one's fingers at right angles to the shifting movement, and at the same time to apply distraction, which makes the shifting movement easier and more effective.

Metacarpophalangeal joints

These joints are almost spherical, and therefore rotation can be used as well as dorsopalmar and laterolateral shifts and (of course) distraction. While with one hand the therapist fixes the patient's palm against his own body or the table, he may carry out any of these shifts with the other. By far the most effective manoeuvre, however, is traction, which can also be used as a thrust (pull). It is a simple method to teach patients for self-treatment.

The carpometacarpal joint of the thumb

This is the only carpometacarpal joint which is highly mobile, and of all the finger joints it is probably the most susceptible to symptoms. Treatment is therefore important. The therapist must first fix the trapezium between the thumb and

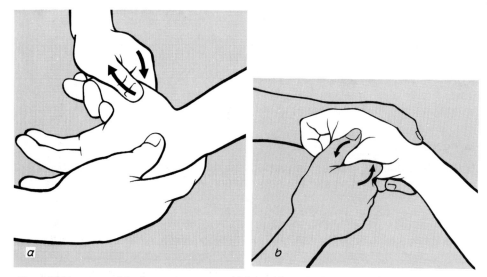

Figure 6.2 Treatment of the first carpometacarpal joint: (*a*) in supination palmar shift of the first metacarpal; (*b*) in pronation dorsal shift; *both* under considerable traction

forefinger of one hand. To find the trapezium he should first palpate the styloid process of the radius; distal to this there is a groove which corresponds to the scaphoid, and then the wrist broadens again; this is the site of the trapezium. With the thumb and forefinger of the other hand, the therapist grasps the first metacarpal bone as close to the joint as possible, so as to examine joint play between the two. For mobilization it is better to grasp the end-phalanx of the thumb with the little finger of the hand that moves the first metacarpal, so as to pull it and thus distract the joint. This can be done with the patient's hand in pronation or supination (the therapist changing hands accordingly). This traction makes the shifting movements of joint play much more effective. If traction is sufficiently strong the therapist can produce a gapping effect by a slight (low-velocity!) thrust in a palmar direction, with the patient's hand in supination, and in a dorsal direction with the hand in pronation. If the therapist is using traction only (with or without a thrust), any fixation of the wrist will suffice; this technique is then very suitable for self-treatment. Mobilization can also be carried out by PR, which is both effective and extremely gentle: while the therapist applies very slight traction, the patient is told to resist with the least possible force for about 10 s, after which he is told to 'let go'. Without increasing the force of his traction the therapist watches the patient relaxing, and repeats the procedure 3–5 times (*Figure 6.2*).

The wrist joints

If palmar flexion is restricted, we must restore joint play by moving the carpal bones in the radiocarpal joint in a dorsal direction. The therapist grasps the supinated hand of the patient close to the radiocarpal joint, fixes the distal end of the forearm against his own knee or the table, and produces a dorsal shift of the wrist (*Figure 6.3*). This technique is well suited for self-treatment. If ulnar flexion is restricted the same technique can be used, but pressure must be applied mainly at the ulnar end of the radiocarpal joint, i.e. against the pisiform bone.

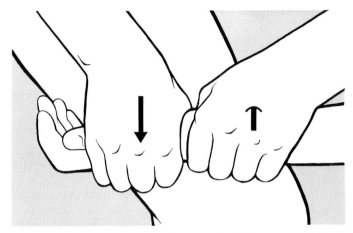

Figure 6.3 Dorsal shift of the carpal bones against the forearm; mobilization of the radiocarpal joint

If dorsal flexion is restricted, joint play must be restored by moving the distal row of the carpal bones against the proximal row, in a palmar direction (*Figure 6.4*). The therapist grasps the patient's hand in pronation, round the proximal end of the metacarpal bones, fixes the distal end of the forearm against his own knee or the table, and produces a palmar shift of the distal row of the carpal bones against the proximal. Again this is an ideal technique for self-treatment. If radial flexion is restricted owing to blockage between the scaphoid and the trapezium, the same technique can be used but the pressure is applied mainly at the radial end of the mid-carpal joint.

There is a simple way to locate the radiocarpal and the carpometacarpal joints exactly: if we extend the wrist against the forearm the skin fold on the dorsal aspect is at the level of the carpometacarpal joint, and if we flex the wrist the skin fold on the palmar aspect is at the level of the radiocarpal joint.

The most specific and also the most important technique is that of shifting one carpal bone against its neighbour, in a dorsal or palmar direction. This is particularly important in the carpal-tunnel syndrome (*see* page 320).

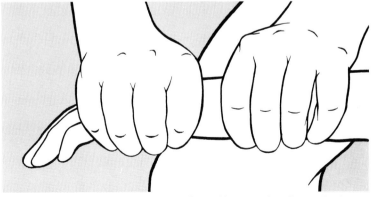

Figure 6.4 Palmar shift of the distal row of carpal bones against the proximal row; mobilization of the mid-carpal joint

The examination technique is simple: one carpal bone is grasped between the thumb and forefinger of each hand, and the therapist moves the two adjacent bones against each other in the dorsal and palmar direction, respectively. For diagnosis it is crucial to use the minimum of force, because under normal conditions friction here is so negligible that the slightest possible pressure will produce some movement. The question of fixation is therefore less important here, although the therapist must support the patient's hand to ensure that it is completely relaxed. If no movement can be felt when this minimum force is applied, there is restriction; the use of greater force renders diagnosis impossible.

This technique can also be used for mobilization, but the following method is preferable, since it provides better fixation. The therapist places both thumbs on the dorsal aspect of one carpal bone and both forefingers (one above the other) on the palmar aspect of the adjacent carpal bone; he then exerts slight pressure, as with pincers, shifting one bone against the other. He then reverses the direction of the shift by placing both thumbs on the palmar aspect and both forefingers on the dorsal aspect of the same two bones (*Figure 6.5*). The movements are rhythmic and repetitive. Obviously, this movement can also be effected with a single hand, the thumb on one and the forefinger on the next carpal bone; in this way the patient can be taught to practise self-treatment.

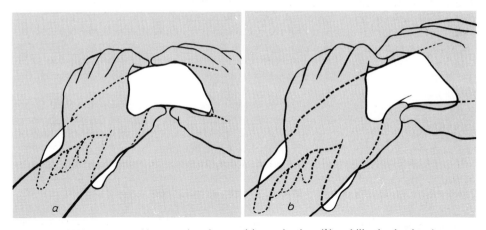

Figure 6.5 Shifting one carpal bone against the next (*a*) examination; (*b*) mobilization by shearing

To locate single carpal bones exactly we must start with one and feel our way to the next. I have already shown how to locate the scaphoid and the trapezium (*see* page 198). The capitate forms the most prominent point of the wrist at palmar flexion. The triquetrum lies below the pisiform. (The latter can be mobilized against the triquetrum to both sides as well as proximodistally.)

This technique can be used both for diagnosis and for treatment, not only for the carpal bones themselves but also for the carpometacarpal joints and the intermetacarpal joints. Technically it is of course most important to place the fingers on adjacent bones; if the therapist places his fingers too close together (on the same bone) by mistake, he will obtain no movement, while if they are too far apart (so that there is a bone in between) there will be too much mobility. The range of shift between two adjacent carpal bones is only slight.

In addition to these shifting techniques there is a distraction technique with high-velocity thrust which is very effective and entirely innocuous if correctly applied (*Figure 6.6*). The therapist stands in front of the patient, who is seated with her arm stretched forward and downward. The therapist places both thumbs on the

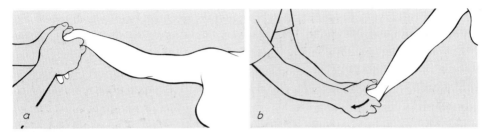

Figure 6.6 Traction high-velocity thrust on the os capitum against the os lunatum: (*a*) finding the os capitum and making contact; (*b*) taking up the slack and making the thrust

patient's distal bone (where restriction has been found), and both hands round the wrist, with the hand in pronation. The slack is taken up by a very gentle pull in the direction of the long axis of the patient's arm, and the wrist is then slightly dorsiflexed over the therapist's thumbs. The thrust is delivered by a sudden pull exactly along the axis of the patient's arm, producing distraction of the joint. There are two mistakes to be avoided: (1) traction must not be released before the thrust is delivered; and (2) no further dorsiflexion at the wrist must occur during the thrust (pull).

The distal radioulnar joint

This is the last joint that can be treated at the wrist, depending for its function on the upper radioulnar joint. For both examination and treatment the technique is broadly that already described for single carpal bones: the therapist grasps the end of the radius and the ulna each between the thumb and forefinger of one hand, producing a dorsal or palmar shift. For treatment he places both thumbs on the dorsal aspect of the radius and both forefingers on the palmar aspect of the ulna, to produce relative shift. After a few repeated rhythmic mobilizations he reverses the pincer movement by placing both thumbs on the dorsal aspect of the ulna and both forefingers on the palmar aspect of the radius.

The elbow

Here mobilization is used mainly for the treatment of painful epicondyles (in combination with muscle relaxation). The most important techniques are distraction and lateral gapping (springing) which is also significant for diagnosis.

DISTRACTION

The patient lies supine, the arm to be treated flexed at the elbow (*Figure 6.7*). The therapist fixes the patient's forearm against his shoulder and places the hand that will perform the traction on the forearm, close to the elbow. With his other hand on the arm, close above the elbow, he fixes the patient's arm to the table from above.

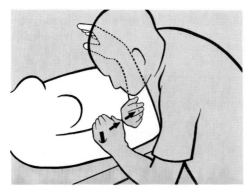

Figure 6.7 Traction of the elbow joint

Traction is carried out along the long axis of the arm by the hand on the forearm; it is greatly enhanced if the therapist presses the thumb of the other hand (close above the elbow) against the hand exerting the pull, and at the same time increases the flexion of the elbow by pressing his shoulder against the patient's forearm; this produces leverage at the elbow, the therapist's thumb serving as the fulcrum.

LATERAL GAPPING (SPRINGING) (*Figure 6.8*)

The patient may be seated or supine, with the affected arm stretched out but not overstretched (the elbow must *not* be locked). The therapist stands facing the elbow (from the radial or ulnar side) and with one hand above the wrist fixes the forearm against his body; with the other hand he takes the elbow from the side, the thumb above and fingers below. Pressing this hand gently against the elbow from

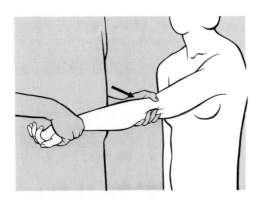

Figure 6.8 Springing the elbow in a radial direction

the side, he takes up the slack, and with a gentle extra push springs the joint, producing gapping of the joint on the opposite side. If the radial epicondyle is painful, as a rule there is no springing (or it is impaired) in the ulnoradial direction, while if the ulnar epicondyle is painful we sometimes find restricted radioulnar springing.

For the purposes of mobilization, springing is repeated rhythmically. The same technique is also used to deliver a high-velocity thrust after taking up the slack (in a radial or ulnar direction). Fast shaking is a useful alternative. For self-treatment *see Figure 6.70,* page 255.

There are two important technical details: the therapist stands at the level of the elbow joint so that the hand springing the joint or delivering the thrust is supported by his trunk, i.e. the movement originates in the therapist's pelvis or even in his legs; and the hand grasping the patient's forearm is there for fixation only, and must not be (mis)used for leverage.

If a high-velocity thrust in a radial or ulnar direction is not successful, a thrust can be applied against the head of the radius with the thumb, from the dorsal aspect, the arm being stretched. This technique may be too violent, and we have introduced instead an equally effective gentle rocking technique. The patient is seated or supine; the therapist grasps the outstretched arm with both hands, just above the elbow, holding it in maximum supination and shaking it gently and rhythmically while the patient is fully relaxed (*Figure 6.9*).

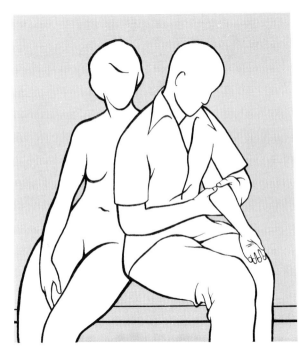

Figure 6.9 Shaking mobilization of the elbow joint into extension

Sachse (personal communication) achieves a similar effect by rhythmic stabilization: with the patient seated and the elbow flexed, the therapist holds the patient's upper arm with both hands, fixing the hand in his armpit, and tells her to extend and flex the arm rhythmically, while he resists the patient's movements.

The shoulder joint

Where we find a typical capsular pattern (*see* page 132), mobilization techniques are practically useless and even the usual traction techniques give little or no results. Surprisingly, what we might call isometric traction brings relief of pain and may even improve mobility. It is best for the patient to stand or to sit (*Figure 6.10*);

the therapist places his right shoulder under the right axilla (or the left under the left), pressing against the patient's thorax. He grasps the affected arm with one hand above the wrist and the other above the elbow, and tells the patient to resist traction very slightly and then to breathe in *slowly*. After about 10 s the patient is told to let go and to breathe out slowly. If relaxation is satisfactory the therapist feels the patient's arm lengthening – but he *must not pull*. This procedure is repeated about three times, according to the degree of relaxation achieved. It is important that the therapist should prop his shoulder against the patient's thorax, not the arm, which is semi-abducted. With the axilla over the top of a cushioned chair-back, this technique is very suitable for self-treatment.

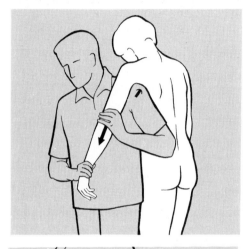

Figure 6.10 Traction of the shoulder over that of the therapist, in the direction of the long axis of the arm; the patient may sit or stand

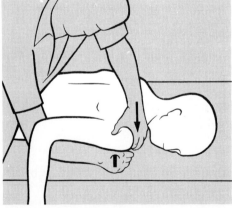

Figure 6.11 Mobilization of the shoulder by ventral shift of the lateral angle of the shoulder-blade (fossa glenoidalis) against the head of the humerus, which is fixed against the table by the therapist's fist

If abduction only is restricted, and we find at examination that joint play is impaired when we spring the head of the humerus against the scapula from above (*see Figure 4.31*, page 134), we restore joint play as follows: the patient lies prone with the arm in abduction; the therapist places his (right) fist under the head of the (right) humerus and stabilizes the patient's arm with his forearm; with his other hand he grasps the fossa glenoidalis and pushes it down (*Figure 6.11*). He then treats the patient supine, in the same way; in this position it is best to mobilize the arm flexed first in external and then in internal rotation, repeating each shift in slow rhythm several times over.

This technique is both easy and effective. Care must be taken, however, to have the therapist's fist located exactly under the head of the humerus, and his other hand at the fossa glenoidalis.

The acromioclavicular joint

To free this joint, the most important technique consists in springing it in a ventrodorsal and a craniocaudal direction (*Figure 6.12*). The patient is supine, the therapist standing by the side of the table. To carry out ventrodorsal springing he places his (right) thenar eminence against the (right) clavicle, fixing the patient's shoulder with his other hand. He now applies gentle pressure against the clavicle from above, and then releases it. If joint play is normal, he will feel the clavicle spring back and will both feel and see movement between the end of the clavicle and the shoulder. This springing is absent in acromioclavicular blockage. To restore it, the therapist repeats this gentle push with his thenar eminence, without ever increasing force, and then releases it. After about five repetitions at the rate of two per second, he usually senses some springing; after 15–20 repetitions (10–15 s) the range no longer increases.

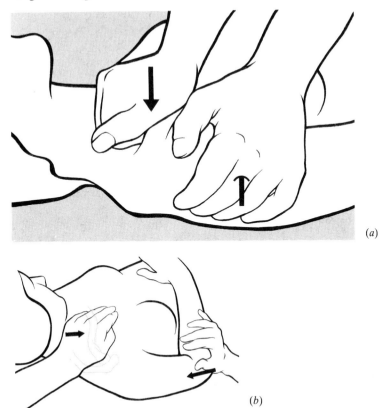

(a)

(b)

Figure 6.12 Mobilization of the acromioclavicular joint by shifting the clavicle against the acromion in (a) a ventrodorsal and (b) a craniocaudal direction

For craniocaudal springing, the therapist at the side of the table fixes the bent elbow from below with his cupped hand, placing the thenar eminence of the other hand on the clavicle from above and giving a slight springing push followed by release, at the rate of two per second. If he neither feels nor sees springing between the clavicle and the shoulder, he repeats the manoeuvre, as for dorsoventral springing.

It appears that it is the springing *back* that frees the joint, and therefore the worst mistake is to increase pressure if no springing has been felt (as though trying to release a spring by pressure on it). Treatment should always be applied in both directions, as movement may be blocked separately in each.

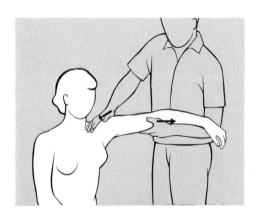

Figure 6.13 Traction–mobilization of the acromioclavicular joint

Another useful technique is that of traction–mobilization (*Figure 6.13*). The patient is seated on a low stool, with the therapist on the side of the lesion, behind the abducted arm. He grasps the arm above the elbow and with the thenar eminence of the other (right) hand on the (left) clavicle he fixes the lateral end of the clavicle by slight pressure from above. He applies traction through the arm, which is slightly raised, abducted and drawn forward, making a gentle movement of rotation until he senses a discreet cracking sound under the hand fixing the clavicle.

The sternoclavicular joint

Simple blockage of this joint without severe arthrosis is a rare condition, and the only technique that seems to give results is ventrodorsal springing. The therapist grasps the medial end of the clavicle between his thumb and fingers and makes a springing movement up and down at the rate of 1–2 per second. He may also, as in the acromioclavicular joint, simply exert and release pressure.

The shoulder-blade

The shoulder-blade lies flat on the thoracic wall and although there is no articulation, it is freely mobile due to the synovial bursae. Although there cannot be blockage of the type found in articulations, there may be some restriction; mobilization can therefore be useful.

The patient lies prone with her head turned towards the therapist at the side of the table (*Figure 6.14*). The therapist grasps the head of the humerus in both hands – one above and the other below – round the patient's shoulder, and carries out a circling movement. With the upper hand he may exert some pressure on the moving scapula from above, or on the contrary he may lift the scapula from the thorax with his fingertips. It is important that the movement the therapist imparts to the scapula over the patient's shoulder should come from the trunk, so that both his hands perform as a single unit.

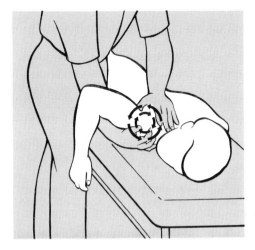

Figure 6.14 Mobilization of the shoulder-blade against the thorax wall (also useful for rib mobilization)

The toes

What has been said about the finger joints is equally valid for the toes. However, the condition that is specific for the foot is pain in the metatarsal joints; here the technique that gives most relief is traction in a slightly plantar direction. For this manoeuvre the therapist grasps the first phalanx of the toe between his thumb and the flexed first phalanx of his forefinger, which is placed under the first phalanx of the patient's toe. With the other hand he fixes the corresponding metatarsal. After taking up the slack he increases traction simultaneously with some plantar flexion, using the first phalanx of his flexed forefinger as a fulcrum. Although there is no real thrust, or only a very low velocity thrust, a click can frequently be heard. This is a simple technique, but care must be taken not to press the joints, which are very tender.

A technique that patients find agreeable consists in spreading the metatarsals fan-wise (*Figure 6.15*). To do this the therapist stands at the foot of the table while the patient sits facing him, on the table, with knees bent and heels resting on the table. The therapist takes the metatarsals in both hands, the thenar above while the fingers form a fulcrum on the plantar aspect; he then spreads the dorsum of the foot.

The tarsometatarsal joints and the joints between the tarsal bones

The term 'Lisfranc's and Chopart's joint' is frequently used for these joints. As a rule it is better to diagnose and treat specifically the joints between single tarsal

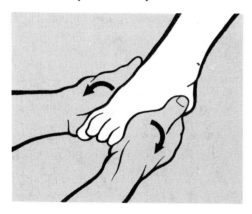

Figure 6.15 Spreading the metatarsals fan-wise

bones as well as the tarsometatarsal joints. A very effective technique for treating Lisfranc's joint (all the tarsometatarsal joints) and Chopart's joint (the articulation between both the cuboid and navicular bone with the talus and calcaneus) together is as follows (*Figure 6.16*). The patient lies supine with the leg bent at the knee, the heel on the table. The therapist stands at the side of the table and clasps the patient's (left) ankle with his (right) hand so as to fix either the talus or the cuneiformia with the cuboid from above. With the other hand at the level of either the cuboid and the navicular, or at the base of the metatarsals, he clasps the instep and after taking up the slack in a dorsal or plantar direction springs the joints in one or the other direction.

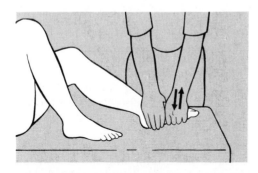

Figure 6.16 Mobilization of the tarsometatarsal and transverse tarsal joints (After Sachse, 1973.)

The following techniques used here correspond to those described for single carpal bones: for diagnosis of joint play the therapist fixes the proximal bone (most frequently a tarsal bone) between thumb and forefinger while the thumb and forefinger of his other hand grasp the base of a metatarsal bone, to examine dorsoplantar shift. To carry out this manoeuvre exactly it is best first to take up the slack in a dorsal direction, springing the joint in the same direction, and then to take up the slack in a plantar direction and again spring the joint in end-position.

For mobilization, however, it is better first to place both thumbs on the plantar aspect and both forefingers on the dorsal aspect of two adjacent bones, to take up the slack by slight pressure, and then by slightly increasing and then releasing pressure (in end-position) rhythmically to mobilize the joint in one direction. The position of the thumbs and forefingers is then reversed to perform mobilization in the same way in the opposite direction.

This is an almost universal technique which may be used for the tarsometatarsal joints, the joints between the cuneiform bones and the navicular, between the navicular and the cuboid and the calcaneus. The most frequent site of restriction is, however, the second, third and fourth tarsometatarsal joints.

After this shifting technique a similarly 'universal' traction technique should be employed (*Figure 6.17*). The patient lies prone, her legs slightly bent at the knee. The therapist puts the fingers of both hands round the patient's instep with both thumbs on the plantar aspect of the distal of two adjacent bones (e.g. on the base of the third metatarsal). He takes up the slack by slight plantar flexion and traction along the long axis of the foot, and can then deliver a thrust by a sudden pull. Recently I have developed a technique that is gentler, more effective, and agreeable to the patient; this consists in simply shaking the foot rhythmically up and

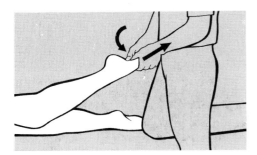

Figure 6.17 Traction manipulation (mobilization) of the tarsal bones by thrust or by rhythmical shaking

down while maintaining traction, rather fast (several shakes per second). This must be done with a relaxed hand, so as to sense the optimum rhythm. A few seconds of this shaking mobilization is sufficient. It can also be used to treat the cuneiform, the cuboid and the navicular.

The subtalar joint

This joint is formed by the talus, the calcaneus and the navicular. To examine joint play and mobilize the joint, the therapist grasps the patient's instep with one hand and cups the other round her heel (*Figure 6.18*); the patient is supine. With this grip

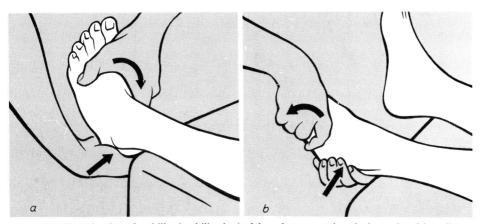

Figure 6.18 Examination of mobility (mobilization) of the calcaneus against the instep in a (*a*) medial and (*b*) lateral direction

the therapist can perform most of the possible movements between the calcaneus and the forefoot: lateral flexion, relative rotation, plantar flexion and dorsal flexion of the forefoot.

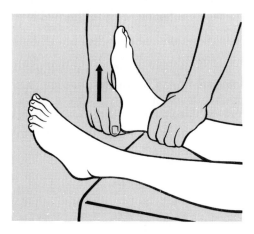

Figure 6.19 Gapping the subtalar joint by pulling on the heel

A very effective traction technique has been developed for the posterior part of the subtalar joint (*Figure 6.19*). The patient is supine with the heel over the free edge of the table; the therapist stands alongside the leg and fixes the distal part of the leg against the table from above. With his other hand he grasps the heel and pulls it slightly upwards to take up the slack, then delivers a thrust by a sudden increase in the force of the pull.

The ankle joint

Here joint play consists in a relative anteroposterior shift of the talus against the fork formed by the distal end of the tibia and fibula. For examination and mobilization the patient is supine, the knee slightly bent and the heel on the table (*Figure 6.20*). The therapist stands alongside the leg and grasps the heel in one hand, supporting the foot with his forearm to hold it at right angles to the leg. He then takes up the slack by a slight push from above and springs it rhythmically in the same direction.

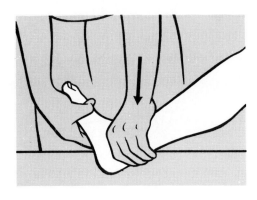

Figure 6.20 Examination of joint play and mobilization of the ankle joint by springing the leg against the heel

There is also a very effective traction technique (*Figure 6.21*). The patient is supine with legs stretched; the therapist stands at the end of the table and grasps the patient's instep with clasped hands, the thumbs parallel on the sole to stabilize the foot at right angles to the leg. He must take care not to hold the foot in maximum dorsiflexion because that would lock the ankle joint. He now takes up the slack by a slight pull along the long axis of the leg, and then makes a thrust in the same direction, as a rule obtaining a 'click'.

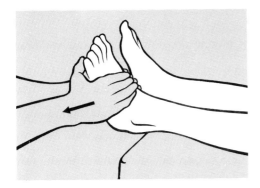

Figure 6.21 Traction manipulation of the ankle joint

An alternative technique is to grasp the forefoot with one hand and the heel with the other, carrying out traction; in this case the subtalar joint is also treated. In both cases the most common mistake is exaggerated dorsiflexion of the foot, and too much force applied to taking up the slack.

The tibiofibular joint

For diagnosis as for mobilization, we move the fibular head on the tibia in an anteroposterior direction, as on the circumference of a circle (*Figure 6.22*). The patient is supine, the knee bent and the foot on the table. The therapist sits so as to fix the patient's toes with his buttocks, grasping the fibular head between thumb

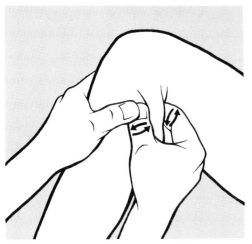

Figure 6.22 Mobilization of the fibular head against the tibia

and forefinger; with the other hand he fixes the tibia below the knee. With his fingers round the fibular head he makes a dorsal and ventral shift round the tibia, to determine which direction is most restricted. For mobilization he takes up the slack in the restricted direction and rhythmically springs the end-position. It is useful to reinforce the thumb at the fibular head with the thumb of the other hand, which follows the rotatory movement round the tibia.

The knee joint

The technique of examination and restoration of joint play begins with the patella: with the leg extended and the quadriceps muscle relaxed, the patella should be freely mobile against the femur in all directions. If there is restriction, there is no real blockage; what we find is some resistance, as though the patella was moving over an uneven or rough surface. This sensation is even more marked if some pressure is applied to the patella from above. While the patient lies supine with the leg stretched at the knee, the therapist grasps the patella between the thumb and fingers of one hand, while the other hand exerts slight pressure from above with the thenar eminence. With both hands acting in unison the therapist now moves the patella so as to sense where the roughness lies; he then slightly increases pressure so as to smooth out the roughness, without causing pain. After a few repetitions he feels that roughness and resistance have subsided. At this moment, too, the patient feels considerable relief. This technique can be taught to patients for self-treatment.

The knee joint can be treated first by (dis)traction techniques (*Figure 6.23*). The simplest is to lay the patient prone on a mat on the floor, the knee bent at right angles. The therapist (standing) puts one foot on the thigh just above the knee and grasps the leg with both hands round the ankle, pulling it in a vertical direction.

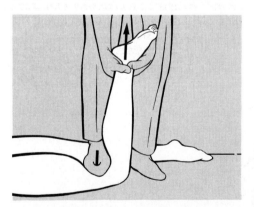

Figure 6.23 Knee traction with the patient prone

As at the elbow, lateral springing to gap the joint on the medial or lateral aspect is an important technique (*Figure 6.24*). The patient lies supine, the leg stretched but not overstretched. The therapist stands by the table alongside the affected knee; with one hand he grips the patient's ankle, lifting it slightly above the table. With the other hand supported by the trunk he exerts slight pressure at the level of the joint space to take up the slack, and then springs the joint medially. In order to spring the joint laterally, the therapist must sit on the table between the patient's legs, facing the knee joint.

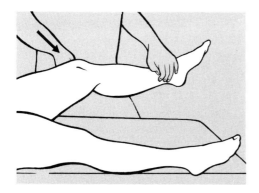

Figure 6.24 Lateral springing (gapping) of the knee joint

To apply a slight thrust, which is sometimes useful, we use this technique but first ask the patient to bend and stretch the knee; while the patient actively stretches the joint the therapist delivers a slight thrust at the knee joint, with his hand, in a medial or lateral direction.

As with the elbow, it is important that the therapist should stand at the level of the knee, so that the hand that springs the joint is supported by the movement of the trunk; the hand that grasps the heel is there for fixation only, and should never deliver a thrust. Fast shaking is a useful alternative.

The hip joint

This joint, as an almost ideal ball-and-socket joint, hardly allows shifting movement; I shall therefore only describe traction techniques. They are the most important and the most effective. Traction may be carried out either along the long axis of the leg, or in the direction of the femoral neck.

In the former case (*Figure 6.25*), the patient is supine with a strap fixing the pelvis. The therapist stands at the foot of the table; a strap passing round his waist is fastened round the patient's leg above the ankle. With both hands on this strap, the therapist takes up the slack by very slight traction, the leg being in 10–15 degrees abduction and flexion at the hip joint. When he feels that the patient has relaxed he delivers a high-velocity thrust by pulling suddenly with both hands and trunk, thus pulling the femoral head slightly out of the socket. (This movement is only of a few mm, as visualized by X-ray.) When traction is released there is a tiny thud.

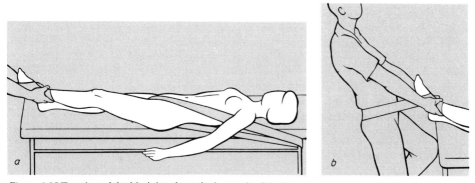

Figure 6.25 Traction of the hip joint along the long axis of the leg, using two straps: (*a*) fixation of the patient with one strap; (*b*) applying the second strap

The following technical details are important: (1) the therapist should take up the slack with as little force as possible, i.e. by waiting for the patient to relax or by beginning with PR; (2) the therapist must not release his pull before giving the thrust; (3) he must not squeeze the ankle with his hands.

I use traction by PR much more often than this high-velocity thrust. As the force used in the former is minimal, strapping is unnecessary. Grasping the patient's heel the therapist tells her to resist traction, i.e. to pull up her leg with minimum force and hold this movement for about 10 s. Towards the end of this isometric phase the patient should breathe in; she is then told to 'let go' and to breathe out. All that the therapist now feels is that the leg lengthens by relaxation, without any further pull. This manoeuvre is repeated 3–5 times.

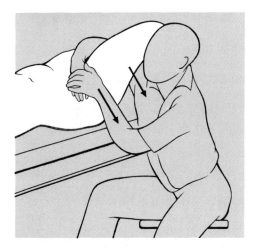

Figure 6.26 Traction of the hip joint along the axis of the femoral neck, over the edge of the table

For traction in the direction of the femoral neck the patient is supine, the buttock on the edge of the table, forming a fulcrum (*Figure 6.26*). The therapist sits on a stool by the side of the table, the patient's leg over his shoulder, with bent knee. He now grasps the patient's thigh with both hands, his forearm in the groin, and gives a slight oblique pull in the direction of the femoral neck. The patient puts up slight resistance by pulling the bent leg in the opposite direction, with the pelvis (i.e. in the direction of the opposite shoulder). This resistance is held for about 10 s during inspiration, after which the patient is told to 'let go' and breathe out. Again, during relaxation the thigh is felt to lengthen slightly. This technique is much less effective when passive pull only is used, with or without the high-velocity thrust.

As the lower extremity is accessible to both the patient's hands, many of the techniques described are useful for self-treatment.

The temporomandibular joint

For treatment, laterolateral movements of the jaw are most convenient, and again PR provides the gentlest and most effective technique (*Figure 6.27*). The patient is seated, with her head turned to one side; the therapist stands behind her, stabilizing the patient's head against his own chest. The patient is told to open her mouth, i.e. to let her chin drop; the therapist cradles the mandible from the side, between two fingers, moving it to the opposite side, towards his chest. When he has taken up the slack he asks the patient to breathe *out* during the isometric phase and *in* during relaxation (*see* page 37). During relaxation the mandible moves in the direction of the affected joint. The procedure is repeated 3–5 times.

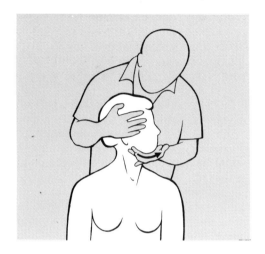

Figure 6.27 Mobilization of the temporomandibular joint

Most frequently, however, movement restriction is dominated by spasm of the masticatory muscles which have to be relaxed. Making use of a respiratory synkinesis – opening the mouth during inspiration, we begin with expiration – the patient opens his mouth, we stand behind him, his head against our chest and put our fingers on the lower incisors, fixing the forehead with the other hand. During inspiration he is told to open his mouth 'as though yawning'. During expiration we give resistance to closing the mouth and during inspiration the patient again opens it. After 3–5 repetitions there is full relaxation and restoration of movement. Conversely, the digastricus can be relaxed by resisting opening of the mouth during inspiration and closing (relaxation) during expiration.

The spinal column

The principles set out at the beginning of this chapter also hold for the spinal column. There are, however, some specific technical points to be dealt with; for instance, it is obviously more difficult to move a single mobile segment than a single extremity joint. Also, it is more difficult to distinguish joint play from function movement in the spinal column. Since it is not possible to move a single segment actively, passive movement represents as it were joint play. This difficulty applies particularly to shifting techniques, and less to distraction. Techniques that produce gapping thus clearly use joint play for their effect (e.g. rotation in the lumbar spine, dorsoventral thrusts in the thoracic spine). Because of this relative difficulty in moving single joints we distinguish specific and non-specific techniques.

There are several ways of achieving specific effect: the ideal way, although not always practicable, is direct fixation of at least one partner (this can always be done in an extremity joint). Another way is to apply 'locking' techniques if leverage is used; this is to great advantage, for example, when moving the head in order to manipulate the cervical spine, or the legs and pelvis in order to mobilize the lumbar spine. To make such a technique specific we must try to 'lock' all the segments except for the one we wish to manipulate. The principle of 'locking' consists in bringing into an extreme position the segments we do *not* move, under a certain degree of tension. The mechanism is either apposition of bony structures or tension of ligaments. Even here, however, we have to take up the slack to make any type of manipulation effective. It can thus be seen that the 'locking' is only relative, and if leverage is forceful treatment will never be specific. Leverage is of course very advantageous, but it must be applied with very little force to make locking techniques effective.

Locking is achieved mainly by a careful combination of side-bending and rotation, making use of spontaneous synkineses. Lordosis in the lumbar spine means that there is side-bending coupled with rotation in the opposite direction; hence we achieve locking by rotation and side-bending in the same direction. In kyphosis the opposite is true, and we therefore have to combine side-bending and rotation in the opposite direction. In the thoracic spine side-bending is always coupled with rotation to the opposite side (in scoliosis rotation is always to the same side) and therefore locking entails side-bending and rotation to the same side. In the cervical spine there is always side-bending and rotation to the same side, and here we achieve locking by side-bending and rotation to the opposite side.

An obvious way of achieving some degree of specificity is by direct contact. Clearly, a vertebra may be fixed by direct contact in at least one direction, for instance by fixation of a spinous process from the side we prevent rotation of that vertebra in the opposite direction. If we exert pressure, spring a vertebra or apply a thrust, some of the force will be effective at the site where it is applied. Indeed, chiropractors believe that a high-velocity thrust applied with sufficient energy acts like a hammer on an uncemented brick wall, throwing one brick out and leaving all the rest in place.

To achieve the maximum specific effect, a combination of leverage and locking techniques with direct contact and fixation is most commonly used. However advantageous these techniques, they are effective only if leverage and locking are applied exactly to the site where the other hand makes contact.

From this it would appear obvious that the hand which makes contact fixes or moves the vertebra in a direction opposed to the direction of leverage applied by the other hand. This is usually true, but there are certain techniques in which both hands move in the same direction, as a single force, the segment below the treated vertebra being fixed by positioning (e.g. the pelvis fixed by the patient sitting astride the table). This type of technique gives considerable leverage, and must depend mainly on locking. It is used most frequently in pure traction techniques, which – although they are without risk and are certainly effective – are of doubtful specific effect unless very gently applied.

There are also unspecific techniques that can be useful in mobilizing longer sections of the spinal column. Such a generally non-specific but widely used technique is that of traction along the long axis of the spine. Its importance and indication have been discussed in Chapter 5 (page 182).

In order to avoid confusion it is important to distinguish between traction along the long axis of the spinal column and distraction of intervertebral joints. This distinction is clearest in the lumbar region, where traction along the long axis acts on the intervertebral discs, whereas distraction of the apophyseal joints is produced by rotation round that same axis. In the cervical spine, on the other hand, traction along the long axis affects the discs and the joints.

Another type of non-specific method is represented by the 'soft-tissue techniques'. These are basically massage techniques, applied mainly to muscles in spasm, using pressure, kneading, or moving the muscles in a direction at right angles to their fibres. However useful these techniques have proved, they are now overshadowed by the techniques of specific muscle relaxation, which will be described in detail later.

The lumbar spine

Traction techniques

Intermittent manual traction is the most important of these methods. If the patient can lie prone it is best if she provides her own fixation by holding on to the end of the table. The therapist grasps both the patient's legs just above the ankle, and with slight traction makes sure that she is completely relaxed. He must then establish the correct rhythm of traction, in order to localize the effect in the low back. If the rhythm is too slow, the patient's whole body will move slightly, up and down, on the table. By quickening the rhythm the therapist will find at which point only the legs and pelvis move while the low back remains still, like a nodal point in a standing wave. When this rhythm has been found, the patient feels the intermittent traction exactly in the low back. This should be done with little force, but once the rhythm is established each pull may be reinforced and occasionally something like a thrust delivered.

Obviously this method implies *manual* traction only. The therapist must avoid squeezing the legs above the ankle.

If the patient cannot stretch out, as is often the case in the acute stage, intermittent traction is carried out in kyphosis (*Figure 6.28(a)*). For this the patient lies on her back with her legs bent at the hip and knee. If the table is adjustable, the patient lies with her pelvis at the end of the table and the therapist stands facing her. If not, the therapist must kneel on the table, his thighs close to those of the patient. The therapist then places the patient's legs on his own iliac crests, fixing them against his body with his arms, and clasps his hands under the patient's bent knees. By straightening up he lifts the patient's pelvis slightly from the table; with correct leverage this is not difficult. It is advisable to let the patient's pelvis sway slightly from side to side in order to obtain complete relaxation, and then to perform intermittent traction by alternately bending and straightening one's trunk.

There are two important technical points: to get good leverage the therapist's hands and thighs must be as close to the patient's thighs as possible; and he must straighten up by increasing lumbar lordosis, not by leaning backwards.

There are two very effective and gentle traction methods that make use of PR. For the first the patient lies prone (*Figure 6.28(b)*), with her head near to the end of the table. The therapist stands at the head of the table and puts the heel of his hand on the patient's buttocks from above. He tells the patient to breathe out slowly and deeply, and feels resistance *increasing*. The patient is then told to take a slow, deep breath, and as he does so the buttocks move down and the lumbar spinal lordosis flattens. This is followed by long, deep expiration and again the buttocks tend to move upwards. The therapist resists this movement, which is followed by relaxation or a caudal movement of the buttocks during inspiration. Resistance to each

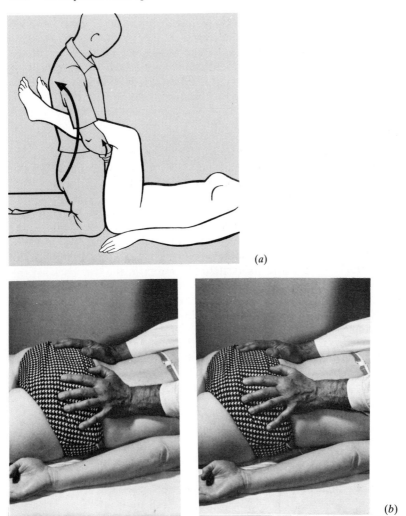

Figure 6.28 (a) Traction of the lumbar spine in kyphosis (supine). *(b)* Isometric traction of the lumbar spine (prone): left, increased resistance during expiration; right, the buttocks move in a caudal direction during inspiration

upward movement of the buttocks during expiration increases the intensity of the traction.

For traction with PR in kyphosis, the patient is prone over the end of the table, her legs hanging down from the hips; the table should be high enough for the feet to be clear of the floor. The therapist stands at the side of the patient's low back, placing the heels of his crossed hands one on the sacrum (from above) and the other from below on the spinous process of a lumbar vertebra, according to the site where traction is required. He now tells the patient to give slight resistance to the traction he applies by a slight push on the sacrum, in a caudal direction, and with the other hand in a cranial direction. The patient is told to breathe out slowly and then to 'let go' and breathe in.

There are many well-known methods of traction performed on special tables, including intermittent traction, but none can compete with manual traction by a skilled therapist. There is one principle that must be stressed, however, both in manual and especially in table traction: *it must not be painful.* If the patient feels discomfort, the therapist must find a position in which traction is well tolerated, or else abandon it.

Manipulation

In manipulation it is useful to begin by using the springing technique described for the examination of retroflexion in individual mobile segments (*see* page 116). The patient lies with both hips and knees flexed. The therapist leans his thigh against the patient's knees, fixing the spinous process of the upper vertebra of the treated segment with one finger, reinforced by the fingers of the other hand placed over it. He now tells the patient to press her knees *very* slightly against the therapist's thigh (but not so hard as to push him away) and to hold this pressure for about 10 s. At the end of this isometric phase the patient should breathe in, after which she is told to 'let go' and breathe out. While the patient relaxes the therapist has the impression that the hands on the spinous process are sinking into a hollow, as the mobilized spinal segment moves into lordosis. The procedure is repeated from this position, about three times (*see Figure 4.10,* page 118).

The most popular manipulative technique is probably that of rotation, with the patient lying on her side (*Figure 6.29*). She should be in a 'neutral' position, i.e. neither in flexion nor extension. The leg that lies on the table is not fully extended

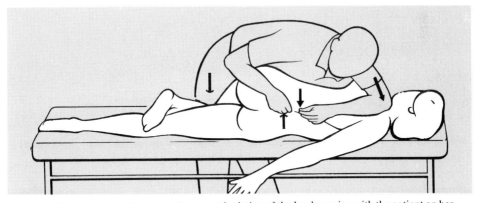

Figure 6.29 Rotation mobilization or thrust manipulation of the lumbar spine with the patient on her side, in neutral position

while the other is bent at the hip and knee, so that the foot is fixed by the slightly bent knee on the table; the other knee is bent and projects over the edge of the table. The therapist stands in front of the patient so as to fix the flexed knee with his thigh. Passing his hand over the patient's hip, he fixes it with his forearm while with the ulnar aspect of the hand he fixes the part of the lumbar spine that is caudal to the lower vertebra of the segment being treated; one or two fingers are used to fix the transverse process of that vertebra. In this way he can completely fix the lumbar spine, up to the segment to be treated. The elbow of the therapist's other arm lies on the patient's shoulder (unless the patient is much taller than the therapist, in which case it lies on the arm below the shoulder) and it is helpful if the patient slings this arm round that of the therapist. With the thumb of the hand coming from the shoulder the therapist establishes contact with the spinous process of the upper vertebra of the segment to be treated. Obviously if this is the lumbosacral segment it is sufficient for the hand passing over the patient's hip to fix the pelvis alone. In order to take up the slack it is best to tell the patient to look in the direction of mobilization (i.e. away from the therapist). With the patient thus positioned, the therapist fixes the shoulder (or arm) from above and tells the patient to look towards him and breathe in slowly; the therapist resists rotation (in the opposite direction from mobilization). The patient is then told to look in the direction of mobilization and to breathe out slowly. In this way the range of rotation automatically increases, a new position is reached and fixed by the therapist, and the procedure repeated about three times. Quite frequently a spontaneous 'click' is heard during relaxation.

A repetitive technique from the extreme position reached by relaxation can be used, as a modification. With his hand over the patient's buttocks to maintain fixation, the therapist tells her to turn to and fro; he may even reinforce the fixing hand by the other (*Figure 6.30*). Or, when the slack is taken up (and end-position is

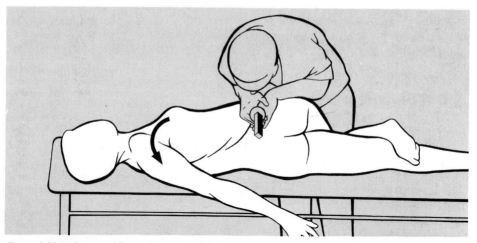

Figure 6.30 Active repetitive mobilization of the lumbar spine with the patient lying on her side

reached), he may make an additional thrust against the shoulder. This is a fully automatic mobilization technique, the patient resisting while looking towards the therapist and breathing in, and relaxing when looking away from him and breathing out. It should be the basic technique used in extension restriction. It produces gapping of the upper intervertebral joint and can be used throughout the lumbar spine and even at the thoracolumbar junction.

The other technique of similar importance is mobilization in flexion (for flexion restriction, *Figure 6.31*). The patient again lies on her side, but in a somewhat kyphotic position, the leg on the table flexed at the hip and knee. The other (upper) leg hangs over the edge of the table (except where the straight leg raising test is highly positive, in which case she bends the leg so as to fix the foot at the knee of the lower limb). The therapist first fixes the pelvis in an oblique position, i.e. not perpendicular to the table but tilted forward so that the weight of the hanging leg enhances kyphosis. The therapist uses his other hand to pull forward the arm on which the patient is lying, so as to increase kyphosis still further. This must be done with great care, so as not to straighten the pelvis, i.e. not to return it to the perpendicular. This position is essential for the success of the technique; the therapist fixes the patient's leg with his thigh, passing his forearm over the hip, the hand pointing in the direction of the caudal vertebra of the segment to be treated. With the elbow of the other arm against the patient's shoulder, the therapist rotates the trunk away from himself, to take up the slack (the patient should be told to look up at the ceiling). The thumb of the hand over the shoulder fixes the spinous process of the upper vertebra from above, by a downward pull with the distal phalanx of the thumb. Again, if the therapist is not tall, it is better for the patient to sling her arm round the therapist's, so that the therapist can exert pressure against the patient's arm below the shoulder.

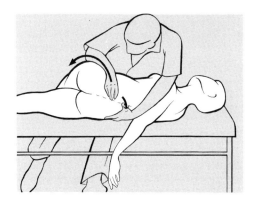

Figure 6.31 Mobilization or thrust manipulation of the lumbar spine with the patient on her side, in kyphosis, the lower leg bent and the upper hanging down over the edge of the table

In this position the patient is told to press her hip slightly against the therapist's hand so as to lift both hip and leg, and to hold this pressure for about 10 s, while breathing in. She is then told to 'let go' and breathe out, and as she relaxes the hanging leg and hip produce further hip rotation and lumbar kyphosis, and the therapist can feel the distance between his hands increasing. This procedure can be repeated 3–5 times. If the slack has been taken up, the hand on the patient's hip may also give a thrust in the same direction. In every case, the thumb on the spinous process must maintain fixation.

How this technique can also be used for muscular relaxation and self-treatment will be described later in this chapter (*see Figure 6.91*, page 273).

The technique produces some degree of rotation and gapping of the joints and effects traction with anteflexion and great muscular relaxation.

There are very many other techniques in use, particularly thrusting manipulation in a dorsoventral direction with the patient prone or on her side, but they do not seem to me to be of such value as to be worth describing here.

The pelvis

The only joint that is treated by manipulation is the sacroiliac. For mobilization excellent results can be achieved with movements in two almost perpendicular planes, the sagittal (nutation of the sacrum in relation to the innominate) and the horizontal (gapping the dorsal part of the sacroiliac joint by springing the ilium against the sacrum). As there are no muscles to move or fix the sacroiliac joint, the simple passive repetitive technique with a minimum of force is always effective, provided there is no structural change present.

For mobilization in the sagittal plane, the patient is prone, while the therapist stands at the side of the table, facing the patient's pelvis, and with crossed hands places one pisiform on the posterior superior iliac spine from below, and the other on the caudal end of the sacrum (*Figure 6.32*). With slight pressure he takes up the

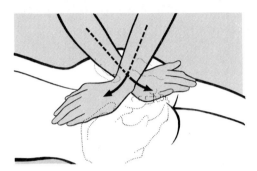

Figure 6.32 Mobilization of the sacroiliac joint, with crossed hands (also used for examination)

slack and can now spring the joint not so much by pressing his hands downwards as by separating them, again with very little force. It is most important that after slightly increasing his pressure the therapist releases it, even if at first there is no response in the blocked joint. After about five repetitions with no increase in force he should begin to sense movement, and mobility is usually restored to normal after about 15 repetitions. The technique should be performed at one or two moves to the second. The following points are important: the pisiform moving the sacrum must be at the caudal end, just above the coccyx, otherwise the lever is too short; taking up the slack implies bony contact – the therapist must move *bone,* not skin. The most serious mistake is to increase pressure before any movement has been felt. Apparently, it is the release pressure that makes the joint spring.

For mobilization in the horizontal plane, a diagnostic technique (*see Figure 4.6,* page 113) can be used, with the patient lying on her side. Once again, all I have said about applying minimum pressure and the importance of releasing it is valid. There is one important detail to be borne in mind: although the therapist moves the anterior superior iliac spine, he must not rotate the pelvis, but only produce gapping of the posterior part of the sacroiliac joint; he must therefore push the iliac spine downwards and backwards with his forearm obliquely pointing in a ventrocraniomedial direction. Using this technique he may also apply a thrust after taking up the slack.

Kubis (1970) has described another thrust technique in the sagittal plane (*Figure 6.33*); the patient lies on her side, the leg on the table stretched and the other bent at hip and knee, with the foot stabilized by the knee beneath it. The therapist stands at the side of the table, facing the patient's pelvis, and fixes the knee with his thigh while rotating the shoulder away from himself. He now makes contact with his pisiform (or the first phalanx of the bent forefinger) pressing on the caudal tip of the sacrum, to take up the slack in a dorsoventral direction, and delivers a thrust in the same direction. There are two important technical points to be noted: the

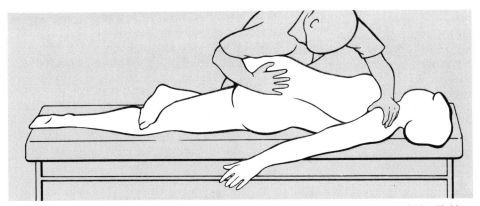

Figure 6.33 Thrusting technique in a dorsoventral direction, against the *tip* of the sacrum (After Kubis, 1969.)

therapist's forearm delivering the thrust must lie in the direction of the thrust, which means that he must bend over the patient; and pelvic rotation must be avoided, the thrust being only dorsoventral.

This technique produces an anterior shift of the end of the sacrum against the ilium which is fixed because the patient is lying on it; the result is a movement of nutation round a frontal axis at S2, acting on the *joint on the side on which the patient is lying*. It is very useful to spring the lower and/or the upper end of the sacrum against the ilium with the patient lying on her side (*see* page 113).

The coccyx

In the majority of cases of a tender coccyx, PR of the glutei maximi (*see Figure 6.97*, page 278) is very effective, and can be administered as self-treatment. It is only in exceptional cases that manipulation per rectum is necessary; even when carefully performed this is unpleasant and even painful. It is a very effective technique, yet the mechanism is still obscure; the sacrococcygeal junction is not a true joint, and there is no movement restriction.

For manipulation the patient lies prone with her heels rotated outwards, or is on knees and elbows. The therapist inserts his forefinger into the rectum, first ascertaining whether the levator ani is not tense on both sides; if it is, he must relax it by massage. Then by moving the coccyx he finds the exact site of the sacrococcygeal synchrondrosis; he may apply counter-pressure with the thumb of the other hand at the end of the sacrum. He may now move the coccyx in a dorsal direction, or simply exert pressure on the sacrococcygeal synchondrosis with the inserted finger and the thumb on the end of the sacrum. After two or three repetitions he must determine whether the coccyx is no longer tender.

The thoracic spine

Here there are no pure traction techniques such as we use in the lumbar and cervical regions. A manoeuvre frequently practised by laymen perhaps provides the nearest thing to traction: the patient (standing or seated) crosses her arms over her chest, with her hands on her shoulders or face. The therapist stands behind her and passes his hands round the patient's body to cup the further elbow, pressing the patient's thoracic spine and ribs against his own chest, to take up the slack. He then straightens up, imparting a thrust to the patient's elbows, in an upward direction, at the same time pressing him closer to his own chest. This unsophisticated and non-specific technique is quite harmless unless the patient suffers from severe osteoporosis.

As stiff increased kyphosis is probably the most frequent disorder in the thoracic region, back-bending mobilization is probably the technique most frequently called for. In order to make full use of the patient's own musculature it is possible to employ not only PR but also the active contraction of the erector spinae during *maximum* expiration.

For the first technique, the patient sits on the table, her legs hanging down and feet crossed; the therapist stands facing her, leaning his thighs against the patient's knees to stabilize her. The patient raises her crossed arms and rests them against the therapist's chest. The therapist puts his arms round the patient, making contact with his fingers on the spinous process of the caudal vertebra of the blocked segment; he first tells the patient to relax, so as to take up the slack by slight pressure on the spinous process, increasing lordosis. He then tells the patient to press her back gently against the fingers on the spinous process, breathing in slowly. A slight increase in kyphosis is inevitable at this stage. The patient is then told to breathe out and relax, trying to achieve maximum expiration. The therapist does not press but uses his fingers to indicate the point into which the patient should breathe; maximum thoracic lordosis is thus achieved. The procedure is repeated about three times. This is a most useful technique for the lower thoracic spine. This technique can be usefully modified as follows: the patient sits facing a wall, leaning both knees and her crossed arms against the wall. The therapist stands behind her, putting the heel of one hand on the spinous process of the caudal vertebra of the blocked segment, after which he proceeds as described above. Not only is this technique very comfortable for the patient, but it lends itself readily to self-treatment, as soon as the patient has realized which segments she must breathe into (*Figure 6.34*).

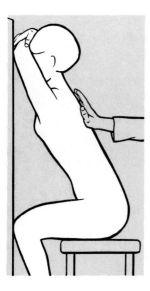

Figure 6.34 Mobilization of the thoracic spine into extension sitting (expiration)

For extension mobilization in the upper thoracic spine (*Figure 6.35*), the patient lies on her side with her hands clasped behind her head; the therapist stands in front of her, his shoulder and upper arm leaning against the patient's elbows, his forearm under the arm lying on the table. If the patient can bring her elbows together in front of her neck, the therapist may grasp them with one hand. The forefinger of his other hand is placed on the spinous process of the caudal vertebra of the blocked segment. He now moves the patient into retroflexion (as at examination), so as to take up the slack. At this point he tells the patient to press her elbows slightly into anteflexion (the therapist resisting) and to breathe in slowly. As in the preceding technique, a slight increase in kyphosis is unavoidable at this stage. After this the patient is told to relax and achieve maximum expiration, especially at the point where she feels the therapist's finger. As expiration reaches the maximum, the thoracic spine moves spontaneously into retroflexion. The procedure is repeated about three times.

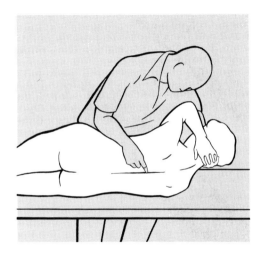

Figure 6.35 Mobilization of the thoracic spine into extension with the patient lying on her side (expiration)

Before proceeding to describe thrusting techniques in the thoracic spine I will deal with mobilization into flexion. Flexion restriction is most often found where the kyphotic arch of the thoracic spine is flattened, which is most frequently the case in the upper thoracic region and also at the thoracolumbar junction.

A very convenient way of mobilizing into flexion is provided by the examination technique (*see Figure 4.14*, page 120). The therapist thus moves the patient into anteflexion with the summit of the arch at the point where his finger is placed; he tells the patient to give some resistance to forward bending, for about 10 s, and then to 'let go'. This procedure is repeated 3–5 times.

Another technique uses a cushion for better fixation (*Figure 6.36*). The patient sits on the table with her arms crossed over her chest. The therapist stands behind the patient, with a small firm cushion between his chest and the patient's back, so placed that the top of the cushion fixes the spinous process of the caudal vertebra of the blocked segment. He now grasps with one hand the *elbow* of the arm lying closer to the patient's chest, while his other hand grips the wrist of the arm that lies above it. By this grip the therapist curves the patient's back so as to make the curve culminate at the top of the cushion, and takes up the slack in anteflexion. He now

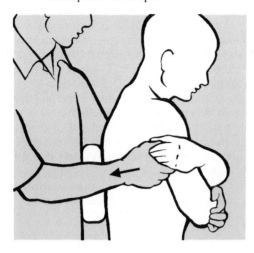

Figure 6.36 Mobilization (manipulation) of the thoracic spine into kyphosis, using a cushion, the patient seated

tells the patient to give slight resistance to this anteflexion, with the elbow of the arm closer to the chest. After about 10 s she is told to 'let go', increasing kyphosis by relaxation until the slack is again taken up. This procedure is repeated 3–5 times.

For the upper thoracic spine, where restricted anteflexion is relatively frequent, there is another mobilization technique which is particularly effective. It is applied on the side of restricted anteflexion (*see* page 108) and here the bulging of the transverse process on the normal side during anteflexion is a useful diagnostic criterion. The patient (*Figure 6.37*) sits on the table and the therapist stands behind her; with one hand he grasps the patient's head, his palm on the occiput on the side of the lesion (i.e. he uses the left hand if the lesion is on the right). He moves the head into anteflexion, side-bending and rotation to the opposite side. With the thumb of the other hand he fixes the transverse process of the lower vertebra of the segment to be treated. To take up the slack with the hand that moves the patient's

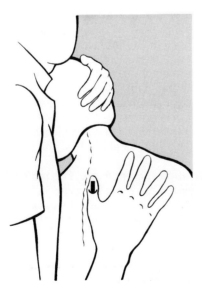

Figure 6.37 One-sided mobilization of the thoracic spine into kyphosis, the patient seated; the transverse process is fixed with the thumb

head, he tells him to look towards the side of mobilization and with his right hand
(if the lesion is on the left) he moves the head into anteflexion, side-bending and
rotation to the right side. He then tells the patient to look towards the side of the
lesion and to breathe in slowly, then to look in the other direction and breathe out.
This procedure is repeated about three times.

The technique in *Figure 6.36* can also be used to deliver a thrust. When the slack
has been taken up the therapist suddenly exerts pressure (pull) simultaneously at
the elbow and the wrist, so as to increase flexion against the edge of the cushion. A
thrust can be delivered by this technique into extension as well as into flexion. This
is done by the therapist not increasing kyphosis by his pull on the patient's arm;
instead he produces extension, or rather dorsal shift of the upper vertebra over the
edge of the cushion, to take up the slack. The thrust follows in the same direction,
during expiration. To apply traction, the operator pulls the patient up.

A closely similar effect can be obtained by a widely used technique, with the
patient supine, her hands clasped behind her neck and both elbows touching in
front of the chin (*Figures 6.38* and *6.39*). The therapist stands by the side of the
table and grasps both elbows with the hand nearer to the patient's head, turning the

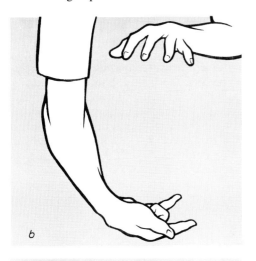

Figure 6.38 Position of the therapist's hands
during manipulation of the thoracic spine with
the patient supine

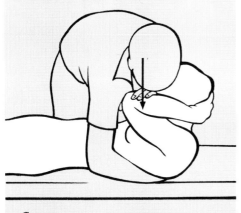

Figure 6.39 Manipulation of the thoracic spine
with the patient supine

patient towards him. He bends the middle finger of the other hand so that the fingertip touches the palm, and applies the middle phalanx of the bent finger to the transverse process of the caudal vertebra of the blocked segment on the near side, and the thenar eminence to the transverse process of the far side, the spinous process lying in the groove between the bent middle finger and the thenar eminence. After this the therapist turns the patient on to her back so that she is lying on the hand making contact at the transverse processes; with the hand grasping the elbows the therapist now brings the thoracic spine into kyphosis, which culminates exactly at the site of the contact hand. He has now two alternatives: (1) he may further increase flexion so as to take up the slack, telling the patient to breathe in and out (this can be repeated as a preparatory mobilization), and deliver the thrust into flexion during expiration; or (2) he may slightly bend the thorax back (or let it fall back) over the fulcrum formed by the hand under the patient's back (but never so far as to let the shoulder-blades touch the table!) in order to take up the slack, asking the patient to breathe in and out slowly (this may be repeated) and then deliver the thrust in the same direction, during expiration.

It may be difficult for the patient to bring her elbows together, in which case instead of clasping her hands she should hold them with the fingertips just touching. Another possible difficulty is that some therapists begin to feel pain in the middle finger; they should use the cushion technique (*see Figure 6.36*), or try a piece of indiarubber in the crook of the middle finger.

Because of their simplicity and popularity direct thrust techniques applied to the thoracic spine, with the patient prone, must be described. No sophisticated locking technique is involved, and there is no question of distinguishing flexion and extension. The thrust must be directed at the caudal vertebra in the blocked segment, producing (like all posteroanterior thrusts) gapping or distraction of the intervertebral facet joints, which are almost in the coronal plane in the thoracic spine. The springing technique described for examination, with the patient supine (*see Figure 4.8*, page 116), can be used after taking up the slack.

Another technique can be used both for mobilization and for a high-velocity thrust, producing some rotation as well. The patient lies prone, and the therapist by the side of the table crosses his hands, placing the pisiform of one hand on the transverse process of one vertebra and that of the other hand on the transverse process of the adjacent vertebra (*Figure 6.40*). He takes up the slack by slight direct pressure and while the patient breathes out he may deliver a thrust to produce gapping of the articulation on the side of the hand moving the caudal vertebra of the blocked segment, in this way restoring rotation to that side. Instead of delivering a high-velocity thrust, he may simply gently increase his pressure, springing the joint while the patient breathes out. This type of mobilization can be carried out as a non-specific treatment, in the rhythm of respiration, in one segment after the other, rather like massage.

Thus far I have been describing techniques dealing with dorsoventral movement (flexion–extension). I shall now deal with side-bending and rotation.

To restore side-bending we use the same technique as for examination (*see (Figure 4.15*, page 121), the only difference being that the thumb is placed on the spinous process of the caudal vertebra to fix it, and not at the interspace for palpation. For mobilization we make use of the alternating muscle facilitation and inhibition described by Gaymans (1980).

The patient is seated on the table, her legs hanging over the side; the therapist stands behind her with one hand round her ribs and the thumb on the side of the spinous process. The other hand is placed on the patient's neck (for the upper thoracic), shoulder (for the mid-thoracic), or under her axilla (for the lower thoracic spine), and bends the patient's trunk sideways so as to take up the slack. If an even segment is being treated, the patient is told to look up and breathe in, the therapist then feeling increased resistance to the side-bending; after a *slow* deep breath the patient is told to relax and breathe out (but not to look down, which would involve bending forward). During this expiration the therapist must *wait* until he feels resistance disappear; the range of side-bending automatically increases. In the odd segments facilitation and inhibition are reversed: the patient is told to breathe out slowly (after breathing in), the therapist feeling resistance to side-bending. When expiration is complete she is told to breathe in slowly, and towards the end of this inspiration resistance to side-bending slackens and the range of movement increases. This procedure is repeated two or three times.

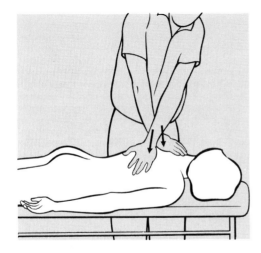

Figure 6.40 Manipulation with crossed hands making contact on the opposite transverse processes of two adjacent vertebrae, with the patient prone

There are several important technical points to note: the therapist must never force side-bending, but wait for it to increase spontaneously, and only *follow* the patient's relaxation with his hands. This usually occurs towards the end of breathing in or out. The effect of this phenomenon decreases in a caudal direction, particularly in those segments where resistance increases during expiration, to be followed by relaxation during inspiration. This is probably because the stability of the thorax as a whole increases during inspiration. The other point to watch, as I pointed out when describing examination technique, is that the hand which stabilizes the thorax from the side must create a strong fulcrum, the palm lying in the axillary line and the therapist's forearm being perpendicular to the lateral chest wall. Even if the patient is broad shouldered and the therapist has small hands, his thumb still reaches the spinous process during side-bending, owing to rotation of the vertebrae. In everyday practice the therapist rarely counts to see whether he is dealing with an odd or an even segment, but simply starts by telling the patient to look up and breathe in; if resistance increases during inspiration and relaxation follows during expiration, he is satisfied. If not, he tries the reverse procedure, beginning with expiration. This technique is very useful for mobilization, but not to deliver a thrust.

For mobilization in rotation the patient should sit astride the end of the table while the therapist stands behind her at the end, passing one arm under the patient's axilla to grasp the opposite shoulder (*Figure 6.41*). A slightly kyphotic position is recommended, to make the spinous processes more prominent. The other hand is placed with the palm against the ribs and the thumb on the spinous process of the caudal vertebra of the treated segment, from the side. To achieve good fixation the therapist's arm is abducted so that the forearm follows the direction of the thumb, and the palm stabilizes the ribs. If fixation is adequate little locking is needed. The patient is now told to look toward the side to which mobilization is being carried out, and the therapist takes up the slack. The patient is then told to look to the *opposite* side, breathing in slowly (the isometric phase), and then to look the other way again, breathing out slowly. During this relaxation phase the range of mobility increases spontaneously. The procedure is repeated two or three times.

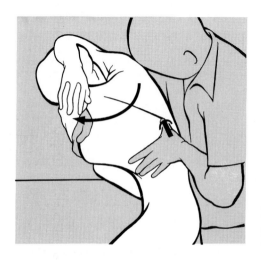

Figure 6.41 Rotation mobilization (manipulation) in slight kyphosis, with the lower vertebra of the treated segment fixed by the therapist's hand and thumb

The following technical points are important: fixation should be such that the thumb on the spinous process of the caudal vertebra remains in place. When the patient looks towards the side of mobilization, therefore, her eyes and head should naturally turn as far as the clasped hands behind her head allow, in the direction of rotation; the trunk, however, should only relax, and not actively press. The trunk must always rotate about its own axis.

The same technique can also be used to deliver a thrust, after the slack has been taken up, i.e. at the end of the relaxation phase, if it is thought advisable. In this case the therapist may increase kyphosis and slightly side-bend the trunk in the direction opposite to that of rotation, to obtain better locking. If the fixation is good, this is not absolutely necessary.

This technique is used mainly in the low thoracic spine and the thoracolumbar region, but it can also be applied to the lumbar spine.

There is another very effective technique to deliver a thrust for manipulation of the thoracic spine into rotation (*Figure 6.42*); the therapist's hand rotating the patient's trunk, and the thumb on the transverse process, act in the same direction. Careful locking is essential. The patient is seated as for the preceding technique and the therapist grasps the far shoulder, with his arm across the patient's chest, from

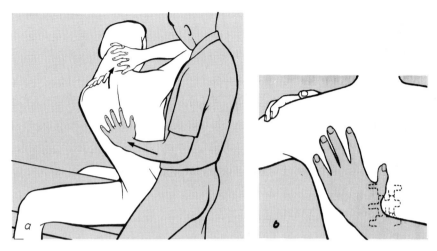

Figure 6.42 (*a*) Rotation (thrust) manipulation of the thoracic spine, the patient seated with her trunk leaning slightly backwards, rotated and bent to the same side, both the therapist's hands acting in that direction. With the patient sitting erect, the same rotation technique can be used to manipulate a rib, contact being made at the angle of the rib instead of at the transverse process. (*b*) Detail of (*a*)

behind. He now obtains locking by side-bending and rotation to the same side, so that the arch so formed culminates at the site of the segment to be treated. Rotation of the trunk must be carried out about the vertical axis of the trunk, the head remaining fixed. This is achieved by the therapist bending the patient sideways, using his elbow on the patient's chest and his hand on the shoulder; he must stand behind the patient with his legs well apart, so that he himself can rotate around the patient. After taking up the slack he delivers the thrust by further increasing rotation at the patient's shoulder, simultaneously giving a push to the transverse process in the same direction.

The following technical points are important: the axis of rotation is the patient's trunk, and his head must not deviate from side to side. Only a little side-bending is needed and is performed by means of the hand across the patient's chest, not by the therapist bending his own trunk sideways. The thrust is delivered by the therapist rotating his own body from the legs and pelvis, so that both his hands act exactly at the same moment. As there is no fixation from below, only very little force must be used. Instead of his thumb, the therapist may use his thenar or pisiform.

A technically simple but not very specific technique for mobilizing the thoraco-lumbar junction has been suggested by Gaymans (unpublished observations), making use of the rhythmical pull of the psoas (*Figure 6.43*). The patient lies on her side, with the upper hip bent at right angles. The therapist stands at the side of the table so as to resist further flexion of the patient's knee with his own thigh. He now tells the patient to look as far to the opposite side as she can, producing rotation of the head and trunk; at the same time the patient pushes her bent knee against the therapist's thigh. Or the therapist may tell the patient to resist with her knee while he himself rhythmically pushes it into extension. Mobilization is obtained by the trunk rotation and the rhythmical pull of the psoas muscle at the upper transverse processes of the thoracolumbar junction in an opposite direction. The technique should be performed at about two pushes per second. This technique is ideal for

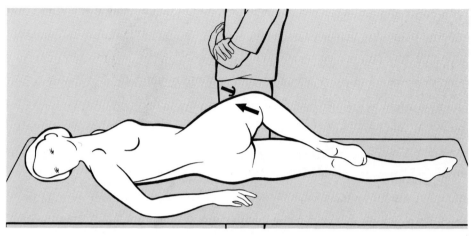

Figure 6.43 Rotation mobilization of the thoracolumbar junction with the patient on her side, looking to the opposite side during rhythmical isometric contraction of the upper psoas

self-treatment, the patient resisting rhythmical knee flexion with her outstretched arm.

All the techniques described for the thoracic spine are applicable from T3 down; the cervicothoracic junction requires techniques that will be described in the section on the cervical spine. Rotation techniques are the methods of choice in the thoracolumbar region, where trunk rotation takes place.

The ribs

The technique I myself use most frequently, particularly for the upper ribs, is a modification of the diagnostic technique of Kubis through the shoulder-blade (*see Figure 4.17,* page 122). It is also used by Mitchell (1979) with the patient supine. As presented here it closely resembles the mobilization technique of the thoracic spine

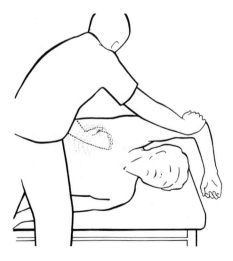

Figure 6.44 Rib mobilization into dorsal flexion during expiration, the patient on her side

into extension (*Figure 6.44*). The patient lies on her side, the upper arm raised over her head, with the elbow bent. The therapist standing at the side of the table puts one palm against the patient's elbow and the fingers of the other hand on the rib to be treated. By pushing the elbow back, using the hand fixing the rib as a fulcrum, he takes up the slack into retroflexion. At this point the patient is told to press against the therapist's hand slightly, slowly breathing in. She is then told to 'let go' and breathe out for as long as possible, directing her breath to the rib in question. When maximum expiration is reached, retroflexion increases spontaneously. This procedure is repeated about three times.

Again, as in diagnosis, the shoulder-blade is no obstacle to the fixation of the rib during retroflexion. The first rib, however, can be neither treated nor diagnosed in this way, while the second rib is the most difficult. The ribs to which this technique is most frequently applied are the third, fourth and fifth. It is technically important to raise the upper arm vertically to obtain a pure movement of retroflexion, as, if this is not the case, one easily obtains rotation, which is highly undesirable. Maximum elevation of the shoulder is therefore necessary; if there is pain in the shoulder this may prove to be an obstacle, and therefore I frequently begin with treatment of the shoulder itself (a necessity in any case if there is a shoulder lesion) before going on to treat the ribs.

Some gentle mobilization may be obtained directly while examining the 'over-take phenomenon' (*see* pages 122–3). The therapist has both thumbs on the relevant rib on either side, resisting rib movement from above, with very little force, during inspiration; he exerts slight pressure from above during expiration (mainly on the side that is 'overtaken', i.e. restricted). As a rule the overtake phenomena disappear.

The technique described for mobilization of the shoulder-blade (*see Figure 6.14,* page 207) can also be used for the ribs. The therapist lifts the shoulder with the hand that has grasped it from below, while the other hand on the shoulder-blade exerts some pressure on the scapula from above, using the medial edge of the scapula as a fulcrum. By moving the scapula up and down, and applying some pressure to the ribs, mobilization can be achieved. If it is correctly applied, the patient finds this technique pleasant.

If we find, on comparing the two sides, that one rib is restricted during *expiration,* the following technique (Greenman, 1979) is useful: the patient lies supine, while the therapist standing at the side of the table places his thumb on one of the upper ribs from above, close to the sternum. The patient is told to breathe in and out; during maximum expiration the therapist lifts the patient's trunk into slight anteflexion and gives a little push on the rib from above, with his thumb. For treatment of a lower rib the therapist's thumb must lie more laterally on the arch of the rib, and during expiration the patient's trunk is not only lifted into anteflexion but also bent to the side of the rib being treated.

If *inspiration* is restricted Greenman (1979) makes use of muscle pull. In the region of the upper ribs he uses the pull of the scalenes, for the middle ribs the pectoralis and for the lower ribs the serratus lateralis. The patient is supine and muscle pull is obtained by side-bending of the patient's head (scalenes), by maximum abduction of the arm (pectoralis) and by raising the arm (serratus), and giving a push with the fingers of the other hand against the angulus costae from below, during inspiration. For this the therapist bends the patient's neck or further arm towards himself, while reaching with his other arm across the patient's neck or chest, his hand on the angle of the rib.

There are three ways of applying a high-velocity thrust. In the first, the patient is supine with her arms crossed over her chest and hands on her shoulders, the arm on the side of the rib to be treated lying uppermost. The therapist stands by the opposite side of the table and grasps the far shoulder or upper arm so as to turn the patient's shoulder towards himself. He now applies the thenar eminence to the angle of the blocked rib (*Figure 6.45*). To do this effectively he must have his thumb in opposition, for only then is the thenar eminence contracted and firm (*Figure 6.46*). With his free hand the therapist now grasps the upper arm lying beneath the

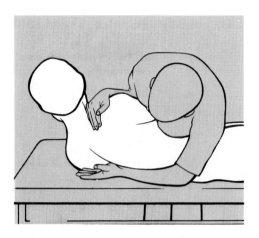

Figure 6.45 Manipulation of the ribs with the patient supine, preparatory phase: the therapist turns the patient towards himself

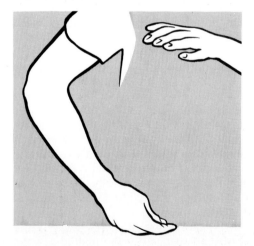

Figure 6.46 Position of the therapist's hands during manipulation of a rib with the patient supine (full opposition of the thumb!)

one he used to turn the patient towards him and turns her away on to the thenar eminence of the contact hand, so that the angle of the rib forms the most prominent point of the back. Having stabilized the patient in this position, the slack is taken up by the patient's own weight, and she is told to breathe in and out. During expiration the thrust is delivered through the upper arm, vertically towards the therapist's thenar eminence lying beneath (*Figure 6.47*).

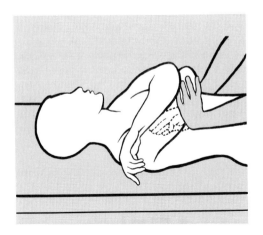

Figure 6.47 Delivering the thrust through the patient's upper arm vertically towards the therapist's thenar (*see Figure 6.46*) in contact with the angle of the rib

The following technical details are important: when he turns the patient away from himself the therapist must turn her over the mid-line, i.e. over the spinal column, and at the same time keep the trunk in flexion. At that point the contact hand must be in maximum supination so as not to make contact between the rib and the bony base of the first phalanx of the thumb, instead of the muscular thenar eminence.

A similar but harder thrusting technique is performed with the patient prone, her head turned to the side of the rib to be treated (*Figure 6.48*). If this is an upper rib, the patient's arm hangs down over the edge of the table in order to produce abduction of the shoulder-blade; otherwise it may lie parallel to the patient's trunk.

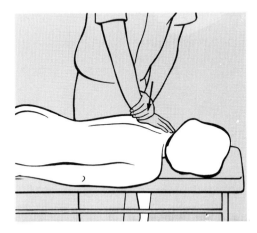

Figure 6.48 Thrust manipulation at the angle of a rib, with the patient prone

The therapist stands at the side of the rib to be treated and applies the pisiform of one hand to the angle of the rib. He may now reinforce this hand by grasping it just above the wrist with his other hand. The slack is then taken up by pressure of both arms and the thrust is delivered during expiration. It comes from the therapist's trunk and shoulders, vertically from above.

For the lower ribs a different thrust is frequently more effective, using a technique closely similar to manipulation in rotation restriction of the thoracic spine (*see Figure 6.42*). For this the patient sits astride the end of the table, while the therapist stands behind her, his feet well apart, and passes his arm under the axilla of the opposite side, to grasp the shoulder on the side of the rib to be treated. The thumb of the other hand is on the angle of the rib, with the forefinger encircling it. By rotating the patient round her body axis the slack is taken up and the thrust follows by the therapist simultaneously increasing rotation at the shoulder while the contact hand on the rib delivers a push or a pull in the same direction.

Treatment of the first rib: as in diagnosis, the treatment of this rib differs from that of all the others. For mobilization I use a technique that is as simple as it is effective: the therapist stands behind the patient seated on the table, and stabilizes the neck or shoulder from the side. He places his other hand on the side of the patient's head, on the side of the lesion, and tells her to resist a rhythmic push (two per second) delivered softly and gently from the side; this produces a rhythmic contraction of the scalenus which mobilizes both the *first* and the *second* rib. This is a technique ideally suited for self-treatment (*Figure 6.49*).

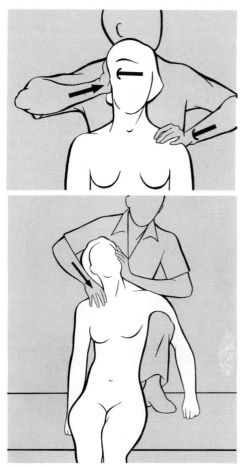

Figure 6.49 Repetitive mobilization of the first and second ribs by isometric rhythmic contraction of the scalenus

Figure 6.50 Springing and thrusting manipulation of the first rib.

In order to deliver a thrust the springing technique is most effective. It is also useful for diagnosis and mobilization. The therapist stands behind the seated patient, supporting her back against his own chest while one hand supports the head; the first phalanx of his other forefinger is placed on the first rib from above; with slight pressure downwards he takes up the slack. Quick repetitive springing can now be applied, or a thrust delivered in the same direction during expiration (*Figure 6.50*).

The cervical spine

Traction

Manual traction can be performed with the patient supine or seated; in the former case the head must project over the edge of the table. The therapist grasps the occiput with the thumb and forefinger of one hand, stabilizing the chin with the other hand from above (*Figure 6.51(a)*). Instead of applying forceful traction, I tell the patient to pull her head down between her shoulders (but *without* either ante-

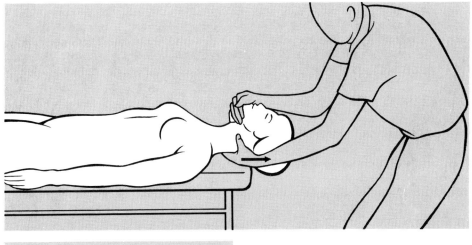

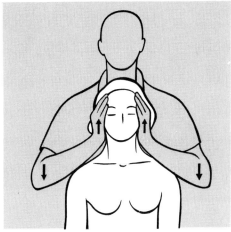

Figure 6.51 (a) Traction with the patient supine: the occiput is cradled between the therapist's thumb and forefinger while his other hand stabilizes the chin; traction is applied by the hand at the occiput; (*b*) traction of the cervical spine with the patient seated: the therapist rests his arms on the patient's shoulders

retroflexion) as gently as possible, and then to breathe in slowly. Then she is told to 'let go' and breathe out slowly. During relaxation the therapist feels the patient's neck lengthen. This is repeated about three times; it is not unusual for relaxation to be unsatisfactory at the first attempt. If the patient is well relaxed and supine it is frequently better *only* to tell the patient to breathe in slowly, then hold her breath and then to breathe out slowly and to relax. As a rule the patient will slightly pull her head in (automatically) during deep inspiration and relax during expiration, the advantage being that if the patient is told to pull her head down between her shoulders she frequently does this too forcibly, and with ante- or retroflexion of her head and neck.

If the patient is seated on the table (*Figure 6.51(b)*), the therapist stands behind her and leans the patient against his chest to facilitate relaxation. He then takes the patient's head in both hands, his palms on the cheeks and thumbs at the mastoid, without exerting pressure. The patient is told to draw her head down between her shoulders, with neither ante- nor retroflexion, using minimum force, and then to breathe in slowly. After full inspiration the patient is told to 'let go' and breathe out slowly. During relaxation the therapist should feel the patient's head moving slightly upwards. Here, too, deep inspiration followed by expiration usually suffices.

Since it employs PR manual traction is both gentler and more effective than mechanical traction. The latter may be applied with the patient supine on a table tilted downwards towards the feet, or sitting, with a sling pulling upwards. It is most important that the pull should be exerted on the *occiput* and not on the *chin*.

Mobilization

SIDE-BENDING

This can be carried out with the patient seated or supine. The phenomenon of alternating fixation and relaxation during breathing in and out can be effectively used for the cervical spine. In the even segments (C0, C2, C4), resistance increases during inspiration and we can therefore achieve greater facilitation by telling the patient *first* to look up and then to breathe in slowly. After this she is told to look down and breathe out slowly, unless we prefer to keep the neck in slight retroflexion (in the lower cervical spine, if the patient is seated), in which case it is better to tell her to 'let go' or 'relax', and then to breathe out. In the odd segments (C1, C3, C5), the patient is only told to breathe out slowly (after taking a short breath), and then to breathe in slowly and deeply.

The technique is exactly the same as that described for examination (*see Figure 4.21, page 126*). The therapist takes up the slack in the segment where he has diagnosed restriction, and feels increasing resistance as the patient looks up and breathes in (in the even segments) or breathes out (in the odd segments). After this he waits until he feels resistance disappear during inspiration or expiration respectively, and encourages the patient to relax into side-bending. If he makes the crucial mistake of forcing side-bending, the effects of spontaneous relaxation will be lost. This technique is applicable for segments C1–C6. The manoeuvre is usually repeated two or three times.

ROTATION

This is carried out with the patient seated. Again the technique is basically that of examination (*see Figure 4.23, page 128*). While the therapist fixes the arch of the lower vertebra of the treated segment between thumb and forefinger, he rotates the head in the direction of mobilization until the slack is taken up. He then tells the patient to look in the opposite direction and to breathe in slowly, and resists the tendency of the patient to automatically turn her head in the direction of her gaze. After inspiration he tells the patient to look in the direction of mobilization and to breathe out, obtaining automatic mobilization in the restricted direction, while he maintains fixation of the lower vertebra. This is repeated two or three times.

It is gentler and usually just as effective if, instead of looking in the opposite direction during the isometric phase, the patient looks up, and during the phase of relaxation looks down (the rest remaining the same).

In the cervicothoracic junction mobilization takes place mainly in lateral flexion. Again the techniques are the same as for diagnosis (*see Figure 4.22* and *6.54a*). Throughout the cervicothoracic junction inspiration increases resistance to side-bending while expiration has a mobilizing effect. The patient is therefore told first to look up and then to breathe in slowly, and after inspiration to *relax* and breathe out. (If she was told to look down, she would bend her head forward and thus 'unlock' the cervical spine). Care must be taken to hold the patient's head in the side-bending position, using the fingers, maintaining retroflexion and rotation to the opposite side while the upper vertebra is fixed by the therapist with the thenar eminence of the same hand. The thumb of the other hand meanwhile fixes the spinous process of the lower vertebra of the segment being treated.

It is technically easier (though less comfortable for the therapist) to carry out this mobilization with the patient lying on her side. He holds the patient as during diagnosis (*see Figure 4.25,* page 130). Standing in front of the patient, the therapist cradles the head and neck in his forearm, with his elbow on the table or slightly above it. He now tells the patient to look upwards, to increase resistance, and to breathe in slowly. After inspiration the patient is told to relax and to breathe out slowly. When the therapist feels the relaxation he has only to move his elbow slightly forward, following the patient's relaxation, and his hand will automatically move the patient's head into lateral flexion, retroflexion and rotation in the direction opposite to the side-bending.

With both these techniques (the patient lying on his side, or seated), it is possible to deliver a thrust after taking up the slack, and thus also after mobilization. If the patient is seated the thrust is delivered by the thumb against the spinous process, the hand holding the head and neck providing the fixation. If the patient is lying on his side, it is the hand cradling the head and neck that delivers the thrust in the same direction as mobilization, while the thumb on the spinous process provides the fixation.

Mobilization of the occiput against the atlas

This is performed by exactly the same techniques as used in diagnosis. In this segment the facilitating effect of inspiration and the inhibitory effect of expiration on muscle activity is the greatest, and this is true for *all* directions.

ROTATION

With the patient seated, the therapist brings the head into maximum rotation, with the minimum of force, taking up the slack and stabilizing the head, in axial rotation, against his chest. He now tells the patient to look up and to breathe in slowly, while he feels increased resistance to rotation. The patient is then told to look downwards and breathe out; during or towards the end of expiration, rotation of the head increases almost spontaneously. In this case looking up and down is better than looking first to one and then to the other side, because less force is produced.

SIDE-BENDING (*see Figure 4.26,* page 136)

After taking up the slack with the patient's head rotated into lateral flexion, the therapist tells her to look upwards and to breathe in slowly; he will feel increased resistance to side-bending. After inspiration the patient is told to look down at her chin and breathe out; towards the end of expiration the patient spontaneously relaxes into lateral flexion. (*See* also gravity PR of the sternomastoid muscle, *Figure 6.77,* page 262.)

RETROFLEXION (*see Figure 4.27,* page 131)

After taking up the slack with the head rotated and in retroflexion, the therapist asks the patient to do no more than breathe in slowly. He will sense increased resistance to retroflexion, then he tells the patient to breathe out slowly and let the head fall back. (In this case, looking up during the first phase would interfere with increased resistance to retroflexion, while looking down during the relaxation phase would interfere with retroflexion.) For relaxation into retroflexion it is wiser not to rotate the patient's head more than 45 degrees: the patient relaxes better and we avoid the odious combination of retroflexion with maximum rotation of the cervical spine.

ANTEFLEXION (*see Figure 4.28,* page 131)

Using the same technique, the therapist bends the head forward to take up the slack; he then tells the patient to look upwards and breathe in. The therapist resists the patient's automatic head retroflexion. After inspiration the patient is told to look downwards and to breathe out slowly; head anteflexion automatically follows. This is repeated two or three times.

After atlas mobilization, the therapist should make sure that the painful spasm of the short extensors crossing the posterior arch of the atlas has disappeared; this is the most important criterion of successful treatment of this segment.

Thrust techniques

With few exceptions, cases of serious complications after manipulation always occurred after high-velocity thrusts had been used in the cervical region. Further scrutiny showed that manipulation had been applied with force, without first taking up the slack. This is an extremely faulty technique, and to make matters worse a combination of maximum rotation with retroflexion was employed. The logical consequence is that of the large number of techniques to choose from, we avoid those that produce too much rotation and particularly rotation in retroflexion. The most important and frequently used techniques are those in which the thrust is delivered in the direction of traction, in a cranial direction; with the apophyseal joints tilted at about 45 degrees from the horizontal plane in the mid- and lower cervical spine, and almost horizontal at C0, C1 and C2, traction produces gapping of the these joints, in addition to distraction of the intervertebral discs.

TRACTION HIGH-VELOCITY THRUST APPLIED TO THE CRANIAL VERTEBRA OF THE BLOCKED SEGMENT, WITH THE PATIENT SUPINE

The patient's head is over the edge of the table, with the therapist facing and cradling it from above with the occiput on his forearm and the fingers on the patient's chin. With the radial surface of the first phalanx of the forefinger of the other hand he makes contact with the transverse process of the *upper* vertebra of the treated segment, side-bending the cervical spine only so far as not to slip over the transverse process (if the upper vertebra is the atlas, no side-bending is needed because the transverse processes of the atlas are longer and naturally jut beyond the others. The lower the transverse process, the further we bend the cervical spine). The patient's head can be very slightly rotated away from the therapist, but care must be taken not to rotate so far that the segments we want to treat are locked. In the position described (*Figure 6.52*), the therapist takes up the slack by giving a slight pull with both hands in a cranial direction, after which the thrust is delivered either (1) with both hands giving a pull (push) in the same direction, or (2) delivering the thrust into traction with a slight lateral flexion towards the therapist. In both cases the two hands must operate as a single unit. The thrust must therefore come from the therapist's trunk, over the shoulders to the hands, whether pure traction is applied or traction with side-bending. This technique can be used for C1–C5.

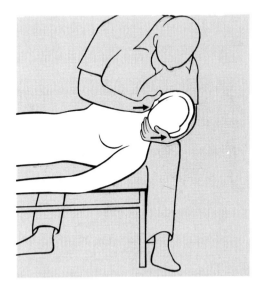

Figure 6.52 Traction–thrusting manipulation of the cervical spine with the patient supine; contact is made at the transverse process of the upper vertebra of the segment treated, or at the mastoid process

For the occipitoatlantal segment the therapist rotates the head so as to lock the atlas/axis at about 45 degrees, and makes contact at the mastoid process. If he wants to apply lateral flexion at the same time, he must bear in mind the rotation of the head, i.e. the side-bending must be at right angles to the sagittal plane of the (rotated) head.

TRACTION LOW-VELOCITY THRUST APPLIED TO THE CRANIAL VERTEBRA OF THE BLOCKED SEGMENT, WITH THE PATIENT SEATED (*Figure 6.53*)

The patient sits on the table with her hands clasped behind her head and the elbows far apart. The therapist stands behind the patient and threads his forearm through the triangle formed by the patient's upper arm and forearm, first on one and then on the other side. He makes contact with both forefingers and middle fingers crossed on the spinous process of the upper vertebra of the segment to be treated.

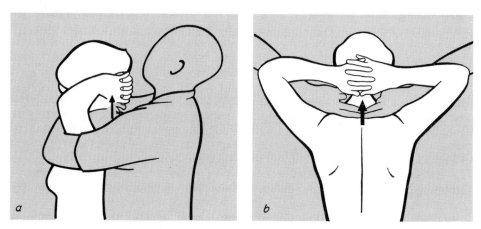

Figure 6.53 (*a*) Traction manipulation of the cervicothoracic junction; (*b*) application of the fingers

The patient is now told to relax and let her head fall forward. The thrust is delivered by the fingers increasing their pressure in a forward and upward direction. This technique is most easily applied to the segments C4–C7. Below this the therapist's fingers become ineffective; they merely produce a slight pull of the cervical spine in an upward direction, while the thrust is given by the operator's breastbone against the spinous process of T1 or T2. Both these traction techniques are safe and if correctly applied are very gentle. However, they are not absolutely specific, because the thrust is given to the *upper* vertebra of the blocked segment, while the lower vertebra is not fixed. Traction may therefore affect some of the more caudal segments; it need not, however, be considered harmful.

ROTATION THRUST WITH THE PATIENT SEATED (*Figure 6.54*)

The patient sits on a low stool; the therapist stands behind her, passing one hand and forearm in front of the patient's face (brow) so that the elbow is in front of the forehead and the hand below the occiput, the little finger clasped round the arch of the upper vertebra of the blocked segment and the occiput comfortable against the therapist's chest. The neck is thus held in a kyphotic position. With the thumb of the other hand, the therapist fixes the spinous process of the lower vertebra of the segment on the side opposite to the direction in which the head is rotated, so as to keep it in neutral position. The arm round the patient's head now rotates it and the upper vertebra of the blocked segment, so as to take up the slack, the thumb of the

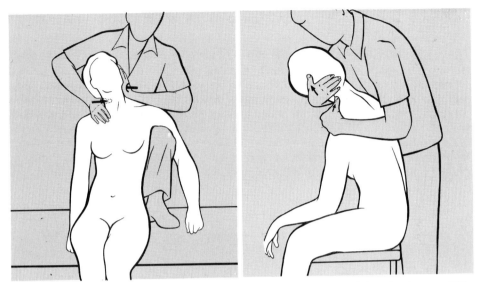

Figure 6.54 (*a*) Side bending mobilisation (manipulation) of the cervicothoracic junction (*see* page 239); (*b*) Rotation thrusting manipulation of the cervical spine with the patient seated, under traction, in kyphosis, withthe therapist's thumb fixing the lower vertebra of the treated segment at the spinous process

other hand holding the spinous process of the lower vertebra in mid-position. The thrust is then delivered with the hand round the patient's head, mainly into traction in a cranial direction, slightly increasing rotation at the same time.

This technique is highly specific, since the lower vertebra is fixed; if this fixation is correct, rotation is only moderate and there is always kyphosis and traction during the thrust. This means that the technique is quite safe.

Self-mobilization

Self-treatment – self-mobilization – constitutes a link between manipulative therapy and remedial exercise. Since the modern mobilization techniques making use of muscular facilitation and inhibition are already based on the active co-operation of the patient, it is logical that the trend should be to teach the patient increasingly how to deal with his problems himself.

To use one's own muscles to move one's spine, even with considerable force, is nothing new. Indeed, the usual movements performed in physical training – somewhat forceful, fast and non-specific – do more harm than good. Movement restriction goes hand in hand with muscle spasm protecting the blocked segment. Forceful movement suddenly applied to that segment is likely only to increase spasm, with the result that the normal and hypermobile segments will be mobilized, while the affected segments will be fixed even more firmly by muscle spasm.

Self-mobilization must therefore be as gentle and slow as the mobilization techniques we use, moving the segment after the slack has been taken up; it must also be as specific as possible. Precise clinical diagnosis and indication are mandatory.

Self-mobilization of the sacroiliac joint (according to Sachse, personal communication; *Figure 6.55*)

The patient is kneeling on the table, close to the edge, her trunk supported on her elbows. One knee is shifted to hang over the edge of the table, with the instep supported just above the heel of the other foot. In this position the patient must relax so that the pelvis slopes obliquely downwards from the ilium, which is supported by the knee on the table. In this way the slack is taken up at the sacroiliac joint of the *supported side*. The moment the patient senses tension in the region of her sacroiliac joint, she makes a very small downward springing movement with the knee over the edge of the table, moving in a vertical direction and thus mobilizing the sacroiliac joint on the supported side. Another very effective technique is

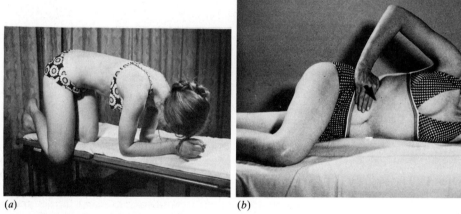

(*a*)   (*b*)

Figure 6.55 (*a*) Self-mobilization of the left sacroiliac joint (After Sachse, unpublished observations); (*b*) self-mobilization of the sacroiliac joint with the patient lying on her side

derived from mobilization lying on the side (*see Figure 4.6* page 113). Lying on her side with her lower leg extended, the patient stabilizes her pelvis with the knee of the upper flexed leg on the table. She now puts the wrist of her upper hand on her upper spina iliaca anterior superior, so as to produce rhythmical springing pressure in a ventrocranial direction; this produces gapping of the sacro-iliac joint (*Figure 6.55(b)*). In itself, this is an easy manoeuvre, the difficulty lying in the need to teach the patient to exert pressure in the correct direction, and not to use force.

Self-mobilization of the (lower) lumbar spine, ante- and retroflexion (*Figure 6.56*)

The patient sits on her heels, supporting herself with outstretched arms resting on her knees. By contraction of the gluteal muscles (glutei maximi) she raises her pelvis, producing kyphosis of the lumbar spine; after relaxation the pelvis falls forward, producing lordosis at the lumbosacral junction. This exercise is important for training correct position of the pelvis while standing (*see* page 285).

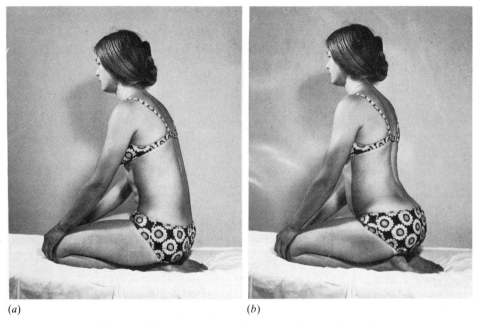

(*a*)   (*b*)

Figure 6.56 Self-mobilization of the lower lumbar spine: (*a*) anteflexion; (*b*) retroflexion

Self-mobilization of the lumbar spine, rotation (*Figure 6.57*)

The patient lies on her side near the edge of the table. The lower leg is stretched out, the upper leg bent at the knee so that the toes are hooked behind the lower leg. If self-mobilization is directed to the low lumbar spine, the toes rest *below* the knee of the supporting leg; if the upper lumbar spine, or up to the thoracolumbar junction is to be treated, the upper leg is supported above the knee and then the lower leg should be slightly flexed at the knee. With the hand that lies uppermost the patient holds the far edge of the table for stabilization, while the other (lower) hand lies on the (upper) flexed knee. The patient should turn her head to the side opposite to that of rotation; she may now exert pressure rhythmically with the hand lying on the knee, once or twice per second, producing repetitive mobilization; or she may exert slight pressure on the knee with this hand, from above, resisting her own pressure for about 10 s while breathing in, and then relaxing and increasing rotation. This manoeuvre is repeated 3–5 times.

There is also a very effective gravity induced exercise for self-mobilization, into rotation and flexion in the lumbar spine, which is identical with PR of the lumbar part of the erector spinae and will be described later (*see Figure 6.91*, page 273).

Self-mobilization into retroflexion and lateral flexion, standing
(*Figure 6.58*)

Here fixation is decisive. The patient may either fix the upper vertebra of the segment to be treated, with the radial surface of her forefinger, from above; or she may fix the lower vertebra with the tips of her thumbs, thus creating a fulcrum. By back or side-bending as far as to the fixation point (fulcrum) she takes up the slack,

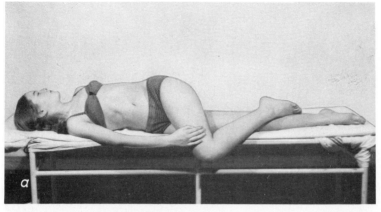

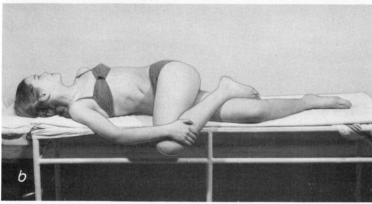

Figure 6.57 Rotation self-mobilization of the lumbar spine, the patient lying on her side: (*a*) lower, (*b*) upper lumbar spine

and then makes a slight repetitive movement, rhythmically springing the segment above or below the thumbs or forefingers respectively. Fixation from above (by the forefingers) is indicated if there is hypermobility above the segment treated, and from below (by the thumbs) if there is hypermobility below. Obviously the lumbosacral segment is always treated from above. It is essential that any forceful movement of large range should be avoided; only the small, specific springing movement should be performed, above or below the fulcrum with the spine fixed below or above respectively, moving once or twice per second.

Self-mobilization of the thoracolumbar spine into rotation

This corresponds to the technique described above (*see Figure 6.43,* page 232). The patient lies on her side with the lower leg stretched out and the upper leg bent both at the hip and at the knee, at about right angles. With her outstretched lower arm the patient fixes the thigh of the flexed leg from above, turning her head and neck into maximum rotation while looking at an object placed behind her back. In this position she exerts rhythmic pressure against the outstretched arm, with her knee, about twice per second. It is the rhythmic contraction of the psoas that produces the mobilization effect.

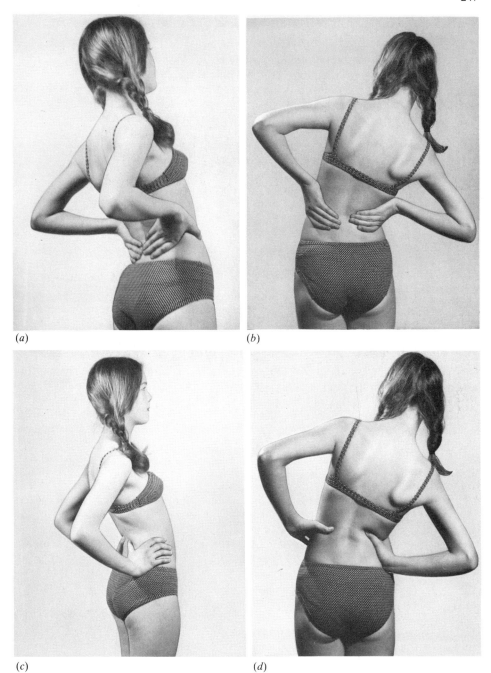

(a)

(b)

(c)

(d)

Figure 6.58 Self-mobilization of the lumbar spine, the patient standing. Fixation of the upper vertebra of the treated segment from above, with the hands: (*a*) back bending; (*b*) side-bending. Fixation with the hands from below: (*c*) back bending, (*d*) side-bending

Ante- and retroflexion self-mobilization of the thoracic spine (*Figure 6.59*)

The patient is supported on both knees and elbows. Moving the thoracic spine into kyphosis she breathes in, then into lordosis while she breathes out to the maximum. The more cranial the mobilization required, the further forward the elbows are placed (and the chest lowered), while for mobilization at the thoracolumbar junction it may be better to perform the exercise on hands and knees.

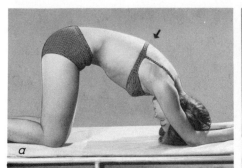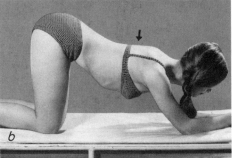

Figure 6.59 Self-mobilization of (*a*) anteflexion and (*b*) retroflexion of the mid- and lower thoracic spine

Rotation self-mobilization in the thoracic spine (*Figure 6.60*)

The patient is again on knees and elbows; she lifts one arm bent at the elbow (the left arm for rotation to the right, and vice versa), rotating her chest to the site of the segment to be treated, so as to take up the slack. She then carries out a small repetitive rotation round that point (at the rate of once per second), using primarily the *trunk rotators* (the impulse should not come from the arms, which is the reason why the arms should not be stretched).

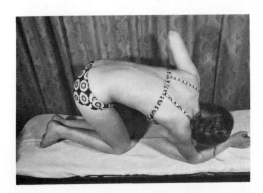

Figure 6.60 Rotation self-mobilization of the mid- and lower thoracic spine

Retroflexion self-mobilization of the thoracic spine during expiration (*Figure 6.61*)

The patient sits on the table with both arms stretched by her side and the hands in supination with the fingers spread fan-wise. She now breathes in lightly, then during *maximum* expiration she bends her thoracic spine backwards, at the same

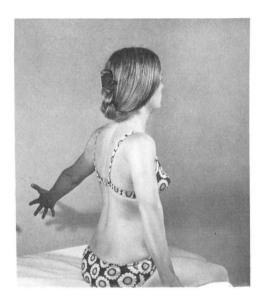

Figure 6.61 Retroflexion self-mobilization of the thoracic spine with the patient seated, using maximum expiration and outward rotation of the arms, with fingers widespread

time increasing supination of the hands. Care must be taken not to raise the shoulders and not to bend either the head or the lumbar spine backwards. If this exercise is correctly performed the patient should feel slight pain in the thoracic spine at maximum expiration and retroflexion. A very good alternative is described on page 224 (*Figure 6.34*).

Anteflexion self-mobilization of the thoracic spine in inspiration
(*Figure 6.62*)

The patient sits on her heels, bending forward so as to have her forehead on the table. In this position she breathes into her back. She easily learns how to direct inspiration into the stiff segments; this should first be checked with the therapist's finger, and then by the patient.

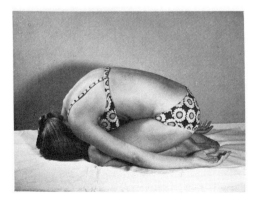

Figure 6.62 Anteflexion self-mobilization of the thoracic spine in inspiration, the patient squatting and bending forward

Inspiration self-mobilization of the upper ribs (*Figure 6.63*)

The patient is seated over the edge of the table with her knees apart, in anteflexion; her head is turned towards the side to be mobilized. One arm hangs between the knees and the other at her side. In this position the ribs to be mobilized bulge slightly and if the patient relaxes her shoulder-blades, she feels some tension at the site (the slack is being taken up). She now breathes into those ribs, separating them during inspiration.

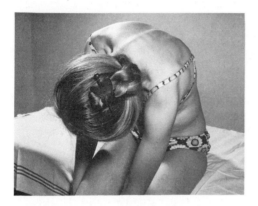

Figure 6.63 Inspiration self-mobilization of the right upper ribs

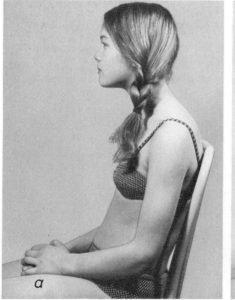 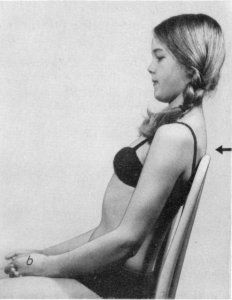

Figure 6.64 Ante- and retroflexion self-mobilization of the upper thoracic spine and the cervicothoracic junction, the patient seated on a chair with the back supported at the lower vertebra of the affected segment: the head and the spinal column is shifted (*a*) forwards and (*b*) backwards

Retroflexion self-mobilization of the upper thoracic spine and the cervicothoracic junction (*Figure 6.64*)

The patient is seated, her back supported by the chair-back at the level of the lower vertebra (spinous process) of the segment to be treated. She now shifts her head and spine backwards, so as to take up the slack at this segment. By repeated rhythmical movements in the same direction she springs the segment into retroflexion, the head moving back horizontally.

Rotation self-mobilization at the cervicothoracic junction (*Figure 6.65*)

Rotation of the outstretched arms with fingers spread wide has some mobilizing effect on the cervicothoracic junction; this effect is enhanced if each arm rotates in an opposite direction, one from supination into pronation and the other vice versa. This alone is not enough, however; the exercise becomes very effective if the head is also rotated, in the same rhythm as the arms and preferably facing the hand that is rotating into pronation (the thumb down). Care must be taken not to lift the shoulders, which should be relaxed. This technique should not be used if there is hypermobility in the upper thoracic region.

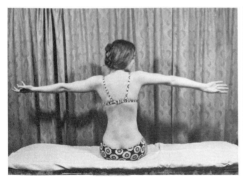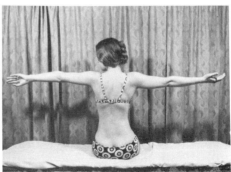

Figure 6.65 Rotation self-mobilization at the cervicothoracic junction, by a combination of rhythmic rotation of the arms in opposite directions, with the fingers spread, and head rotation in the direction of the pronated arm

Self-mobilization of the first rib

This corresponds to the technique described above (*see Figure 6.49,* page 236); the patient simply uses her own arm, resisting with head and neck the rhythmical impulses given by her hand.

Retroflexion and rotation self-mobilization of the cervical spine (*Figure 6.66*)

With the ulnar surface of both hands the patient fixes the lower vertebra of the segment to be treated. Now she either shifts her head back so as to take up the slack and then springs the segment into retroflexion by a small repetitive movement (*see* also retroflexion self-mobilization of the upper thoracic spine and cervicothoracic

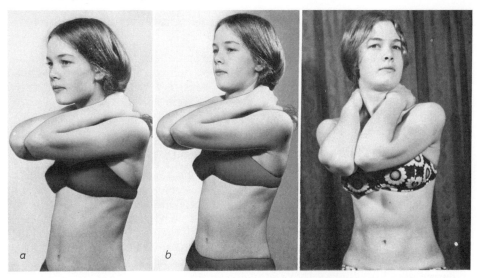

Figure 6.66 Rhythmic repetitive self-mobilization of the cervical spine, with the arch of the lower vertebra fixed by the ulnar edge of both hands: (*a*) forward shift; (*b*) backward shift; (*c*) rotation

junction); or she rotates her head to take up the slack and then makes rhythmical rotation movements springing (mobilizing) the segment into rotation. Instead of springing the segment into rotation, she may (after taking up the slack) look up, breathing in slowly, and then to the side of the desired mobilization while slowly breathing out, automatically increasing the range of rotation. The exercise is repeated three times.

Side-bending self-mobilization of the cervical spine

The patient may either place the palm of her hand against the side of her neck, so that the thumb is supported by the clavicle and the ulnar surface forms a fulcrum at the transverse process of the lower vertebra of the affected segment, using her other hand to bend the head to that side to take up the slack (*Figure 6.67*), a technique that is only suitable for segments C1–2 and C2–3. Or she may put her third and fourth fingers round her neck from behind, fixing the arch of the lower vertebra of the segment; with the other hand passing over the crown of her head she pulls it away from that side, over the fulcrum formed by her fingers, to take up the slack (*Figure 6.68*). In both positions PR is now applied, making use of the principle of alternating facilitation and inhibition during inspiration and expiration (*see* page 238). When treating an even segment the patient first looks up and breathes in slowly, and then relaxes while looking down and breathing out. For an odd segment she begins by breathing out slowly, relaxation taking place during inspiration. The exercise is repeated three times; care must be taken that side-bending is performed strictly in the coronal plane. With her fingers round her neck the patient may achieve good fixation down to C5, or to C6 if her neck is slender. The fingers should go round the posterior arch from behind one transverse process to the next.

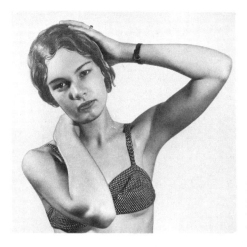

Figure 6.67 Side-bending self-mobilization of the upper cervical spine: while one hand side-bends the head to the opposite side, the other fixes the transverse process of the lower vertebra of the treated segment

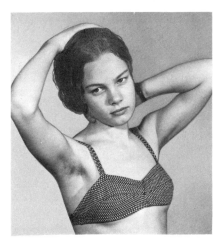

Figure 6.68 Side-bending self-mobilization of the mid- and lower cervical spine: one hand fixes the vertebral arch while the other reaches over the crown to bend the head sideways

Ante- and retroflexion self-mobilization between occiput and atlas
(*Figure 6.69*)

The patient turns her head so as to lock atlas/axis. To mobilize into anteflexion, she pulls her chin in to take up the slack, breathing out sharply through the nose, looking down, and making a brisk movement into anteflexion at the same time. To mobilize into retroflexion she lifts her chin to take up the slack, looks up and breathes in sharply, making a brisk but slight movement into retroflexion. Care must be taken not to move the cervical spine below the axis.

LATERAL FLEXION SELF-MOBILIZATION BETWEEN OCCIPUT AND ATLAS

The best technique is identical with gravity induced PR of the sternocleidomastoid muscle (*see Figure 6.77*, page 262).

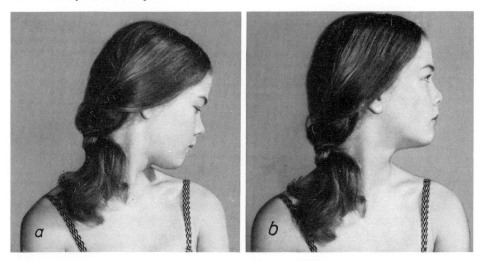

Figure 6.69 Self-mobilization between atlas and occiput with the head rotated (*a*) into anteflexion and (*b*) into retroflexion

Self-mobilization of the extremity joints

Obviously, self-treatment can also be applied to the extremity joints. This is particularly true for the lower extremities, because the patient has both hands free. I shall therefore deal only with a few instances of treatment of the upper extremity joints.

SELF-MOBILIZATION OF THE ELBOW IN A RADIAL DIRECTION (*Figure 6.70*)

The patient grasps the edge of a table, with the arm stretched in supination so that the thumb lies parallel with the edge of the table. The other hand grasps the elbow from the ulnar side, gapping (mobilizing) it by repeated rhythmical pushes in a radial direction.

MOBILIZATION OF ONE CARPAL BONE AGAINST THE NEXT (*Figure 6.71; see* also *Figure 6.5(b)*, page 200)

The tip of the thumb is placed on one carpal bone (e.g. the os capitatum) and the tip of the forefinger on its neighbour (in this case the os lunatum), producing a slight shearing pressure resulting in a small shift. If the fingers change position, the shift will take place in the opposite direction.

TRACTION OF THE FINGERS, INCLUDING THE FIRST METACARPAL

The distal phalanx is grasped by the little finger of the other hand, while the thumb and forefinger grasp the first phalanx or the metacarpal of the thumb. Traction and even mobilization can be applied to the metacarpophalangeal joints and the carpometacarpal joint of the thumb.

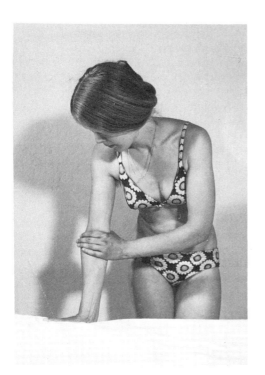

Figure 6.70 Self-mobilization of the elbow in a radial direction

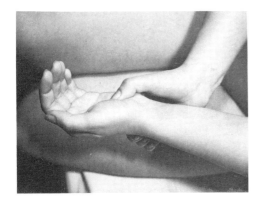

Figure 6.71 Shearing self-mobilization of carpal bones, using thumb and forefinger

SELF-APPLIED TRACTION AT THE SHOULDER

This can be performed over the padded back of a chair, preferably by the technique of isometric traction and relaxation, the other hand grasping the arm above the elbow. The patient resists her own (slight) traction and breathes in against the back of the chair; she then relaxes and breathes out, distraction resulting from relaxation (*see Figure 6.10,* page 204).

REMEDIAL EXERCISE

The main task of remedial exercise in disturbed function of the locomotor system is to correct faulty movement patterns (stereotypes) that are relevant to the patient's complaints. The most important pathogenic mechanism, to be treated first, is motor imbalance between muscle groups, manifested by faulty movement or posture.

The plan of treatment is as follows: first, the hyperactive muscles showing increased tension (spasm, trigger points, shortening) should be relaxed; *after* this, the weak (inhibited, flabby) muscles should be trained. This order is mandatory, in particular if the muscles with increased tension are the antagonists of the weak muscles. Only if this imbalance improves is it possible – as a rule – to re-integrate the activity of the individual muscles into correct muscle patterns.

There are some general principles to be observed: it is most important not to tire the patient. At first 20 minutes may be the tolerated limit, increasing later to 50 minutes. The process of learning how to use inhibited muscles and correcting movement patterns is particularly tiring for the beginner; this is easily recognized by the therapist, as the patient's performance begins to deteriorate rapidly. It is obviously best to begin with simpler tasks and to train more complex movements later. Thus it is best if the patient first trains lying on the floor, and only later under the influence of gravity; again, it is easier for the patient to be seated, since it is much more difficult to fix the pelvis correctly while standing.

What the patient is taught must be practised at home, so that at a later stage she need not visit the physiotherapist so frequently. Finally, those activities should be trained that correspond to the daily activities required of the patient at work, etc.

Post-isometric muscle relaxation

PR as described by Mitchell (1979) is the most prominent of the mobilization techniques using muscular facilitation and inhibition. As it obviously acts on muscles with increased tension, I began to use it preferentially for the treatment of these muscles. This is at variance with Mitchell himself, who writes: 'Isometric contraction . . . can be used for articular mobilization techniques. When isometrics are used for joint mobilization, maximal contractions are not desirable since they tighten, or freeze, the joints. Moderate contractions are much more appropriate for joint mobilization . . . . When a muscle and its fasciae must be stretched, hard maximal contractions are useful. . . .'

In my experience, however, this method is as advantageous for muscle relaxation as it has proved to be for joint mobilization. The procedure I recommend is as follows: the muscle is first brought into a position in which it attains its maximum length without stretching – taking up the slack in the same way as in joint mobilization. In this (extreme) position the patient is asked to resist with a minimum of force (isometrically) and to breathe in. This resistance is held for about 10 s, after which the patient is told to 'let go' (relax). It is now essential to wait until the therapist senses that the patient has indeed relaxed, after which he can usually obtain a greater range of movement by pure relaxation, taking up the slack again. During relaxation the patient should breathe out slowly, while the therapist makes use of this phase for so long as he feels a spontaneously increasing range of movement. This may last 10 s or even longer, but the process should never be interrupted, for relaxation is the real goal. If relaxation proves to be unsatisfactory, however, there is a simple and reliable way of improving it: by lengthening the isometric phase to as much as half a minute. However, if relaxation has been satisfactory from the start, it is possible to shorten the isometric phase. The procedure is repeated 3–5 times; the ground gained each time should not be lost during the following phase. If relaxation is good, the therapist senses that tension is so to speak 'thawing away', in which case repetition adds nothing to the result.

We not only combine isometrics with inspiration, and relaxation with expiration; for instance, head or trunk rotation is facilitated by eye movements, so we make use of this effect, asking the patient to look to one side during the isometric phase (this is resisted) and then to look in the direction of relaxation. Recently, Zbojan (personal communication) showed that the force of gravity could be used during both the isometric and the relaxation phase; during the latter this has the great advantage that the patient is utilizing the force of gravity for self-treatment in the most natural way, from the outset (gravity induced PR).

The effects of treatment can be ascertained not only in the muscle treated, where trigger points and tension ('fibrositis') should have disappeared; pain points, situated most frequently where the tendon is attached to the periosteum, will also have disappeared. At times, these pain points are more likely to be the result of referred pain, in which case PR is as effective as local anaesthesia or needling.

This method is highly specific: in large muscles those fibres must be treated where increased tension is found and that are attached to the pain point (e.g. pain points on the ribs). One reason for failure is insufficient specificity. This method is useless where there is no increased muscle tension. Therapeutic failure may also be due to an underlying cause producing renewed muscular tension, such as joint blockage or visceral disease in the corresponding segment.

Theoretically, Sherrington's post-isometric (medullary) inhibition cannot explain the effectiveness of this method, because of the long latency period. Compared with the classic method of Kabat (1965), not only is resistance much weaker, but active stretch is also avoided. The explanation of the excellent results furnished by this method may be sought in the fact that (1) during resistance of minimal force only very few muscle fibres are active, the others being inhibited, while (2) during relaxation the stretch reflex is avoided, a reflex which is brought about even by passive and non-painful stretch. On the other hand, there are situations in which the patient experiences some pain during PR and yet goes on relaxing (e.g. in 'ligament pain'), and yet after the procedure there is analgesia. This method demonstrates very clearly the close interrelation between tension and pain, and relaxation and analgesia.

This method is comparable with the 'spray and stretch' method of Travell (1976) but places greater emphasis on relaxation. Indeed, stretch does not seem essential, since it is merely the proof of successful relaxation. In some of the gravity induced techniques, and in relaxation of the glutei, no stretch takes place. Stretch seems to be required only where there is true muscle contracture due to fibrotic change, i.e. if there is no mere disturbance of function.

To show the effectiveness of our method, 351 painful muscle groups or muscle attachments were treated in 244 patients. There was immediate analgesia in 330 instances, while there was no effect only in 21.

Treatment of individual muscles and points of attachment

The techniques described here are useful not only for therapy, but also for diagnosis. For treatment of masticatory muscles *see* page 215.

Tension in the region of the posterior arch of the atlas (*Figure 6.72*)

Tension and tenderness of these muscles, i.e. the short extensors of the craniocervical junction, can be palpated only with the patient supine, her head in anteflexion. For treatment the patient sits on the table, with the therapist behind her, and leans against his chest. The therapist places both thumbs on the patient's

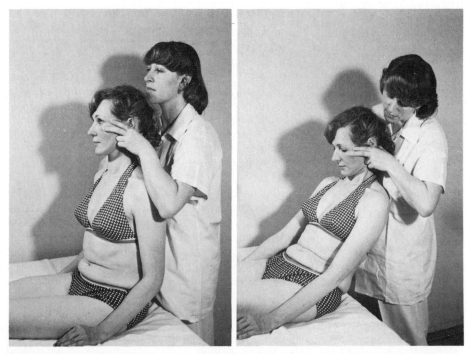

Figure 6.72 Post-isometric muscle relaxation of tension in the short extensors of the craniocervical junction: (*a*) resistance; (*b*) relaxation of tension in the short extensors of the craniocervical junction

occiput, with his fingers on the malar bones from above. To take up the slack, the therapist tilts the head slightly forward so as to draw the patient's chin in to her neck. He then tells the patient to look up and breathe in slowly, while resisting the patient's tendency to raise her head; the patient is then told to look down and breathe out slowly, leaning back and bringing her chin ever closer to the throat (she must *not* bend forward). This manoeuvre is repeated about three times. For self-treatment, the patient (*Figure 6.73*) uses her own hands, placing her fingers on the occiput and her thumbs on the malar bone. In order to bring the chin in towards the throat during relaxation, the patient must lean backwards over a low chair-back.

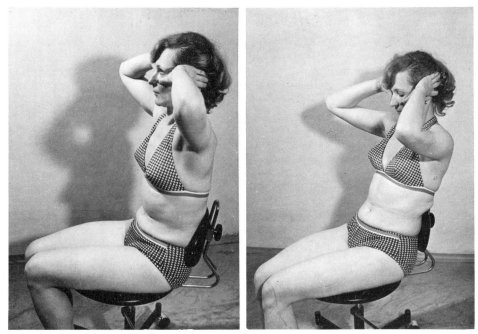

Figure 6.73 Self-treatment of tension in the short extensors of the craniocervical junction (*see Figure 6.72*)

Tension in the levator scapulae (*Figure 6.74*)

The typical pain points are on the lateral surface of the spinous process of C2 and on the superior border of the scapula. For treatment the patient is supine with her head at the end of the table and the elbow of the flexed arm raised above her head. The therapist exerts pressure on the scapula by pressing in a caudal direction against the elbow, fixing it with his thigh. Using both hands he now bends the head to the opposite side until he feels resistance. This is felt sooner on the side of

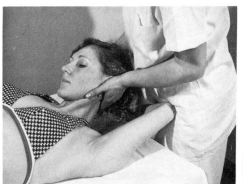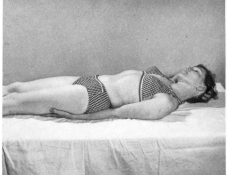

Figure 6.74 (*a*) Examination and post-isometric relaxation of tension in the levator scapulae, with fixation of the scapula pushed down by the therapist pressing his thigh on the patient's elbow. (*b*) Self-treatment with the shoulder fixed by the patient lying on her forearm

increased tension than on the other side. After taking up the slack in this way, he tells the patient to look towards the side that is being treated, and slowly to breathe in, while he resists the automatic tendency to turn to that side. He then tells the patient to 'let go' and breathe out, and during the ensuing relaxation he slightly moves the head sidewards and forwards. He may also tell the patient to pull one elbow up slightly, while he resists the movement, after which he again moves the head sideways and forward. This is repeated about three times.

For self-treatment, the patient pulls her shoulder down as far as she can and fixes it in this position by placing her supinated hand under her buttocks. Her other hand passes behind the head, with her fingers on the ear, to draw the head over to the side, *without* rotation, thus taking up the slack. The patient now looks in the direction of the side to be treated, resisting the automatic tendency to move her head towards that side, and breathes in. During relaxation her hand moves her head to the opposite side, while she breathes out. This technique, slightly modified, may be used by the therapist when the patient cannot lift her arm owing to shoulder pain.

Tension in the upper part of the trapezius muscle (*Figure 6.75*)

The upper trapezius should be treated if tender and taut. The patient is supine, while the therapist fixes the shoulder from above with one hand, side-bending the head and neck with the other hand so as to take up the slack. He then asks the

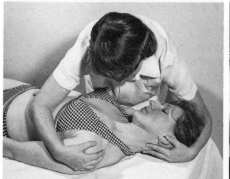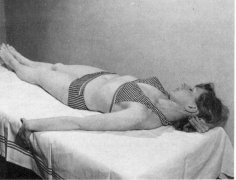

Figure 6.75 (*a*) Examination and post-isometric relaxation of tension in the upper part of the trapezius. (*b*) Self-treatment

patient to look towards the side away from which the head is bent, resisting the patient's automatic tendency to move towards the side of the lesion; the patient must be told to breathe in during this manoeuvre, and to breathe out during relaxation; meanwhile the head is moved further to the side until the slack has again been taken up. Resistance may also be given against the shoulder, from above; in this case the patient is told to lift her shoulder against the pressure of the therapist, with the least possible force; after about 10 s she should 'let go'. The therapist should then bend the head and neck sideways again, to take up the slack. In both cases the procedure is repeated about three times.

For self-treatment the patient grips the edge of the table with the hand on the side of treatment. With her other hand she reaches over the top of her head to draw the head sideways, thus taking up the slack. She then looks to the side of the painful muscle and breathes in; she then relaxes while increasing side-bending of the head with the other hand.

Tension in the scalene muscles (*Figure 6.76*)

In most cases tension of the scalenus does not cause direct pain but is of great clinical significance. As a rule the scalenes are tense if the other upper fixators of the shoulder girdle are tense; they play a decisive role in faulty respiration, causing the patient to lift her thorax. Tension in the pectorales and pain points at the

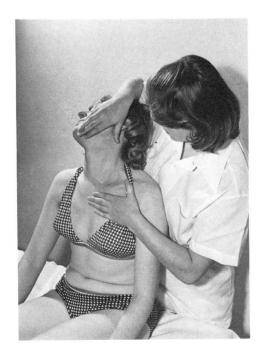

Figure 6.76 Examination and post-isometric re-laxation of the scalenus

sternocostal junction of the upper ribs seem to be connected with tension of the scalenes. This may explain why tension of the scalenes seems to produce a sensation of oppression in many patients, who thus feel great relief after PR. Blockage of the first rib goes hand in hand with reflex spasm of the scalenus on the same side, which is abolished by treatment of the first rib. A painful Erb's point can be abolished by PR of the scalenus.

On examination, tension in the scalenus causes restriction of oblique retroflexion of the head rotated to the opposite side. If there is marked cervical lordosis, tension of the scalenes may restrict side-bending of the head with the patient seated, simulating tension in the upper part of the trapezius.

For examination, as for treatment, the patient sits on the table, while the therapist stands behind her and supports the shoulder on the side to be treated, with one hand fixing the upper ribs of the same side by pressure on the patient's chest. With the other hand the therapist turns the patient's head to the other side, bending head and neck backwards so as to take up the slack. He now tells the patient to look to the side of treatment, resisting automatic movement with minimal pressure on the patient's temple, telling her to breathe in slowly; the therapist resists this inspiration by pressing his hand against the patient's chest. After full inspiration the patient is told to 'let go' and breathe out, letting the head and neck drop into retroflexion (there must be *no* pushing). This procedure is repeated about three times. There is perhaps no muscle that better lends itself to relaxation than the scalenus. Self-treatment by the patient is possible, but since the cause of tension in the scalenes is faulty respiration, correction of this fault is the treatment of choice.

Tension in the sternocleidomastoids (*Figure 6.77*)

There is frequently a pain point at the medial end of the clavicle and at the transverse process of the atlas. There are however numerous trigger points to be found in the course of the muscle (the clavicular as well as the sternal division), particularly below the mastoid process, referring pain to the face and cranium. Tension in the sternocleidomastoid muscle may also produce tension in the subclavicular part of the pectoralis muscle.

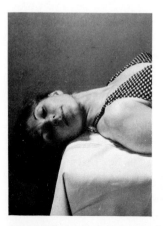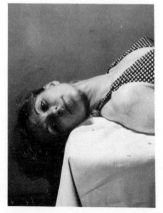

Figure 6.77 Gravity induced post-isometric relaxation of the sternocleidomastoid muscle. Left: with her head turned to the side over the edge of the table, the patient breathes in and looks up, automatically contracting the sternocleidomastoid and slightly lifting her head. Right: she breathes out and relaxes, thus letting the head drop

For treatment of this condition, gravity induced PR is the most effective method. The patient lies supine, with her head rotated and resting over the edge of the table, the chin supported by the edge of the table, acting as a fulcrum. If the left sternomastoid is to be treated, the head is rotated to the right. In this position the patient is told to look up and to take a slow deep breath; during deep inspiration the sternomastoid muscle slightly contracts, lifting the head, which is pivoted on the edge of the table. During slow expiration the patient relaxes, the top of the head is lowered, and a slight stretching of the sternocleidomastoid ensues. This manoeuvre is repeated about three times.

This technique gives excellent results in the treatment of a blocked atlanto-occipital joint, and can be used for self-treatment of this joint. It has a marked analgesic effect on painful or tender transverse processes of the atlas.

Tension in the pectoralis major

Increased tension (shortening) of the upper (subclavicular) part of the pectoralis (*Figure 6.78*) results in a forward-drawn position of the shoulders. For both examination and treatment, the patient is supine, her arm abducted at right angles.

(a)

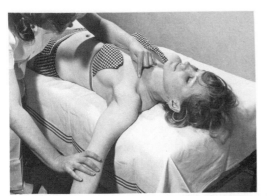

(b)

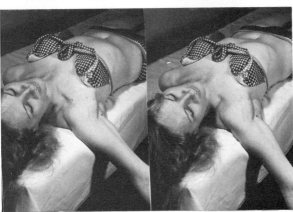

Figure 6.78 (a) Examination and post-isometric relaxation of the subclavicular part of the pectoralis; (b) Gravity induced post-isometric relaxation (self-treatment) of the subclavicular part of the pectoralis: left, inspiration and slight raising of the arm; right, expiration and relaxation, letting the arm fall

The therapist stands at the side of the affected muscle; with his forearm he fixes the patient's sternum from above and palpates the tendon with his fingers; it should not be tense even at maximum abduction. The other arm brings the patient's arm into maximum abduction over the side of the table, to take up the slack. For treatment the patient is told to lift her arm against the therapist's hand, using little force, while breathing in slowly. Once the patient has found the correct direction of abduction, the force of gravity is sufficient to hold it, and the patient is ready for self-treatment: she is told to lift the fully abducted arm about 2 cm, breathing in slowly. She then relaxes and breathes out slowly, repeating this procedure about three times. She should not relax suddenly, as this would cause brusque stretching.

If the lower part of the pectoralis muscle is tense, full elevation of the arm is restricted (*Figure 6.79*), and the tendon in the axilla is taut on palpation, as well as tender. Fixation and treatment are similar to that prescribed for the upper part of the muscle. Once the patient has understood the correct position and direction, gravity induced PR is carried out by the patient herself.

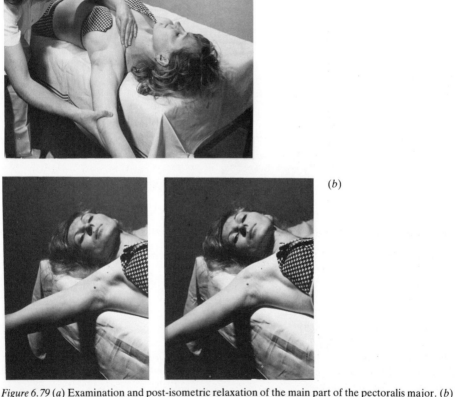

(*a*)

(*b*)

Figure 6.79 (*a*) Examination and post-isometric relaxation of the main part of the pectoralis major. (*b*) Gravity induced post-isometric relaxation (self-treatment) of the pectoralis major: left, inspiration and slight raising of the arm; right, expiration and relaxation, letting the arm fall

Pain points on the ribs (*Figure 6.80*)

These points are found most frequently in the mid-axillary and mid-clavicular line, and their treatment is of particular importance. These pain points are the points of attachment of fibres of the pectoralis muscle with increased tension. For treatment of pain points in the mid-clavicular line the patient lies supine; for those in the mid-axillary line she lies on her side, the lower leg (on the table) stretched out while

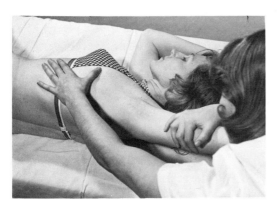

Figure 6.80 Specific treatment of pectoralis fibres attached to a pain point on a rib

the upper is flexed for stabilization. The therapist lifts the patient's arm to produce tension in those fibres that are directed towards the pain point. This can be palpated with the thumb at the pain point, and often is visible to the eye. Once the correct direction has been established, the therapist takes up the slack by maximum elevation of the patient's arm. He then tells her to press gently against the hand holding the arm up, and to breathe in against the thumb (or thenar eminence) on the pain point. This is followed by relaxation of the arm into further elevation, and expiration. After about three repetitions the therapist feels that the tension has disappeared, and this usually means that the tenderness at the pain point, too, has been abolished.

Painful lateral humeral epicondyle

In addition to blockage at the elbow there is usually tension in the supinator, in the extensors of the hand and fingers, and in the biceps. If the supinator is tense (*Figure 6.81*) there is restricted pronation on the affected side. For treatment the patient may be supine or seated, with the elbow flexed and fixed by the therapist against the patient's trunk. He stands facing the patient and brings his forearm into pronation in order to take up the slack. The patient is then told to supinate with minimal force, the therapist resisting for about 10 s, after which he tells the patient to 'let go'; when relaxation is achieved, the therapist brings the forearm further into pronation until the slack has been taken up once more. After 3–5 repetitions there is usually no difference between the two sides, and pain should be reduced. For self-treatment the patient performs the same movements with her arm as the therapist did.

If the extensors are in tension, the flexion of both wrist and fingers is restricted on the side of the tension. For treatment (*Figure 6.82*) the therapist places his palm on the back of the patient's hand and his fingers over the flexed fingers, taking up the slack into flexion of the fingers and hand. He then tells the patient to press her fingers slightly into extension; after resisting this pressure for about 10 s the therapist tells the patient to 'let go', increasing flexion of the wrist and fingers as far as relaxation allows. The procedure is repeated about five times. For self-treatment the patient places her thenar eminence and thumb over her flexed fingers, bringing her wrist into flexion. She then continues as does the therapist.

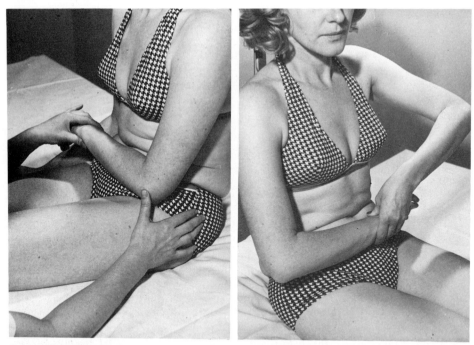

Figure 6.81 (*a*) Examination and treatment of tension in the supinator. (*b*) Self-treatment

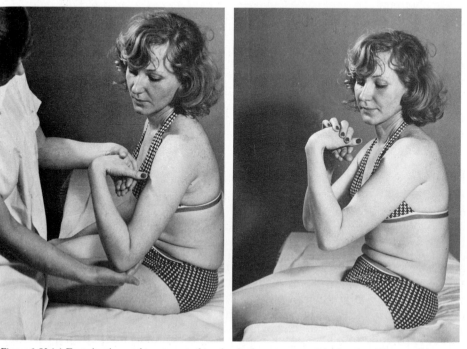

Figure 6.82 (*a*) Examination and treatment of tension in the extensors of the hand and fingers. (*b*) Self-treatment

If the biceps is in tension, extension of the elbow is (slightly) restricted. For treatment (*Figure 6.83*) the therapist extends the patient's elbow so as to take up the slack and asks her to exert slight counter-pressure for about 10 s, followed by relaxation into extension. This is repeated 3–5 times. For self-treatment the patient uses her own knee as a fulcrum; she may also use gravity induced PR by alternately lifting the forearm about 2 cm, holding this position for about 20 s, and then relaxing into extension.

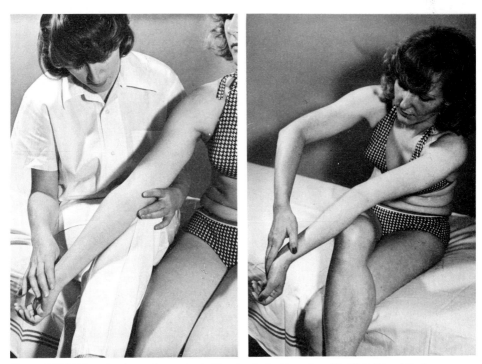

Figure 6.83 (*a*) Examination and treatment of tension in the biceps brachii. (*b*) Self-treatment

Painful medial humeral epicondyle

In this condition tension is felt in the flexors at the forearm. For treatment (*Figure 6.84*) the patient sits facing the therapist, with her elbow flexed and the hand in dorsiflexion at the wrist. The therapist threads his fingers between the patient's thumb and forefinger, from the radial to the ulnar side, with his thumb on the dorsal surface of the hand acting as a fulcrum. He thus takes up the slack into pronation by slightly pressing his fingers against the ulnar side of the patient's palm. He then tells the patient to resist this movement by slight counter-pressure into supination. After about 10 s the patient is told to 'let go', increasing pronation and dorsiflexion during relaxation. This procedure is repeated 3–5 times.

For self-treatment the patient holds the affected hand in the same way, but with her other hand she grasps the ulnar aspect of the hand being treated, on the palmar side, placing her thumb on the dorsal aspect as a fulcrum so as to take up the slack into pronation. She then repeats the therapist's movements.

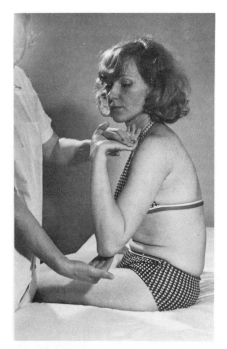 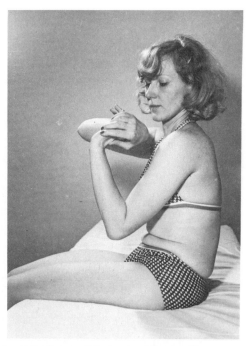

Figure 6.84 (*a*) Examination and treatment of tension in the flexors of the hand and fingers. (*b*) Self-treatment

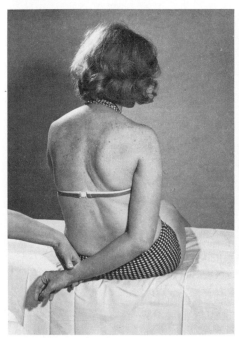 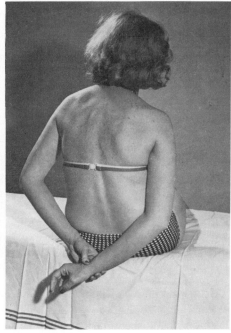

Figure 6.85 (*a*) Examination and treatment of tension in the biceps if the long tendon is painful. (*b*) Self-treatment

Painful long biceps tendon

For treatment (*Figure 6.85*) the patient sits in front of the therapist with her hand behind her back, the dorsal aspect of this hand passing over the buttock on the opposite side. The therapist grasps this hand, bringing it into pronation to take up the slack. In this position the patient is told to apply slight counter-pressure (into supination), resisted for about 10 s by the therapist. The patient is told to 'let go' and relax into pronation and simultaneous extension at the elbow. This is repeated 3–5 times. For self-treatment the patient deals with her own hand in exactly the same way.

Tension in the supraspinatus muscle

In this condition, abduction against resistance is painful. For treatment the therapist stands behind the patient seated on the table (*Figure 6.86*) and brings the patient's flexed arm into adduction in front of his chest, to take up the slack. In this position the patient is told to exert slight counter-pressure into abduction and to breathe in; the therapist resists this pressure for about 10 s, when the patient is told to breathe out and 'let go'. During this relaxation phase the therapist brings the arm further into adduction. This is repeated about three times. For self-treatment the patient does exactly the same using her own hand.

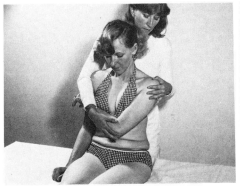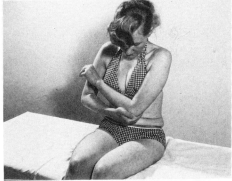

Figure 6.86 (*a*) Examination and treatment of tension in the supraspinatus. (*b*) Self-treatment

Tension in the infraspinatus muscle

In this condition external rotation against resistance is painful. Here gravity induced PR is most advantageous (*Figure 6.87*). The patient lies supine with her arm in abduction over the side of the table and the elbow bent at right angles, the forearm pointing towards the hip. By relaxation the slack is taken up in internal rotation at the shoulder. The patient now lifts the forearm about 2 cm, holding it for about 20 s, then relaxing into internal rotation for another 20 s. This is repeated about three times.

Tension in the subscapularis muscle

If this muscle contracts adduction and internal rotation result, i.e. the 'frozen shoulder' position. It appears that there is indeed a close relationship between the muscle and this condition, and that painful spasm of the subscapularis, with trigger points, accompanies frozen shoulder from the outset. Direct palpation is essential for diagnosis. For this the patient is supine with the upper extremity in slight abduction. The therapist grasps the patient's hand and gives axial traction while with the fingers of the other hand he penetrates over the edge of the latissimus dorsi on to the ventral aspect of the scapula with the subscapularis muscle and its trigger points. The moment he touches the muscle, the patient will react on the affected side. Here, too, gravity induced PR is the treatment of choice. The patient is supine, her arm abducted as far as her condition allows, the elbow flexed at right angles and the forearm in external rotation (*Figure 6.87(b)*), relaxed so as to take up the slack by the weight of the forearm. She now raises her arm about 2 cm and

(*a*)

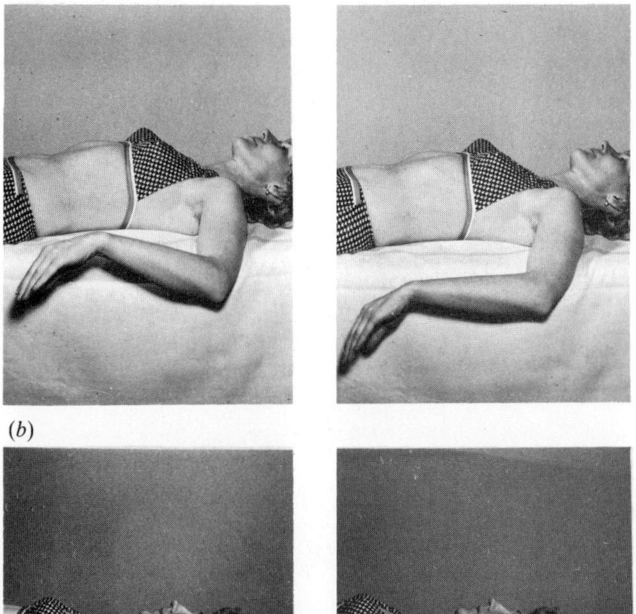

(*b*)

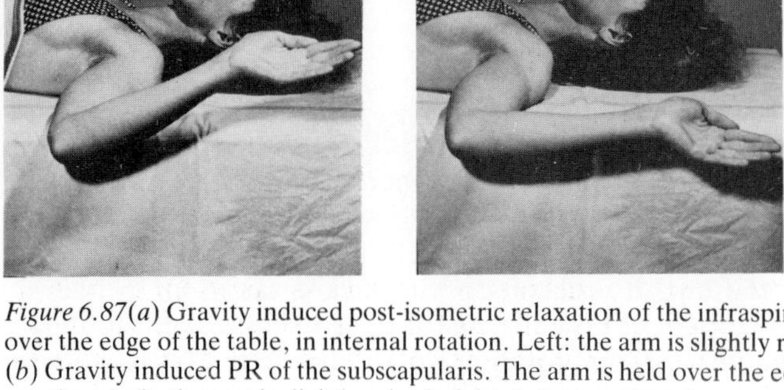

Figure 6.87(a) Gravity induced post-isometric relaxation of the infraspinatus muscle: the arm is held over the edge of the table, in internal rotation. Left: the arm is slightly raised; right: it drops, relaxed; (*b*) Gravity induced PR of the subscapularis. The arm is held over the edge of the table, in external rotation. Left, the arm is slightly raised; right, it drops, relaxed.

holds this position for at least 20 seconds, then relaxes into external rotation. If spasm is so severe that external rotation is too little for gravity to be effective in the supine position, the patient may lie on the affected side. The procedure must be repeated three to five times. This is one of the few effective methods for dealing with a frozen shoulder.

Tension in the erector spinae

Increased tension and pain, including trigger points, are very frequent in all parts of the erector spinae muscle. If the muscle is shortened, full stretch is obtained by anteflexion, side-bending and rotation to each side.

Treatment of the cervical and upper thoracic part of the erector spinae

Here gravity induced PR is useful and simple (*Figure 6.88*): the patient lies prone, her head only slightly over the end of the table and turned towards the side of intended treatment, so that it is supported between the chin and the mastoid process. If the cervical part of the muscle is to be relaxed, the head is only very

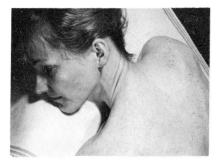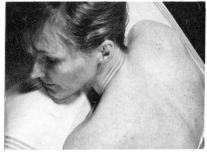

Figure 6.88 Gravity induced post-isometric relaxation of the cervical and upper thoracic erector spinae; the rotated head over the edge of the table is (left) slightly raised (inspiration) and (right) relaxed, it drops (expiration)

slightly lifted, so that the cervical part contracts; this position is held for a while, the patient slowly breathing in. Then she relaxes, slowly dropping her head. If the upper thoracic part of the muscle is to be treated, the head is raised further, until contraction is felt. Again the patient breathes in slowly, while during expiration she relaxes and drops her head over the edge of the table. This is repeated about three times.

The erector spinae of the cervicothoracic junction and in the upper thoracic region is also treated with the patient seated in front of the therapist. For the cervicothoracic junction (*Figure 6.89*) the therapist fixes the shoulder on the side of treatment with one hand, while the other passes round the patient's head to bend it

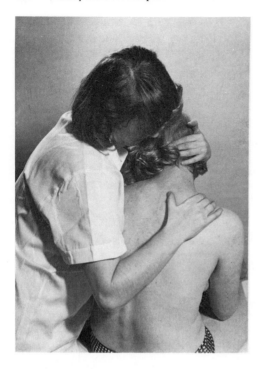

Figure 6.89 Post-isometric relaxation of the cervicothoracic part of the erector spinae with the patient seated

forward to the side and into rotation away from the affected side, until he has taken up the slack. The patient is then told to look in the opposite direction; the therapist resists the automatic counter-pressure while the patient breathes in slowly. The patient is then told to look to the side of rotation and to breathe out. This is repeated about three times.

For treatment of the upper thoracic erector spinae the technique is the same, except that the therapist does not fix the shoulder, but the upper ribs, similarly as in restricted anteflexion of the upper thoracic spine (*see Figure 6.37* page 226).

Treatment of the lower thoracic and upper lumbar part of the erector spinae

The patient is seated (*Figure 6.90*), her hands clasped behind her neck. The therapist stands behind him and threads his arm under the axilla of the patient to the shoulder on the opposite side (the side of treatment), so as to obtain anteflexion, side-bending and rotation. The summit of the curve thus obtained should correspond to the point of maximum tension (trigger point). In order to achieve this the therapist supports the patient with his thigh, which acts as a fulcrum, placing his knee on the table on the side towards which the patient is bent and rotated. After taking up the slack in anteflexion, side-bending and rotation, the patient is told to look in the opposite direction and to breathe slowly into the top of the curve, while the therapist resists the automatic tendency for her to turn to the opposite side. After this, the patient is told to look towards the side of rotation and to breathe out, automatically relaxing over the therapist's thigh. This is repeated about three times, the free hand checking muscle relaxation.

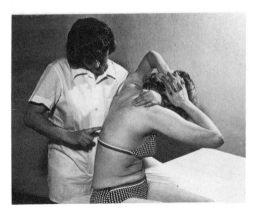

Figure 6.90 Post-isometric relaxation of the thoracolumbar part of the erector spinae, with the patient seated

Treatment of the low lumbar erector spinae

Gravity induced PR is most suitable, since it is also a method of self-treatment (*Figure 6.91*). Since the position is identical with that used for mobilization of the lumbar spine into flexion (*see Figure 6.31,* page 221), this technique can also be used for self-mobilization of the lumbar spine. The patient lies on her side in kyphosis, the lower leg bent at the hip and knee, the upper hanging over the edge of the table, bringing the pelvis into a forward-tilted position; she looks up at the ceiling in order to rotate the head and shoulder in the opposite direction from that of the pelvis. In this position the patient relaxes and the weight of the leg hanging down is sufficient to take up the slack of the low lumbar erector spinae. The patient

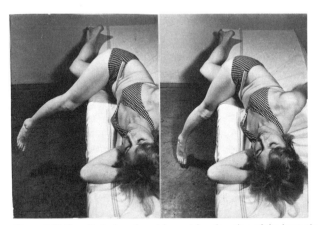

Figure 6.91 Gravity induced post-isometric relaxation of the lower lumbar erector spinae with the patient on her side: left, the leg hanging over the side of the table is slightly raised (inspiration); right, the leg drops in relaxation (expiration)

then lifts the leg about 2 cm, breathing in slowly; during expiration she lets the leg fall slowly, increasing lumbar kyphosis and pelvic rotation. This technique may be usefully applied in the treatment of pain at the spinous processes, most frequently between L4 and S1; the painful side must lie uppermost. Here it is helpful if the therapist first fixes the tender spinous process from above, to give the patient the exact feel of the direction of the pull of the hanging leg.

For self-treatment of the erector spinae while seated, the following technique is effective (*Figure 6.92*): with her hand on the top of her head the patient brings head and trunk into a position of anteflexion, side-bending and rotation, treating the erector spinae on the convex side. The curve should culminate at the point where treatment is indicated. After taking up the slack, the patient looks in the opposite

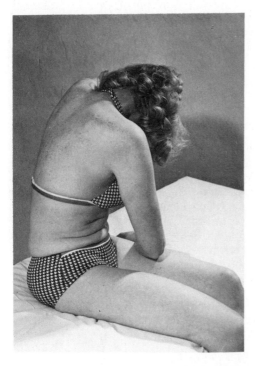

Figure 6.92 Self-treatment of the erector spinae, sitting: the hand on the head induces anteflexion, rotation and side-bending of the trunk, the curve culminating at the point where treatment is required

direction from the rotation, resisting automatic movement in the reverse direction by the hand on his head, while slowly breathing in. She then looks in the opposite direction (that of rotation) and breathes out, automatically producing relaxation. The procedure is repeated about three times. Where gravity induced PR is used no other self-treatment is needed.

Pain close to the medial angle of the scapula and at the spinous process of T5 and T6

Pain close to the medial angle of the scapula with a pain point at this site is the rule in radicular syndromes in the upper extremity and is also frequently found in non-radicular cervicobrachial syndromes. The painful spinous process of T5 or T6 is typical of interscapular pain as described by Maigne (1969). The treatment is similar for both conditions, achieving contraction and relaxation of interscapular muscles, mainly of the middle part of the trapezius (*Figure 6.93*). For this purpose the patient's elbow is adducted and lifted (or lowered) so as to bring about tension in those fibres which lead horizontally from the scapula to the interscapular pain

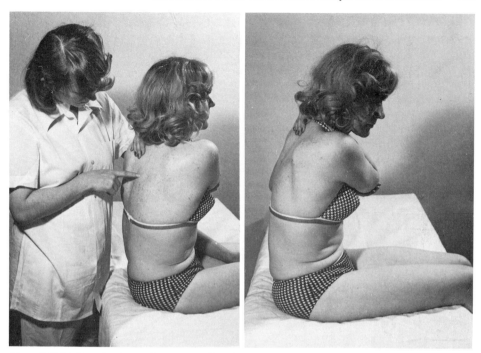

Figure 6.93 (a) Examination and treatment of tension in the interscapular musculature (parascapular pain point or pain at the spinous process of T5). (*b*) Self-treatment

point, or obliquely down to the spinous process of T5 or T6. If some tension is obtained (the slack taken up), the patient seated in front of the therapist is told to give slight counter-pressure with her elbow and to breathe into the painful area. She is then told to 'let go' and to breathe out slowly. In self-treatment the patient uses her other hand against her elbow, in the same way as the therapist.

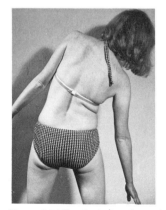 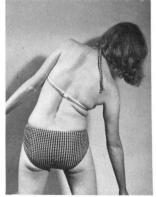

Figure 6.94 Gravity induced post-isometric relaxation of the quadratus lumborum with the patient standing with legs apart, bending sideways: left, trunk slightly raised during inspiration and looking up; right, increased side-bending during expiration, looking down and relaxing

Tension in the quadratus lumborum

This may interfere with side-bending of the trunk, and cause pain at the lowest ribs and on the iliac crest. It is treated very simply by gravity induced PR (*Figure 6.94*): the patient stands with her legs apart and relaxes into maximum side-bending (taking up the slack). On looking up while taking a slow deep breath, her quadratus lumborum automatically contracts, slightly raising the trunk; when the patient looks down and breathes out slowly, the muscle relaxes and side-bending increases its range. Trigger points are easily felt at the waist.

The iliopsoas muscle

Increased tension in the psoas muscle is felt through the abdominal wall, parallel to the spinal column, while tension of the iliacus is parallel to Poupart's ligament in the innominate. For treatment (*Figure 6.95*) we use the same position as for examination (*see Figure 4.42,* page 153), employing gravity induced PR. The patient is told to lift her knee slightly (about 2 cm) and to breathe in slowly, and then slowly to let the knee drop while breathing out. By extending the knee and letting the leg drop the m. rectus femoris can be relaxed as well (self-treatment).

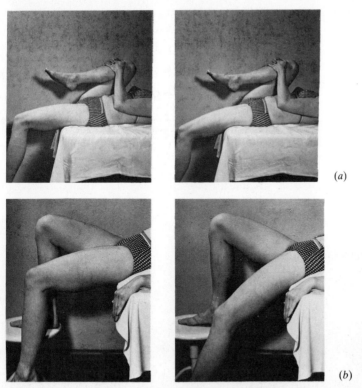

(a)

(b)

Figure 6.95 (a) Gravity induced post-isometric relaxation of the iliopsoas: the patient lies supine with her buttocks at the edge of the table, drawing one knee to the chest while the other leg hangs over the edge of the table: left, the leg is slightly raised; right, she lets it drop, in relaxation; (*b*) Gravity induced PR of the rectus abdominis: the patient lies supine with her buttocks at the edge of the table, her legs hanging over the edge. One is supported by a stool while the buttock of the free-hanging leg is raised by a cushion. Left: the leg is slightly raised at the knee; right: she lets it drop, in relaxation

Tension in the rectus abdominis

Increased tension in the straight abdominal muscles may manifest itself in trigger points causing referred pain simulating visceral disease, as well as low back pain. It may cause a forward-drawn posture and back bending restriction. Direct palpation of the trigger points is not easy, although increased tension is not difficult to sense. It is, however, very easy to palpate the tender points of insertion on the upper aspect of the pubic symphysis and the lower aspect of the xiphoid process and the adjacent parts of the lower ribs.

For treatment gravity induced PR is most effective: the patient is supine with her buttocks at the end of the table, her legs hanging over the edge. A stool is placed under the foot of the side which is not being treated; the patient is then turned to that side, so that a cushion can be inserted under the buttock of the side to be treated, lifting this side of the pelvis and abdomen. In this position the patient relaxes to take up the slack by the weight of the hanging leg. She then lifts the knee of that leg about 2 cm, holding it slightly raised during slow inspiration. After this she holds her breath, before breathing out slowly. This manoeuvre is repeated about three times (*Figure 6.95(b)*). This technique acts mainly on the insertions at the symphysis. If we wish to act primarily on the xiphoid process, it is better for the patient to raise her head and shoulders and breathe in, then letting the head and shoulders drop while slowly breathing out. This exercise can be used for self-treatment, the patient performing it two or three times a day.

Lumbosacroiliac 'ligament' pain

When ligament pain is tested, increased tension is usually found on the affected side, together with movement restriction into adduction (*see* pages 113–4). In this condition PR is the treatment of choice (*Figure 6.96*): the patient is supine, the therapist at the opposite side of the table to the leg to be treated. The patient flexes that leg at the hip and knee; the therapist grasps the knee, bringing it into adduction and flexing the hip so as to find the position in which there is the greatest resistance to adduction and the most pronounced pain, whether this pain corresponds more to the iliolumbar or to the sacroiliac ligament. When the therapist has taken up the slack into adduction in that position, the patient is told to resist the

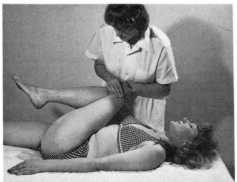
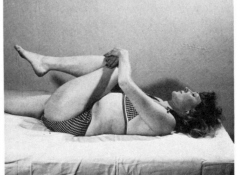

Figure 6.96 (a) Examination and treatment of tension in muscles in cases known as ligament pain. (*b*) Self-treatment

pressure of his hand, slightly, for about 10 s, and then to 'let go'. During relaxation, adduction is increased (this may be painful!) and when the slack has been taken up again the procedure is repeated from the newly gained position, 3–5 times. For self-treatment the patient uses her hands, one maintaining flexion at the hip while the other moves the knee into adduction.

Painful (tender) coccyx

This condition is most frequently due to increased tension in the gluteus maximus and the levator ani. PR of the gluteus maximus is the treatment of choice (*Figure 6.97*): the patient is prone, with the heels rotated outwards. The therapist crosses his hands, placing one on each buttock at the level of the anus. As a rule he feels increased tension but there is no tenderness. The patient is told to press her buttocks together with very little force and to maintain this pressure for about 10 s, then to 'let go'. During relaxation the therapist feels the tension in the muscles diminishing. This is repeated 3–5 times, and palpation of the coccyx is then easier and usually painless.

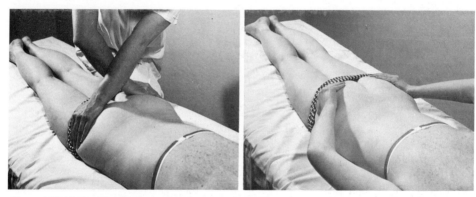

Figure 6.97 (*a*) Examination and treatment of tension in the gluteus maximus, for tenderness of the coccyx. (*b*) Self-treatment

For self-treatment the patient is supine, with her hands under her buttocks, feeling increased tension as she presses the buttocks together, and relaxation afterwards. As the gluteus maximus contracts and relaxes, so does the levator ani.

If this method fails, the cause is usually tension in the piriformis, which must then be treated. In exceptional cases there is no increased tension, and the coccyx then has to be treated per rectum.

Tension in the piriformis muscle

This is palpated as painful resistance above and medial to the greater trochanter. For treatment (*Figure 6.98*) the patient is prone with the knee bent at right angles. The therapist rotates the patient's leg outwards (i.e. internal rotation at the hip) to take up the slack, and tells the patient to give slight counter-pressure, which he resists for about 10 s before telling her to 'let go'. During relaxation, internal

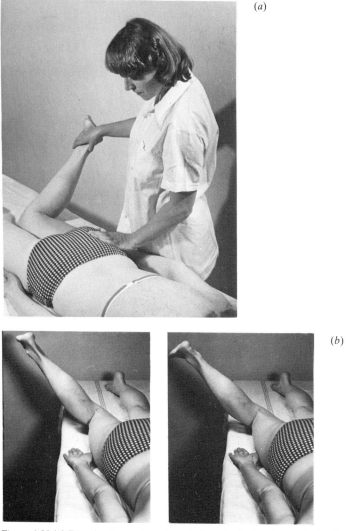

(a)

(b)

Figure 6.98 (*a*) Examination and treatment of tension in the piriformis. (*b*) Gravity induced post-isometric relaxation of the piriformis with the patient prone, the bent leg in internal rotation: left, the leg slightly raised; right, relaxation, the leg drops slightly

rotation at the hip increases. This procedure is repeated 3–5 times. For self-treatment gravity induced PR is most useful: when the slack has been taken up in internal rotation, the patient lifts the leg slightly, holds this position for about 20 s, and then lets the leg fall outwards, relaxing for another 20 s.

Tension in the rectus femoris

Both examination and treatment correspond to the femoral nerve stretch test equally characteristic for a radicular syndrome at L4 and for blockage at the L3/4 segment. For treatment (*Figure 6.99*) the patient is asked to exert slight pressure

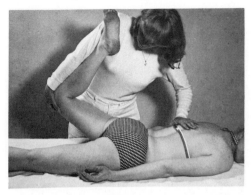

Figure 6.99 Examination and treatment of tension in the rectus femoris

with the back of the heel against the therapist's arm, maintaining this pressure for about 10 s; during relaxation the therapist increases hip extension and knee flexion simultaneously, to take up the slack. This is repeated about three times. Some pain may be felt even if only relaxation is obtained.

Pain at the ischial tuberosity

This symptom requires gravity induced relaxation of the hamstring examined by the straight leg raising test. The patient lies prone, her legs hanging over the edge of the table. She lifts the leg for 20 seconds and drops it relaxing for another 20 seconds.

Pain at the head of the fibula

This is due to tension in the biceps femoris, and less frequently to blockage of the fibular head. The patient is supine (*Figure 6.100*), the therapist at the end of the table. With his right hand he grasps the right foot (or the left with his left), his

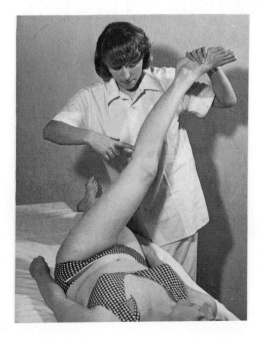

Figure 6.100 Examination and treatment of tension in the biceps femoris, for tenderness of the fibular head

thumb at the heel and little finger at the little toe, to be able to rotate the foot inwards. He then raises the stretched leg, moving it into adduction 'at the same time, and rotates the foot inwards until the slack has been taken up. From this position the patient is told to exert very slight pressure against the therapist's hand, pressing towards external rotation. The therapist resists for about 10 s before telling her to 'let go'. During relaxation he increases internal rotation of the foot, straight leg raising and adduction, to take up the slack, before repeating the procedure 3–5 times. Frequently, pain is felt at the fibular head during relaxation.

A painful greater trochanter

This is due to tension, mainly in the thigh abductors, and is most frequent in painful conditions of the hip joint. Isometric traction of the hip should first be applied. If the pain persists, the following technique should be adopted (*Figure 6.101*): with the patient supine, the leg on the painful side is brought into maximum adduction (taking up the slack) below the other leg, which is flexed. Standing on the far side,

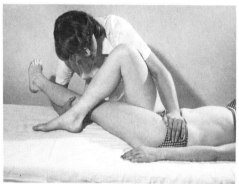
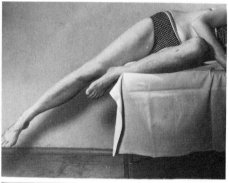

Figure 6.101 (*a*) Examination and treatment of tension in the abductors, for a painful trochanter major. (*b*) Gravity induced post-isometric relaxation (self-treatment) with the patient lying on her side at the end of the table, the lower leg flexed, the upper hanging over the edge of the table: left, upper leg slightly raised; right, the patient has let the leg drop, relaxed

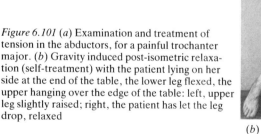
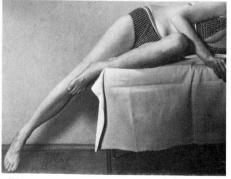

(*b*)

the therapist fixes the pelvis on the side of the lesion, from above, while his other hand moves the leg into adduction to take up the slack. The patient is told to exert slight counter-pressure, into abduction, for about 10 s, then told to 'let go', and the procedure repeated 3–5 times.

Gravity induced PR is most useful for self-treatment. The patient lies on her side at the end of the table, the lower leg flexed at the hip and knee, the upper hanging over the edge of the table. When the patient relaxes, the slack of the abductors is taken up by the weight of the hanging leg. The patient is then told to lift that leg about 2 cm and hold it in this position for about 20 s, and then to let it fall slowly and relax for another 20 s. This procedure is repeated about three times.

Tension in the adductors

Tension here causes pain in the pes anserinus on the tibia; this is again a sign of hip lesion, which should be treated first. If pain persists the following technique should be tried (*Figure 6.102*): the patient is supine, close to the edge of the table; the therapist brings the leg on the lesioned side over the edge of the table, into maximum abduction and extension, taking up the slack. This movement is resisted by the patient for about 10 s, before the patient relaxes, and the procedure is repeated 3–5 times.

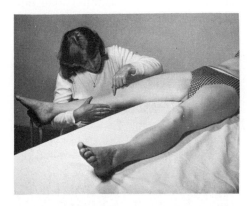

Figure 6.102 Examination and treatment of tension in the adductors for pain at the pes anserinus

Tension in the short adductors is shown by a positive Patrick's test. If the tension is not due to some underlying factor, we use gravity induced PR. The patient is as during Patrick's test and relaxes the abducted and flexed lower extremity into abduction, under the influence of gravity. She then raises the knee about 2 cm and holds this position for at least 20 seconds; she then relaxes into abduction again for at least 20 seconds. The procedure is repeated three to five times, and the whole exercise should be performed two or three times a day.

Tension in the toe extensors

This is felt as pain on the anterior aspect of the tibia. With the patient seated or supine (*Figure 6.103*), the therapist places his hand over the toes to bring both foot *and* toes into maximum plantar flexion, to take up the slack. The patient is told to resist slightly for about 10 s then to relax, and the procedure is repeated 3–5 times. She may perform this manoeuvre herself.

A painful Achilles' tendon

This is a sign of tension in the soleus muscle. For treatment the patient lies prone, with the knee on the lesioned side flexed (*Figure 6.104*). The therapist palpates the tendon to make sure which side of it is painful, and then brings the foot into dorsal

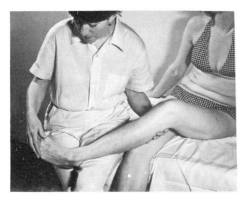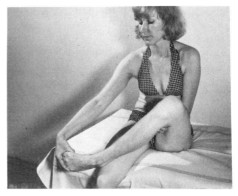

Figure 6.103 (*a*) Examination and treatment of tension in the extensors of the foot and toes. (*b*) Self-treatment

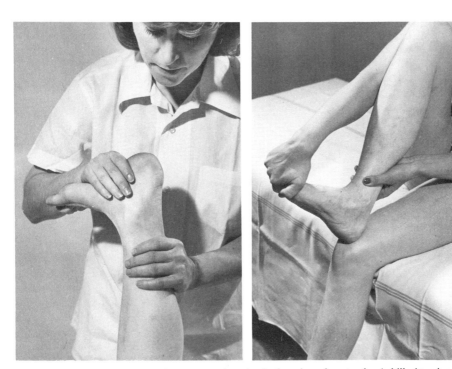

Figure 6.104 (*a*) Examination and treatment of tension in the soleus, for a tender Achilles' tendon. (*b*) Self-treatment

flexion so as to create tension at the painful side, with the foot either in pronation or in supination. After the slack has been taken up, the patient is told to exert counter-pressure with minimum force for about 10 s, then to relax; the procedure is repeated 3–5 times. For self-treatment the patient is seated, using both hands.

A painful calcaneal spur

This condition is due to increased tension in the muscles attached to the plantar aponeurosis. In treating this condition (*Figure 6.105*) it is first necessary to treat movement restriction between the tarsal bones, etc. The patient is prone, with knees bent. The therapist grasps the foot, with one hand round the heel and the

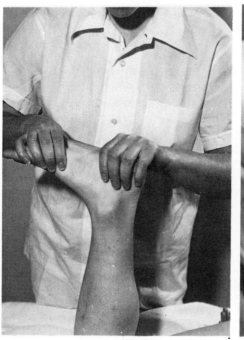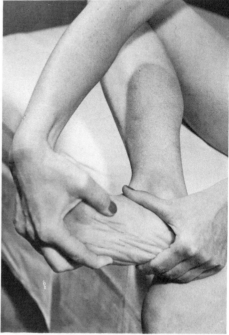

Figure 6.105 (*a*) Examination and treatment of tension in the plantar aponeurosis for a tender calcaneal spur. (*b*) Self-treatment

other round the distal part of the foot, producing dorsiflexion mainly of the metatarsals, and even of the toes, in relation to the calcaneus, until tension is felt in the sole. The patient is then told to flex the extended toes, with little force, against the therapist's resistance, making as it were a 'hollow' foot. This is held for about 10 s, then the patient is told to relax and the procedure repeated 3–5 times.

It is most important to avoid plantar flexion of the foot. For self-treatment the patient sits with the affected foot supported by the other knee, using her hands to grasp the foot just as the therapist does, or makes the 'hollow' foot while standing and then relaxes (for 20 seconds).

Training weak muscles

As explained above (*see* page 146), there is no true paresis in our patients, weakness being the result of inhibition and disuse. It is therefore up to the patient to learn how to use these weakened muscles again. There are various facilitation methods that are useful for the purpose and these will be dealt with separately.

They have one feature in common, which is that the patient must be made aware of the inhibited muscle; she must feel it. This means that for a certain period the patient learns conscious control of the muscle, until correct function is again automatic.

The gluteus maximus

If we find this muscle weak, for instance if it contracts little, or only towards the end of the movement, in hip (hyper-) extension, prone (*see Figure 4.35,* page 147), the most effective automatic facilitation is to perform hyperextension with the foot in outward rotation. If even this fails, the patient is first told to contract the buttocks consciously and then to extend the hip while keeping the glutei contracted. In severe cases, particularly if the lumbar erector spinae is hyperactive, it is important to reduce lumbar lordosis. For this the patient should place both forearms (or a cushion) under the abdomen, and contract the abdominal muscles. She then consciously contracts one buttock, lifting that leg very slightly so as *not* to contract the lumbar erector spinae and not to bring the lumbar spine into lordosis. The patient may be told to 'lift her leg and stretch it as far as possible', at the same time.

Having learned this, the patient is then taught to use both the glutei to tilt the pelvis back (the most important postural function). The technique needed here is that used for self-mobilization of the lower lumbar spine into ante- or retroflexion (*see Figure 6.56,* page 245).

The gluteus medius

For facilitation the following method is most effective: the patient lies on her side, and since the gluteus is weak, she makes a 'false abduction' as described in *Figure 4.36* (page 148). After this the therapist performs maximum abduction, correctly, and lets the leg drop suddenly. At that moment the gluteus medius automatically contracts. The therapist repeats this manoeuvre, and now the patient herself palpates the automatic contraction of the gluteus medius with her own fingers. Once she has become aware of this contraction, and has 'got the feel of it', she is told to contract the muscle consciously, checking with her fingers (feedback) and thus achieving correct abduction, i.e. abduction using simultaneously both the gluteus medius and the tensor fasciae latae.

The recti abdominis

The test for this muscle is for the patient to sit up from the supine position, keeping the legs bent at the hips and knees. For co-ordinated contraction of the glutei maximi the patient may press her heels against a hard cushion or other obstacle; it is a grave mistake to fix the foot from above. If the patient cannot do this, without her lumbar erector spinae being too short, the abdominal muscles may be trained by the patient sitting with bent knees, and lying down slowly with her spine in kyphosis and her neck in anteflexion, the contracted abdominal muscles allowing the vertebrae to touch the table one after the other (eccentric contraction) (*Figure 6.106*). The exercise must be stopped if the patient's feet are lifted from the table. After a few days or weeks of practice, the patient will be able to lie down correctly in this way, and then she will also be able to sit up by the same method.

The following exercises also train co-ordinated contraction of the glutei maximi and the abdominal recti.

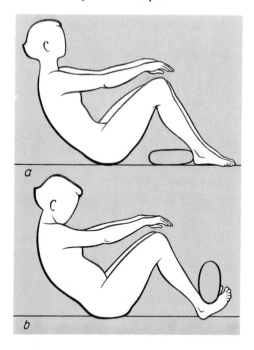

Figure 6.106 Training the recti abdominis by lying down from a sitting position, keeping the knees bent: (*a*) correct and (*b*) faulty

The 'pelvic see-saw' (*Figure 6.107*)

The patient is supine with knees bent and feet on the table. By contracting her erector spinae she brings her lumbar spine into lordosis, and breathing quietly she relaxes the erector spinae while contracting both the abdominal muscles and the glutei maximi, bringing the lumbar spine flat on the table. Once she has mastered

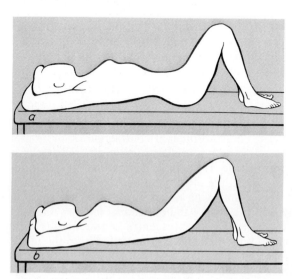

Figure 6.107 The 'pelvic see-saw': (*a*) bringing the lumbar spine into lordosis, supine; (*b*) lifting the pelvis and lumbar spine from the table, in kyphosis, and returning it to the previous position

this phase the patient, with her lumbar spine still flat on the table, puts her knees together and lifts in kyphosis first the pelvis and then the lumbar spine, up to the low thoracic region, in caudocranial order. The lumbar erector spinae must be kept relaxed, the recti abdominis and glutei maximi contracted and the knees together. The patient then lies down again, reversing the order of the exercise, from the thoracic spine to the pelvis.

The lower part of the trapezius muscle

This muscle plays a key role in the correct fixation of the shoulder. The following exercise should be carried out to facilitate contraction (*Figure 6.108*): the patient sits on her heels and bends forward to rest her forehead on the table in front of her; the arms may be either along the trunk or above the head, relaxed. In this position

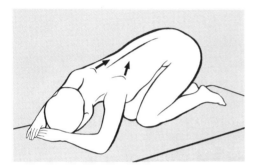

Figure 6.108 Squatting on her heels, trunk bent over thighs, the patient contracts the lower part of the trapezius

the medial border of the shoulder-blade diverges from the spinal column in a caudal direction. The therapist tells the patient to draw her shoulder-blade in a caudal direction, by contracting the lower part of the trapezius. Correctly performed, this movement brings the medial border of the shoulder-blade parallel with the spinal column, the lower angle being pulled in a caudal–medial direction. Once the therapist has palpated good contraction of the lower part of the trapezius, the patient should also palpate it with the thumb or index finger of her own furthermost hand (feedback). The shoulder-blades must *not* be drawn together.

Once the patient has mastered this procedure, she learns to do it lying prone, flat on the table, checking the contraction with her finger. She can then contract both the lower trapezii, lying with both arms by her sides in internal rotation. She lightly lifts both arms, then her head and neck, keeping the neck in line with the thoracic spine, the mandibles at right angles to the neck. If the lower trapezii are contracted, the upper trapezii remain relaxed owing to reflex inhibition. The patient first relaxes the neck, then the arms and lastly the shoulder-blades.

Once the patient has learned to contract the lower part of the trapezius while prone, she can do the same upright (sitting or standing), again first checking up on the contraction with her fingers.

The serratus lateralis

To train this muscle (*Figure 6.109*), the patient is on hands and knees, with her weight mainly on the *hands,* which are in internal rotation, the fingers pointing at each other. The shoulder-blades must be kept well apart and the thoracic spine held

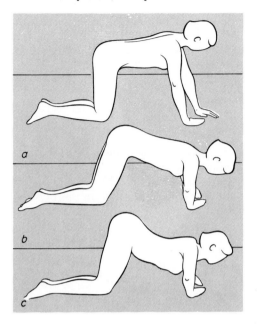

Figure 6.109 The patient on hands and knees for examination and training of the serratus lateralis: (*a*) first position; (*b*) arms bent (correct); (*c*) faulty position with arms bent

in a straight line. The patient is then told to bend her arms at the elbows. Correct fixation of the trunk and shoulder girdle is most important: the shoulder-blades must be kept apart (by the serrati) and fixed from below by the lower part of the trapezii. The neck is held straight, in prolongation of the thoracic spine. Contraction of the abdominal muscles is necessary to keep the trunk straight; this is made easier if the patient breathes out while bending her arms.

On hands and knees (*Figure 6.110*) with a book resting on the occiput has a similar effect, training correct fixation of the shoulder girdle by contraction of the serrati laterales and the lower part of the trapezii, as well as by co-ordinated contraction of the neck extensors *and* deep flexors, the upper part of the trapezii remaining relaxed and the recti abdominis contracted. The back and neck should be as flat as a board.

The deep flexors of the neck

The simplest exercise is head anteflexion against resistance: the patient is seated, her chin supported from below by the cupped hands, giving resistance to head anteflexion (isometric as well as isotonic resistance may be used).

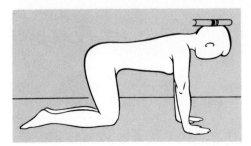

Figure 6.110 On hands and knees with a book on the occiput – correct position

A very effective exercise consists in drawing the chin in to the neck while sitting, with the thoracic spine bent backwards over the low back of a chair (*Figure 6.111*), repeating the movement several times. This movement may also be carried out supine, with the head hanging over the edge of the table.

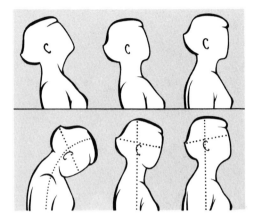

Figure 6.111 Training the deep neck flexors by drawing the chin in with the thoracic spine bent backwards over the low back of a chair

Training for some of the most important stereotypes (movement patterns)

Standing on both feet

For correct stance, fixation and co-ordination of the muscles of the pelvic girdle is essential. After training the individual muscle groups the following exercises may be useful.

STRAIGHTENING UP FROM SITTING ON THE HEELS TO KNEELING (*Figure 6.112*)

The patient is seated on her heels, the trunk erect. From this position she straightens up into kneeling with the aid of the muscles of the thighs and the glutei. To keep the spinal column straight, co-ordinated contraction of the abdominal and

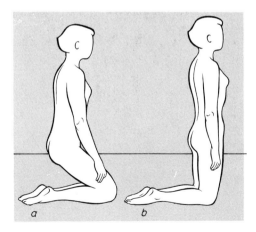

Figure 6.112 (a) Straightening up from sitting on the heels with trunk erect, to (*b*) kneeling position

back muscles is essential. Some resistance by the therapist, on the top of the patient's head, is useful for correction. In this way co-ordination of all the muscles essential for correct standing is trained.

STANDING AGAINST A WALL

The patient stands with her back against a wall. In this position she corrects the position of her pelvis and observes correct respiration. The abdominal muscles should never be entirely relaxed, and yet respiration should not be forced. Correct position of the pelvis should be maintained by the glutei. To facilitate the glutei the patient should rotate her feet symmetrically outwards against the resistance of the floor, the contracted glutei tilting the pelvis backwards.

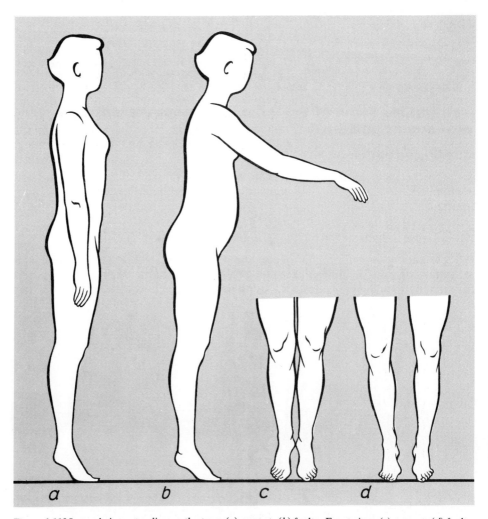

Figure 6.113 Lateral view, standing on the toes: (*a*) correct; (*b*) faulty. Front view: (*c*) correct; (*d*) faulty

STANDING ON THE TOES (*Figure 6.113*)

The patient holds her heels together, the feet at an angle of about 30 degrees. The abdominal and gluteal muscles are contracted, but the position of the trunk and pelvis also depend upon the position of the feet. The centre of gravity of the patient's body is in front of her scaphoid. The knee should be stretched but not pushed back. The patient should hold this position for a few seconds without losing balance and then slowly lower her heels to the ground. The centre of gravity of the body shifts back; the muscles of the arch of the foot as well as those of the pelvic girdle should be kept in moderate contraction.

In this way the patient learns to control her feet, ankles, pelvis, trunk and head.

Standing on one leg, or walking

This is useful to correct asymmetry, because it is an asymmetrical function. Correct standing on one leg is essential for walking, which entails alternate standing on each leg. Some asymmetry is frequent, and as a rule we can distinguish the supporting leg, the one on which the subject puts more weight when standing at ease. The asymmetry should not be too marked, however.

Alternate forward and backward shifting of the legs, supine (*Figure 6.114*) – The patient is asked to shift her slightly abducted leg in the direction of its long axis, 'into the distance'. There is contraction of the gluteus medius and at the same time there is alternating contraction of the internal and external rotators of the hip. The abdominal and gluteal musculature provides fixation of the pelvis and lumbar spine. In this way the patient learns to fix her pelvis and trunk during leg rotation.

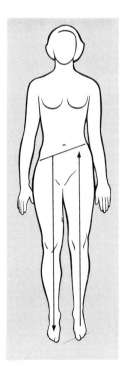

Figure 6.114 Alternate forward and backward shifting of the legs, supine

Rotation of the hip with the leg in abduction (*Figure 6.115*) – The patient lies on her side with the upper leg abducted and pushed (as in the preceding exercise) 'into the distance'. The other leg is pulled up by the quadratus lumborum to produce pelvic obliquity. The gluteus medius of the upper leg is contracted while the abdominal and gluteal musculature fixes the pelvis. In this position the patien‹ rotates the foot and the leg.

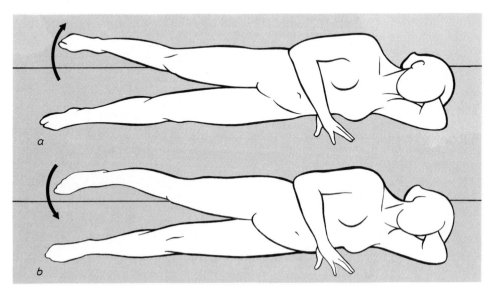

Figure 6.115 Alternating rotation of the hip in abduction, with the patient on her side: (*a*) external and (*b*) internal rotation

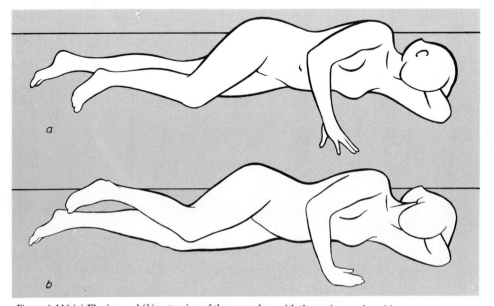

Figure 6.116 (*a*) Flexion and (*b*) extension of the upper leg, with the patient on her side

Flexion and extension of the upper leg, lying on the side (Figure 6.116) – The patient is in the same position as for the preceding exercise; she lifts (abducts) the stretched upper leg. During leg flexion at all joints (dorsal flexion of the ankle, bending hip and knee) there is also slight kyphosis of the lumbar spine, and during extension with all the extensors active, the lumbar spine moves into slight lordosis. Correct contraction of the abdominal muscles and the glutei should prevent hyperlordosis during extension. The therapist can help the patient by giving some resistance (during flexion) to the knee or the big toe; and during extension, to the heel, or to the big toe from above.

These exercises teach the patient co-ordination during walking.

Standing on one leg (see Figure 4.65, page 168) – The patient first stands on both legs, and then puts her weight on one leg. She now has to fix both hip and pelvis. She then lifts the other leg by bending the hip and knee almost at right angles. She should be able to keep her pelvis horizontal without losing her balance. Correct fixation of the pelvis and trunk are required, for which the key muscle is the gluteus medius; the patient should palpate it on the side of the supporting leg. If she feels this contraction she should check up with both hands on the crests of the ilia, to make sure that the pelvis is horizontal.

Sitting *(see Figure 4.58, page 164)*

Sitting erect on the floor, for trunk rotation (Figure 6.117) – The patient sits on her ischial tuberosities, the legs parallel and slightly bent, her hands clasped on the occiput. By co-ordinated contraction of the trunk musculature, the spinal column is held erect; correct fixation of the shoulder-blades is also essential. From this

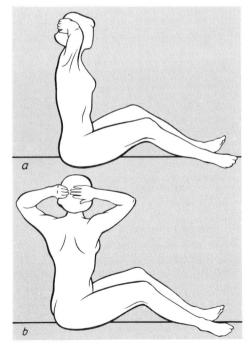

Figure 6.117 (a) Sitting erect on the floor. *(b)* Trunk rotation

position the patient carries out axial rotation, bending neither backwards, forwards nor sideways. Good facilitation can be obtained if she looks to the side of rotation and upwards, breathing in during rotation to the side and breathing out during rotation back to neutral position. (All that holds for trunk rotation while seated can be applied during trunk rotation standing, with legs apart.)

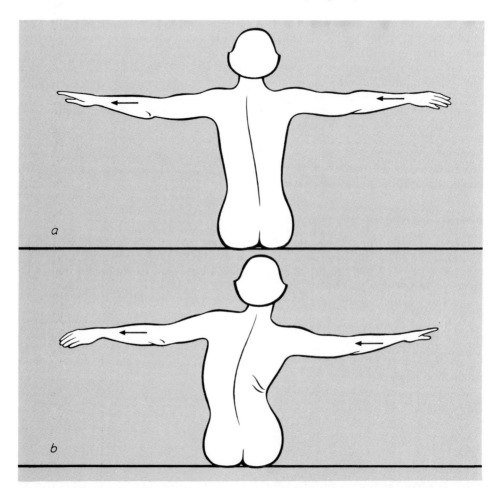

Figure 6.118 Lateral movements of the thorax with the patient seated: (*a*) correct and (*b*) faulty

Lateral movement of the thorax, sitting (Figure 6.118) – The patient is seated, preferably in front of a mirror, and moves her thorax to the side in the direction of the arms, which are held horizontally. She does this by correct control of her trunk musculature, chiefly the abdominal muscles, keeping the trunk straight and avoiding a crooked position. The therapist can facilitate this exercise by effecting resistance against the patient's ribs, first from one and then from the other side. Upright posture is also facilitated by breathing *out* on moving to the side and *in* while returning to neutral position; this is due to contraction of the oblique abdominal muscles.

Controlling the pelvis while seated – The patient sits on a stool, facing a mirror (*see Figure 4.58*, page 164). She first intentionally relaxes her abdominal and gluteal muscles, bringing the lumbar spine into lordosis. She then slowly contracts the gluteal and abdominal muscles to cause lumbar kyphosis. The shoulder girdle should move as little as possible during this exercise.

Brügger's relief position (*Figure 6.119*)

In a number of publications Brügger points out the deleterious effect of sitting in a kyphotic position, overloading the intervertebral discs, pressing on the sternum and the pubic symphysis and causing a forward-drawn neck, with hyperlordosis of the craniocervical junction. This creates increased tension in most of the postural musculature.

For maximum relief he has the patient adopt the following position: seated on the edge of a stool with the knees apart, resting her weight on her legs, she completely relaxes gluteal and abdominal muscles; the pelvis is tilted forward,

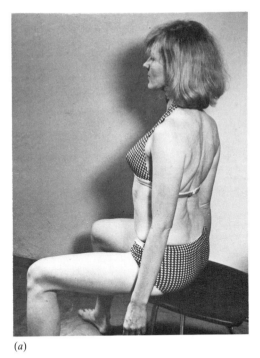

(*a*)

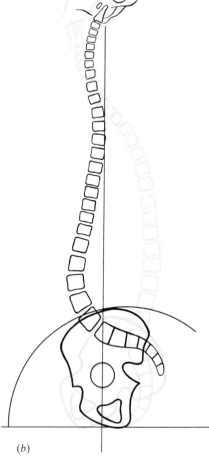

(*b*)

Figure 6.119 (*a*) Brügger's relief position. (*b*) The usual kyphotic position (shading) and the relief position (black)

creating maximum lumbosacral lordosis with the abdomen protruding. Once the patient has found this position, the upper lumbar, thoracic and cervical spine straighten up, and all the postural musculature relaxes; the entire spinal column is apparently in balance.

It is simple to test the immediate effect of this manoeuvre: while in the usual kyphotic position even moderate pressure on the upper trapezii, the pectorals, biceps, brachioradials, quadriceps and calf muscles is unpleasant if not positively painful; whereas in the relief position it is painless, and even as the therapist palpates them all of these muscles remain relaxed.

Whatever the theoretical implications of this rather extreme sitting position, it may represent a compensation for sitting in kyphosis, the position most people adopt if they relax their muscles without proper support. The fact remains that it frequently gives relief in particular to patients who easily 'flop' into a kyphotic sitting posture and are tense. It is useful to profit from this position for patients who seem to be able to relax in this way, even if only temporarily. Interestingly, the position greatly facilitates normal respiration.

Stooping

Preparation: uncurling from sitting on the heels (Figure 6.120) – This is a useful preparatory exercise. The patient sits on her heels, relaxed, and breathing quietly, with her hands on the floor in front of her knees; she is in a lordotic position with the pelvis tilted forward. By contraction of the gluteal and abdominal muscles the

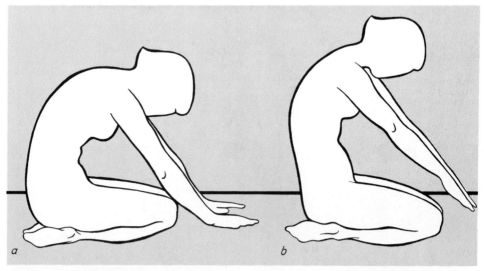

Figure 6.120 Uncurling from sitting on the heels: (*a*) with hands on the floor; (*b*) straightening up

pelvis is tilted back and the lumbar spine brought into kyphosis. By co-ordinated contraction of the abdominal and back musculature, and fixation of the pelvis by the glutei, the patient lifts her arms from the ground while the lumbar and thoracic spine curl up in succession. The pelvis may also be raised from the ground (*see Figure 6.112,* page 289).

Ante- and retroflexion of the spinal column while standing – Another preparatory exercise for stooping consists in training correct 'curling up' of the spinal column. Standing erect, the patient contracts her abdominal and gluteal musculature to fix the pelvis, and anteflexion begins with the head and neck followed by the thorax and abdomen, the pelvis remaining in the original position. The patient cannot usually reach further than to her knees, with her hands. From this position she straightens up, beginning with the lumbar spine.

Lifting an object from the ground (see Figure 4.60, page 165) – The patient puts one foot forward and bends trunk and knees simultaneously. In this way the load is evenly distributed between leg, pelvic and trunk musculature. To return to erect position, both knees are stretched while the gluteal muscles straighten the pelvis and the abdominal muscles control the uncurling of the spinal column. To facilitate the abdominal muscles, the patient may breathe out against resistance, or may press her fingers to the floor. This forces the abdominal muscles to contract, and this contraction should be maintained as the patient straightens up, keeping her chest as close as possible to the thighs or pelvis, to avoid leverage by the trunk. The patient may check up on her abdominal muscles by palpating with one hand (feedback).

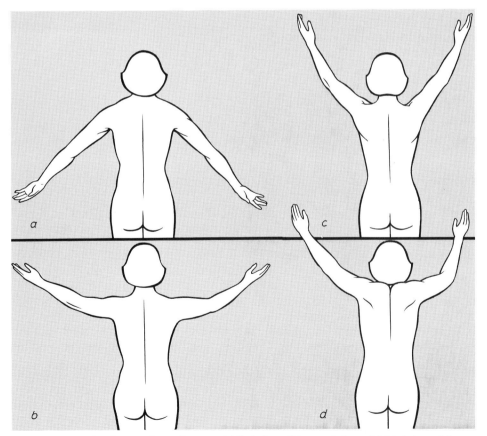

Figure 6.121 Moving the arms forward, prone: (*a*) first phase; (*b*) second phase; (*c*) third phase; (*d*) faulty

Lifting the arms

The principle here is to improve fixation of the shoulder girdle by the lower fixators of the shoulder-blade (serratus anterior and the lower trapezii), and to relax the upper fixators which are attached at the cervical spine.

Moving the arms forward, prone (*Figure 6.121*) – The patient is prone, both arms stretched out, palms downwards, and the forehead on the floor. The pelvis is fixed by the gluteal and abdominal musculature. The therapist brings the shoulder-blade into correct position by contraction of the lower part of the trapezius. The palms are now flat on the floor. Keeping the shoulder-blade well fixed, the patient raises her head slightly, moving her outstretched arms forward in such a way as to turn the palms forwards while keeping the ulnar surface of the hands on the floor. The lower fixators of the shoulder-blade remain contracted, while the upper fixators are relaxed.

Raising and lowering the shoulders (*Figure 6.122*) – The patient is seated, erect, the arms hanging down; one shoulder is raised by contraction of the upper fixators, resisted by the therapist. The patient relaxes deliberately, and finally pulls first one and then the other shoulder down, by the lower fixators. This exercise should be carried out first on one side, and then on both sides together. It teaches the patient control of contraction and relaxation of the relevant muscles.

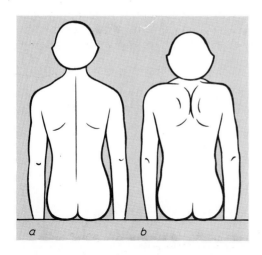

Figure 6.122 Raising and lowering the shoulders to train (active) relaxation of the (upper) trapezius: (*a*) relaxed first and end-position; (*b*) shoulders raised

Raising and lowering the shoulders, with arms raised (*Figure 6.123*) – This exercise is similar to the preceding one but the patient must learn to keep her arms raised even when the upper fixators are relaxed. For this, correct fixation of the thoracic spine with the abdominal muscles is important. We recommend training first one side, and then both together.

Lifting both arms, sitting – The patient sits erect on a stool, before a mirror. She now fixes the shoulder-blades from below, as firmly as she can, to avoid activating the upper fixators. Maintaining this fixation, she slowly raises her arms as far as she can without activating the upper fixators, i.e. at first only up to 90 degrees and finally to 180 degrees. This fixation should also be maintained when lowering the arms.

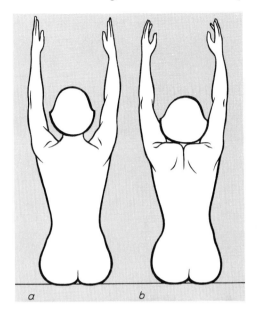

Figure 6.123 Lifting the arms, seated: (*a*) first position; (*b*) lifting the shoulders

Lifting the arms above the head (*Figure 6.124*) – The patient sits erect on a stool, raising her arms above the head as she does, for instance, when combing her hair. Care must be taken to fix the shoulder-blade correctly, to relax the upper fixators and to control the position of the head.

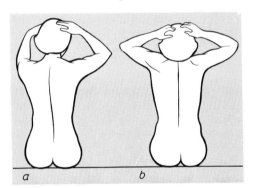

Figure 6.124 Lifting the arms over the head: (*a*) correct and (*b*) faulty

Sitting erect, turning the head (*see Figure 4.63*, page 167) – The patient sits erect on a stool, turning her head. There should be axial rotation of the cervical and thoracic spine, the shoulder-blades fixed from below, the upper fixators relaxed. In this way co-ordinated head rotation is achieved.

Correct weight carrying (*see Figure 4.64*, page 167)

For correct weight carrying, the proper fixation of the shoulder-blade is essential, as during lifting of the arms. Here, however, it is also important to relax the subclavicular part of the pectoralis to move the shoulder joint back, in relation to the spinal column. Co-ordinated contraction of the interscapular muscles is therefore necessary. The moment the patient succeeds in bracing her shoulders back, the weight she carries ceases to affect the cervical spine and the upper fixators of the shoulder girdle remain relaxed.

Breathing

The most serious fault here is lifting the thorax during inspiration. During examination, with his hands on both sides of the patient's thorax (*see* page 169), the therapist may encourage the patient by exerting some pressure during expiration and by releasing this pressure during inspiration to produce widening or narrowing of the thorax. Usually, this does not suffice.

The first step in treatment should be relaxation of the scalenes, where they have been found shortened (*see* page 261). In severe cases the manoeuvre described by Sachse (1975) is advised: the patient, seated or supine, is asked to press her flexed elbows downwards against resistance, while breathing in deeply. For self-treatment she may press her elbows down on the arms of an armchair.

If the patient lifts her thorax more on one side than the other, this usually reveals weakness of the lower trapezius on the side of increased lifting, which must be treated separately.

We then try to make correct breathing automatic, by the method of Gaymans (1980): the patient sits erect on a stool, both feet on the ground (high heels are prohibited!). The head is erect, i.e. the eyes look at an object placed at eye level, while the tip of the tongue presses against the hard palate about one finger's breadth *behind* the teeth. The hands lie in the lap, clasped in supination, the fingertips exerting slight pressure on the back of the hands, or with the fingers over the thumb in supination in front of the abdomen; in *no* case may the shoulders be raised. To facilitate inspiration the patient may lift his toes, while to facilitate expiration he presses his toes against the floor. This exercise should first be performed in front of a mirror, to make sure the clavicles do *not* move up and down.

An alternative is Brügger's relief position (*see* page 295), and possible combinations.

Once the patient has mastered correct respiration, she gets a feeling for the right way to breathe, i.e. how to broaden the thorax from the waist upwards without these facilitating manoeuvres, so that she can breathe correctly during her daily activities. According to Gaymans (1980), high heels constitute a serious impediment to correct respiration. Abdominal respiration must be practised with the patient supine.

If the patient is unable to breathe into the thoracic spine while prone, the same facilitating position should be adopted as for self-mobilization of the thoracic spine into flexion (*see Figure 6.62,* page 249).

It is also important for the patient to relax her facial muscles and the muscles controlling the tongue and jaw. Such is the importance of correct respiration that any gross fault is bound to jeopardize the rest of the motor patterns and even thwart the effect of mobilization techniques.

Supports

So far I have dealt mainly with techniques that restore or correct mobility; it is outside the scope of this book to deal with immobilization techniques. It is useful, however, to recommend simple supports that can be made by patients at home.

One is a soft cervical collar of latex foam (*Figure 6.125*), fitted to the shape of the neck. The soft material, placed round the neck to form a tube, becomes a soft and yet sufficient support for the cervical spine; covered in some soft material, it can be secured by tape and protects the patient from jolting in public transport vehicles.

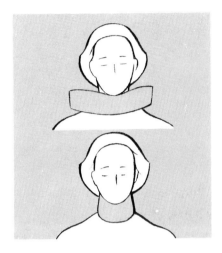

Figure 6.125 Soft supporting collar

Hypermobile patients with marked lumbar kyphosis when seated should carry an inflatable cushion with them, to use when they lean against a chair-back, etc. (*Figure 6.126*). The cushion should be only slightly inflated, and fitted to the top of the kyphosis, fixed by braces or a belt. This is of particular value for car drivers; it is not only easily adapted to each individual case, but also adapts itself to the patient's movements.

Hypermobile patients who frequently suffer from low-back pain in bed ('ligament' pain) may profit from a firm pelvic belt, fixed between the pelvic crests

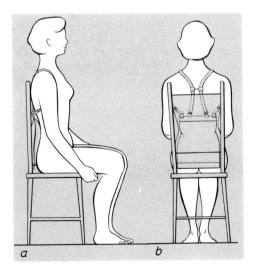

a   *b*

Figure 6.126 Inflatable supporting cushion for lumbar kyphosis: (*a*) lateral view; (*b*) back view

and the greater trochanters. It should be sufficiently broad, and lined with a material that does not irritate the skin. It must be fastened firmly (*Figure 6.127*). The effect is noticeable only after it has been worn for a few weeks. Patients with flabby abdominal muscles, often accompanied by obesity, should wear a firm belt or (in the case of women patients) firm elastic panties.

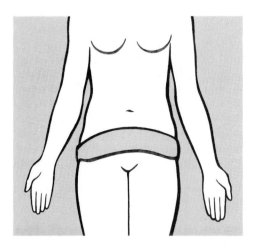

Figure 6.127 Pelvic belt (After Cyriax, 1977.)

Hints on reflex therapy

There are innumerable methods employing reflex mechanisms (*see* Chapter 5) which cannot be described here. Probably the method most popular with doctors is local anaesthesia. As shown in Chapter 5, there seems to be little difference between the effect of local anaesthesia and dry needling, provided the right technique is employed. This is in good agreement with the results of Frost *et al.* (1980), who found in a double-blind test that physiological saline solution was, if anything, more effective than local anaesthetic. The crucial technical point is that the needle must touch the pain point. It is not enough for the patient to feel pain; this pain must be sufficiently intense for the patient to react, and the therapist should search the painful area to find the most painful spot. Only then can full and immediate relief be felt, a relief that is just as intense as if an anaesthetic had been used, but without the accompanying anaesthesia. (This must always be tested.) It is a technical advantage of dry needling that the position of the needle can be corrected if no analgaesic effect has been obtained. Once local anaesthetic has been applied, of course, no correction is possible. If the pain point has not been reached, the therapeutic effect of local anaesthesia is usually slight, once the anaesthesia wears off.

If, however, nerve block is indicated (i.e. nerve root infiltration), then the application of local anaesthetic is necessary. These are well-known and widely published techniques which will not be dealt with here.

Skin stretching

A method of reflex therapy that seems particularly useful yet is little known is skin stretching. In effect it is comparable with some forms of connective-tissue massage, but has the advantage of being more accurate as diagnosis, and entirely painless as therapy (unlike connective-tissue massage).

As explained in Chapter 4 (page 138), an area of the skin may be held between the fingertips or with the ulnar aspect of the crossed hands, from the little finger to the wrist (according to the size of the area), and stretched with the minimum of force so as to take up the slack. On further stretching a springing resistance can be felt. If there is a hyperalgesic zone the slack is taken up sooner and there is much less springing. If the therapist then holds the stretched skin in end-position, resistance weakens until normal springing is restored. The hyperalgesic zone can then as a rule no longer be detected. If pain is due to this hyperalgesic zone, this method is quite as effective as needling, electrostimulation and other similar methods. Moreover, it is entirely painless and can be applied by the patient himself. If we mark the area on the skin, the effect can be measured, and Berger (personal communication, 1982) has constructed an electrical instrument that stretches the skin rhythmically with a constant force that can be recorded (*Figure 6.128*).

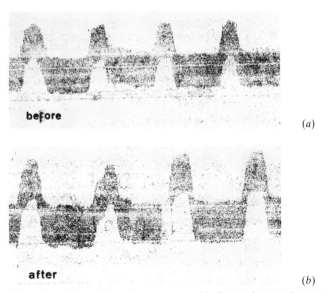

before   (*a*)

after   (*b*)

Figure 6.128 Dermatotensiogram recorded by Berger (personal communication): (*a*) before skin stretching, poor elasticity; (*b*) increased (normal) elasticity after stretching

7

Clinical aspects of disturbed function of the locomotor system

In this chapter the general principles of theory, diagnosis and therapy will be applied to specific clinical entities or syndromes, in which disturbed function of the locomotor system and of the spinal column in particular plays a significant role. It should be remembered that familiar clinical pictures such as back pain, low-back pain, shoulder pain, headache etc. have rarely been considered from this point of view, hence there is little on the subject to be found in the literature (Cyriax, 1977; Mennell, 1952). Nevertheless, this approach must be used to show the practical application of all that has been put forward in the preceding chapters. It is of great consequence for medical theory that this new approach has revealed unsuspected features in these familiar clinical entities. This has been made possible because the therapeutic measures we use are highly specific; nevertheless, they can only be called upon and applied to the best advantage if the clinical diagnosis has been drawn up accurately. As the number of doctors working in this field rapidly increases, the body of clinical data grows apace.

Backache

In backache, at least, the significant role of the spinal column is beyond doubt. However, the problem is traditionally treated mainly or even exclusively morphologically, which gives the impression that all we have to do is to find the underlying inflammatory, degenerative, metabolic or neoplastic disease, or malformation, or at least a gross mechanical obstacle like disc herniation. Before turning to the diagnosis of disturbed function such traditional disorders undoubtedly have to be excluded, or their relevance assessed, but once this has been done we need the diagnosis of disturbed function for the vast majority of patients 'without any specific diagnosis' (*see* page 11). As these conditions form the subject of all classic textbooks of rheumatology or orthopaedics, however, we may pass them by and devote our attention to our main subject.

For anamnesis, refer to the beginning of Chapter 4. Here, too, a part is played not only by the factors acting upon the mechanical functioning of the spinal column, but also by those that affect the (autonomic) nervous system – metereological influences, cold or heat, infection, hormonal changes (including menstruation) and last but not least, psychological factors.

For precise clinical analysis back pain is far too ill defined, and it is necessary to treat the various sections of the spinal column (the back) one by one. The first subject will be low-back pain.

Low-back pain

The dermatome chart shows that in this region a great number of segments converge, from the thoracolumbar junction to the sacral segments (*see Figure 4.32*, page 141f), with the possibility of referred pain from the whole of this vast region. Also, the most powerful forces (muscles) act here, where the trunk has its greatest mobility and where the movement of the lower extremities must be transferred to the trunk. All of this explains the great vulnerability of the region and is a pointer to the many possible pathogenic factors that have to be borne in mind, and whose relevance must be assessed in every case. The most important disturbances of function causing certain types of low-back pain and their respective therapies will now be reviewed. It may be useful to add that the term 'low-back pain' includes pain radiating to both sides, towards the hips, buttocks or groin, or even to the thighs, and that this pain is usually asymmetrical.

LOW-BACK PAIN DUE TO LIGAMENTAL AND MUSCULAR OVERSTRAIN

In this type of low-back pain not only need there be no morphological lesion but the spinal column as such may be functioning normally, at least at the outset. As this first category is not homogeneous, some further definition is required: the cause of strain may be exogenic, like excessively heavy physical labour, or more frequently work performed under conditions causing overstrain by faulty posture or bad movement patterns. More frequently, even, this overstrain is due to faulty statics and/or movement patterns acquired during ontogenesis, such as difference in leg length, juvenile osteochondrosis, muscular imbalance, hypermobility, obesity etc., the common denominator being muscular and ligamental overstrain.

Symptoms
Discomfort and pain are usually the consequence of activity, postural even more than dynamic, and they increase as activity continues. Often it is postural strain that is more disagreeable than movement. Thus, any position that has to be held for any length of time is registered as a strain, patients feeling the need to change position, even in bed. In severe cases there is pain (stiffness) in the morning, which is gradually overcome, only to be followed later by pain as a sign of fatigue.

Clinical signs
These consist in changes both in body statics and in faulty movement patterns, and should be analysed in each case. The typical imbalance in the lumbosacral region is between the gluteal and the abdominal musculature on the one hand, and the hip flexors and the back muscles on the other. This is frequently made worse by hypermobility which results in what is called 'ligament pain' (pages 113–114). The hyperactive erector spinae as well as the iliopsoas can be tender. The most typical tender periosteal points are the spinous processes, in particular the last two and the posterior sacroiliac spine. If there is marked asymmetry there may be pain on the iliac crest and the lowest ribs, as in statically imbalanced scoliosis and/or spasm of the quadratus lumborum. Baastrup's phenomenon, osteochondrosis of the spinous

processes, has frequently been thought to play a role, because of the tenderness of the spinous processes. However, this type of pain is usually found in hypermobile younger patients without osteochondrosis, and where there are typical X-ray changes no pain or tenderness is found on the spinous processes.

Therapy

If exogenic strain is the main cause, we should try to correct posture and faulty movement patterns at work. If the underlying cause is faulty statics and muscular imbalance, correction of statics and/or remedial exercise are indicated. In the hypermobile a support during static loading is important, particularly in public transport vehicles. Where obesity is a relevant factor, weight reduction is essential. For immediate relief of pain, relaxation of muscle tension, of trigger points in muscles and of insertion points is most useful (PR); alternatives are needling or local anaesthesia. Finally it is important to remember that muscular imbalance may stem from movement restriction at the craniocervical junction, which must not be left untreated in cases of low-back pain.

A TENDER COCCYX

This condition may accompany the preceding one. It must not be thought identical with coccygodynia; it is low-back pain due to a tender coccyx of which the patient is often unaware. In an earlier paper I showed that only one-fifth of the patients with a tender coccyx experienced coccygodynia; the majority suffered only from low-back pain. Nor is injury the most frequent cause; this is found in about one-fifth of the cases, and rarely in cases of relapsing tenderness of the coccyx.

Symptoms

Low-back pain, particularly when sitting; there may be constipation and even dyspareunia. Pain may be referred to the groin and hips, but this is not very characteristic.

Clinical signs

The diagnostic sign is a *very* tender (painful) tip of the coccyx which causes a reaction to the slightest touch; this is usually the ventral rather than the dorsal aspect. As a rule the tender coccyx is kyphotic, which makes palpation more difficult. Another important sign is hypertonus ('*défense musculaire*'!) of the gluteus maximus, and sometimes of the piriformis. There may be a positive straight leg raising test, Patrick's sign and spasm in the iliaci, and there is often a HSZ visible on the sacrum in the form of a fat cushion.

Therapy

The treatment of choice is PR, including self-treatment of the gluteus maximus and sometimes also of the piriformis. Manipulation per rectum is only exceptionally necessary, one of the grounds for it being hypotonus of the glutei, causing tenderness of the coccyx because the patient is as it were sitting on an 'unprotected' coccyx.

From the clinical findings as well as from the therapeutical results it can be assumed that tension in the gluteus maximus and the levator ani is the main cause of a tender coccyx. At examination per rectum we find trigger points in the levator ani; both voluntary contraction and relaxation of the gluteus maximus during PR accompany contraction and relaxation of the levator ani. This conception is corroborated by the clinical experience that increased tension in these muscles as well as a tender coccyx, particularly with a tendency to relapse, are linked with psychological tension, relaxation of the glutei also having a very favourable effect on psychological tension.

One final warning: it is important not to miss a tender coccyx, for it can constitute the most relevant finding in low-back pain, and if untreated is one of the most frequent causes of therapeutic failure.

A PAINFUL HIP JOINT

Like pain originating in the coccyx, the patient frequently feels a painful hip joint as low-back pain. A painful hip joint should not be equated with coxarthrosis, although it may (but need not) be the initial stage of that disease. In 59 cases of painful hip with no (43) or very slight (16) changes at X-ray examination, low-back pain was the most frequent complaint (33) (Lewit, 1977). For this reason examination of the hip joint (like that of the coccyx) is routine procedure in cases of low-back pain, and a painful hip joint may be the only relevant clinical finding.

Symptoms
Pain is usually caused by walking, especially by walking on hard ground (paved paths), by long standing, and by lying on the painful hip; otherwise, pain is relieved by lying down. The pain is usually felt in the low back and the hip; it may radiate in segment L4 towards the knee and also to the groin. Sometimes pain localized at the knee is the only complaint!

Clinical signs
There is a positive Patrick's sign. The extreme range of movement of the hip joint is painful if slight force is applied (springing), or it may be reduced; in particular, internal rotation may be restricted (*see* pages 135–136); extreme active abduction with the patient lying on his healthy side is painful. Typical pain points are found at the femoral head palpated in the groin, the insertion points of the abductors at the iliac crest and – most important of all – at the trochanter major. There is also adductor spasm with trigger points and a tender attachment at the *pes anserinus* (it is this that the patient interprets as pain in the knee). The hip flexors may also show spasm (tension) and therefore the lesser trochanter is also tender on deep palpation. (This procedure, however, is most disagreeable to the patient, and I do not find it essential.) The posterior sacroiliac spine is also frequently tender. In more severe cases, usually those with established coxarthrosis, there is flexion at the hip and compensatory lumbar hyperlordosis.

Therapy
The choice of treatment depends largely on the part played by coxarthrosis in the patient's condition. We are concerned here only with the treatment of disturbed function, which can also be improved in cases of coxarthrosis. The classic pharmacotherapy and physiotherapy (spa treatment), and surgical intervention in the severest cases, cannot of course be dealt with here.

The most important technique is traction, either by thrust or by PR. The high-velocity thrust is useful in hypermobile patients with not too much muscle spasm. In the majority of cases isometric traction constitutes the routine procedure (*see Figure 6.26*, page 214). Its effect depends mainly on the degree of relaxation of all muscle groups related to the hip joint. It is therefore the most effective type of conservative treatment.

If there is imbalance of the muscles of the pelvic girdle, most frequently weakness of the glutei, particularly of the abductors, with hyperactivity in the hip flexors and adductors, it is important to relax the taut muscles and train the weak ones. In coxarthrosis a well-planned regimen is essential, setting down how much walking the patient is allowed to do, preferably on soft ground with thick crêpe rubber soles and carrying a stick on the side not affected; regular exercise in the supine position should be performed, and swimming and cycling are to be encouraged. Loads should be carried on the affected side.

BLOCKAGE OF THE JOINTS OF THE LUMBAR SPINE AND OF THE SACROILIAC JOINTS

Low-back pain due to blockage of apophyseal joints and to blockage of the sacroiliac joints share a common therapeutic approach and also have some clinical features in common.

Symptoms

If the state is acute there is severe movement restriction, and straightening up usually presents more difficulty than stooping; there may be pain on sneezing or coughing. In more chronic cases there is usually stiffness after rest lying down or sitting, which improves on movement. Back bending is more frequently restricted than stooping, and the most characteristic complaint is difficulty in straightening up after stooping. Pain is usually asymmetrical and may radiate to the hips, buttocks, lower abdomen, groin, lower extremities, and towards the thoracic spine.

Clinical signs

Typical signs of blockage are found in all the joints affected, including tenderness and resistance to springing (*see* page 107). The more specific signs are given in *Table 7.1*; the thoracolumbar junction is formed by the segments T10–L1; segment L2/3 is affected only in exceptional cases.

Note: A positive straight leg raising test is due to spasm of the hamstrings while the femoral nerve stretch test is positive in spasm of the biceps femoris, just as Patrick's sign is caused by spasm of the adductors. The characteristic muscle spasms for each segment are very important features of the clinical picture of each type of blockage: spasm of the psoas for the abdominal pain in thoracolumbar lesions; spasm of the rectus femoris for pain from the thigh to the knee in lesions of L3/4; piriformis spasm for pain in the buttocks in L4/5 lesions; iliacus spasm for pseudogynaecological symptoms (algomenorrhoea) in lesions of L5–S1.

LOW-BACK PAIN DUE TO DISC LESION

The cases grouped under this heading are those in which there is *no* radicular syndrome, and in this condition, of course, disc herniation is the most likely diagnosis.

TABLE 7.1. Clinical signs of blockage of the joints of the lumbar spine and of the sacroiliac joints

Sign	*T/L*	*L3/4*	*L4/5*	*L5–S1*	*Sacroiliac*
			Segment		
Lack of pelvic rotatory synkinesis	++	+	+	+	++
Straight leg raising: hamstrings spasm	–	–	+	+	+
Femoral nerve stretch test: spasm of rectus femoris	–	+	–	–	–
Spasm of thoracolumbar erector spinae	++	–	–	–	–
Spasm of lumbar erector spinae	–	+	+	+	–
Psoas spasm	++	–	–	–	–
Piriformis spasm	–	–	++	–	–
Iliacus spasm	–	–	–	++	–
Painful iliac crest	++	+	–	–	–
Painful greater trochanter	–	+	–	–	–
Painful posterior superior iliac spine	–	+	+	+	+
Pain radiating in L4 segment (hyperalgesia)	–	++	–	–	–
Pain radiating in L5 segment (hyperalgesia)	–	–	++	–	–
Pain radiating in S1 segment (hyperalgesia)	–	–	–	++	++
Patrick's sign (adductor spasm)	–	+	+	+	++
Tenderness of the symphysis	+	–	–	+	++
Tenderness of both ends of sacroiliac joint	–	–	–	+	++

Symptoms

Unless acute, the course is as a rule more severe than in the conditions already dealt with, that is to say, attacks last longer and the condition has a tendency to relapse. Pain at coughing, etc. is more prominent. The posture that is particularly harmful is that of slightly bending forward, as over a wash-basin while shaving, where contraction of the erector spinae is at its maximum and there is therefore maximum pressure on the disc. Another characteristic complaint is of pain when turning over in bed.

Clinical signs

In acute cases we see the characteristic analgesic position adopted in acute root lesion (*Figure 7.1*), i.e. kyphosis and lumbar scoliosis, most frequently towards the side of the lesion (*see Figure 3.8,* page 55). Stooping is severely limited and the straight leg raising test markedly positive (in lesions at the L3/4 segment it is the femoral nerve stretch test that is positive). All movement disturbing the analgesic posture is severely restricted. If the patient is capable of lying prone springing of the lumbar spine is very painful, particularly at the site of the lesion. Nevertheless, if blockage of individual segments is examined this may be absent.

In the more chronic cases it is stooping that is usually most impaired while the patient is standing, but with the patient seated anteflexion may be normal. Another diagnostic sign is the painful arc (Cyriax, 1977) (*see* page 115). The straight leg raising test, and the femoral nerve stretch test in L3/4 lesions, may be markedly positive, much more so than when there is only joint blockage. A most useful diagnostic sign is pain on springing the lumbar spine if blockage is absent or if it persists after blockage has been treated.

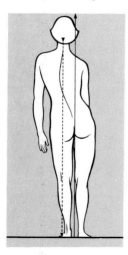

Figure 7.1 Typical posture in acute disc lesion ('sciatic scoliosis')

Therapy

In acute cases complete rest in the relief position is recommended; traction may be attempted (by hand) in this position, because it may procure immediate relief (*see Figure 6.28,* page 218). If pain continues in the relief position epidural infiltration with local anaesthetic may bring about immediate relief. This may and should be combined with the usual pharmacotherapy, aspirin (unless contraindicated) remaining one of the most effective drugs. In the chronic cases traction is again very important so long as it gives relief. Most important here is the establishment of a suitable regimen, avoiding the most dangerous causes of strain such as the forward-bent position, jolting in vehicles, etc., and combined with judicious remedial exercises; the lumbar region should also be well protected against chill.

PELVIC DISTORTION (*see* also page 111 and *Figures 3.12* and *3.13* (page 62)

Even if found in cases of low-back pain, this condition is always secondary. Although in itself a highly characteristic sign, the clinical picture corresponds to the lesion, which is causative and must be treated. If treatment is correct the pelvic distortion subsides spontaneously. In young people in particular, however, it is a hint that there is a lesion in the craniocervical junction that requires treatment.

COMBINED LESIONS

The analytical approach to the individual disturbances presented here is an advantage, as it gives a schematic and clear picture of lesions that have a common pathogenesis and therefore a common therapy. In practice, of course, they are rarely found isolated, or if so it is only after other disturbances have been eliminated by treatment. A combination of disorders is the rule, because all the structures involved in low-back pain are closely related, so that if one link does not function properly, others are likely to suffer.

In low-back pain due to overstrain muscular imbalance and faulty statics may produce ligament overstrain and frequently pain in the spinous processes, for instance through hyperlordosis. But joint blockage in any segment, too, is frequently the result of muscular imbalance, faulty statics or both. On the other hand, it may also be the cause of the imbalance. This is no less true of the painful coccyx resulting from hypertonus of the glutei, quite frequently associated with ligament pain and, on the other hand, frequently associated with sacroiliac lesions and lesions of the hip. Again, lesions of the hip are very often associated with blocked sacroiliac joints. All of these disorders of function in the strict sense of the word may be and often are connected with disc lesions, complicating them, blockage at the segment of disc lesion being the rule rather than the exception.

Only an analysis of this interlocking can make a logical and consistent therapeutic approach possible. Obviously in principle a disturbance of function is more likely to be remedied by adequate therapy than a structural lesion such as disc protrusion. On the other hand, pain originating in the disc or severe blockage may make remedial exercise or static correction impossible because of muscle spasm.

It will therefore be advisable to attack blockage and spasm first and to tackle disc lesion by traction, if required and possible. Some may ask whether disc lesion does not constitute a contraindication against manipulation. On the other hand, blockage is quite frequently the reason why a patient with disc lesion reacts badly to traction, i.e. to one of the most effective ways of treating her condition. The answer is to use the gentlest techniques and if possible to deal with spasm and blockage simultaneously. This is possible, thanks to the PR mobilization techniques ('muscle energy techniques'). It is thus good policy, except in some very acute disc lesions, to start by treating blockage in the most adequate way, to treat disc lesion if present, and then to improve muscular imbalance and faulty statics, and to treat the residual pain (hyperalgesic zones, pain points) by the best method to suit the case.

Pain in the thoracic spine

Since the thoracic spine is less mobile than the cervical or the lumbar spine it is less frequently the site of primary lesion. On the other hand, pain in the thoracic region is often referred pain from the viscera, and lesions of the thoracic spine are often secondary to visceral disease. This must always be borne in mind in order to avoid mistaken diagnosis. There is, however, one important condition affecting the thoracic spine primarily, i.e. juvenile kyphosis with stiffness of the thoracic spine ensuing in adult life, and this unfavourably affects both the cervical and the lumbar spine.

Patients complain mostly of pain between or below the shoulder-blades. Here, again, pain in the dorsal region may be distinguished between that due only to overstrain (whether exogenic or caused by muscular imbalance) and that caused by faulty statics. Exogenic overstrain in this region is most frequently due to a kyphotic sitting position. The typical muscular imbalance is a short pectoralis and weak lower fixators of the scapula. On the other hand, hypermobility can also be linked with pain, particularly in a flat back in the upper thoracic region. The therapy is clear. For its very favourable effect I advocate Brügger's relief position (*see Figure 6.119*, page 295). There is a special type of pain described by Maigne (1964) as 'dorsalgie interscapulaire' in which the spinous processes of T5 or T6 are very tender on palpation and in which findings in the thoracic region are otherwise negative; the primary lesion is in the lower cervical spine and must be treated. Maigne and le Corre (1969) also described painful muscle spasm in this condition, forming an oblique band passing from the tender spinous process to the shoulder. This can be treated by PR (*see Figure 6.93*, page 275).

Blockage in the thoracic region affects not only the intervertebral apophyseal joints but also the joints between the vertebrae and the ribs, causing the same type of pain. In both cases, if the lesion is acute, pain may be worse during deep breathing, but this feature is of course more prominent in rib lesions, where it is useful to know whether breathing in or out causes the greatest pain. The importance of exact differential diagnosis as against pleurisy is obvious.

Both for diagnosis and for therapy the techniques described in Chapters 4 and 6, respectively, are essential and need not be repeated here.

Muscle spasm of the erector spinae is frequently found in the thoracic spine even without blockage, or after blockage has been treated, and in such cases PR of the thoracic erector spinae is most rewarding (*see Figures 6.88–6.90,* page 271).

Finally, it is important to note that lesions of the thoracolumbar junction quite often cause pain and muscle spasm in the dorsal region. Pain at the xiphoid process is often secondary to a lesion of the 7th or 8th rib, and to tension in the abdominal muscles.

Neck pain

Unlike low-back pain, neck pain is clinically simpler, although the 'cervical syndrome' is more complex than the clinical pictures of lesions of the lumbar spine and pelvis.

Here, too, we can distinguish between pain caused only by overstrain (either exogenic or due to muscular imbalance) and that caused by faulty statics. The commonest type of chronic overstrain of the neck is caused by working with the head bent forward. A forward-drawn position of the head due to faulty statics may cause similar complaints (*see Figure 3.37,* page 90). The typical muscular imbalance in the region of the shoulder girdle has been described in Chapter 4 (page 171).

Symptoms
First discomfort and then pain caused by overstrain, usually after working in a sitting position. Another complaint is similar pain provoked by jolting in buses, tractors and similar vehicles.

Clinical signs
Signs typical of muscular imbalance (if present), faulty posture which must be examined in a *relaxed* sitting position without a support. Faulty breathing by lifting the thorax should not be overlooked. The most typical periosteal pain points are the lateral edge of the spinous process of C2 (more frequently on the right) and the upper edge of the shoulder-blade. The most important muscular trigger points are in the upper trapezius, the levator scapulae and the sternocleidomastoid. (Any spinous, articular or transverse process may of course be tender on palpation.)

Therapy
Head anteflexion must be avoided; remedial exercise must include correction of faulty breathing patterns. A supporting collar is useful in jolting vehicles (*see Figure*

6.125, page 301). PR of muscles with trigger points and painful insertions is effective. It is important to provide correct back support when sitting (*see Figure 6.126*, page 301).

ACUTE WRY NECK

One of the most frequent causes of neck pain is, of course, blockage of mobile segments of the cervical spine; this has to be diagnosed by the methods given in Chapter 4. Blockage is also the most frequent cause of what is called *acute wry neck*.

Symptoms
The condition presents most frequently after rest in bed with the neck in an unsuitable position, sometimes after driving a car with the window open, or again after a sudden jerk of the neck; the patient complains of pain and stiffness, usually only on one side of the neck, frequently radiating towards one shoulder or the occiput.

Clinical signs
Not only is the head held very stiffly, it is usually also rotated and inclined. Rotation and bending to the opposite side is most restricted, but anteflexion and retroflexion also suffer. The most frequent cause is blockage of the segment C2/3, in exceptional cases C1/2 or C3/4. It is, however, important to realize that another segment is usually involved, most frequently C5/6, or sometimes occiput/atlas. These segments require treatment, but are better diagnosed after treatment of C2/3, because acute pain and spasm make diagnosis difficult. The typical pain point is the lateral aspect of the spinous process of C2 on the convex side. A pain point between the upper medial edge of the scapula and the spinous processes in the middle part of the trapezius should be looked for: this is a sign of possible complication by a cervicobrachial or radicular syndrome.

Therapy
The first step is isometric traction with the patient seated or supine (*see Figure 6.51*, page 237), which should bring immediate relief; this is followed by gentle mobilization of C2/3. We should then treat the second segment which is usually involved. Residual muscle spasm, most frequently in the trapezius, is treated by PR.

There is a possible diagnostic pitfall in relapsing acute wry neck: the initial stage of a spasmodic torticollis. In such cases, while pain becomes less at each relapse, rotation and inclination of the head become worse and we see the typical spasm of the sternocleidomastoid on one side and the splenius on the other, whereas true blockage becomes less and less marked.

Most cases of neck pain in which blockage is not acute are linked with other forms of the cervical syndrome, as will be described later in this chapter. It is unusual if neck pain is not combined with pain in the region of the shoulder, i.e. dermatome C4, to which pain radiates from about as many structures as into the low-back region. In addition to the large C4 dermatome there is a characteristic hyperalgesic zone in blockage of the craniocervical junction below and posterior to the mastoid process.

Pseudoradicular and other pain due to disturbed motor function of the lower extremities

The reader should take note of what I have already said about pseudoradicular pain in Chapter 2 (page 40). In listing the clinical signs of blockage of lumbar mobile segments, the segment of radiating, i.e. pseudoradicular, pain was included. Clinical experience shows that as in true radicular syndromes, we encounter pseudoradicular syndromes only in L4, L5 and S1. In the L4 pseudoradicular syndrome pain radiates down the ventral aspect of the thigh towards and even below the knee; in L5 syndromes pain radiates down the lateral aspect of the lower extremity to the ankle and in S1 syndromes down the dorsolateral aspect of the lower extremity towards the heel. In the L4 syndrome the femoral nerve stretch test and in the L5 and S1 syndromes the straight leg raising test can be positive, but not to the degree seen in true radicular syndromes. Besides pain, there may be hyperalgesia and dysaesthesia in each segment. The muscles in spasm characteristic for each pseudoradicular syndrome have been given in the list of signs of blockage of individual segments of the lumbar spine (*see* page 309).

Which structures are most frequently affected if we find the pseudoradicular syndromes described above?

The pseudoradicular syndrome L4 is caused by a lesion either in the mobile segment L3/4 or in the hip joint, and for this reason it may be difficult to distinguish a painful hip without clear coxarthrosis from an L3/4 lesion or a combination of both disorders, which is quite frequent – patients in whom we have to treat both the hip and the L3/4 segment. Since pain radiates towards the knee, and spasm of the adductors (Patrick's sign) also produces pain at the attachment point – i.e. the pes anserinus on the tibia – pain at the knee is also common.

The pseudoradicular syndrome L5 is caused mainly by lesions of the mobile segment L4/5 with typical spasm of the piriformis. This spasm – trigger point – in the piriformis frequently persists even after successful treatment of the L4/5 segment, or after it has spontaneously returned to normal, and can then be the cause of a pseudoradicular syndrome. A not infrequent complication of this syndrome is a painful fibular head due to tension in the biceps femoris (hamstrings, straight leg raising!).

The pseudoradicular syndrome S1 is caused not only by the lumbosacral segment but also by lesions of the sacroiliac joint. Another structure that may radiate pain in this segment is the sacroiliac ligament or a painful tuber ossis ischii, the attachment point of the hamstrings. Again, this syndrome is frequently complicated by pain at the fibular head.

A structure that can complicate *all three* pseudoradicular syndromes is the coccyx: there may be a positive Patrick's sign and straight leg raising test, spasm of the iliacus or the piriformis, and pain may even simulate hip pain.

Another structure referring pain to the low back and causing back bending restriction and in some cases even a forward drawn position of the thorax relative to the pelvis, is a painful pubic symphysis due to increased tension of the abdominal muscles.

In addition to pseudoradicular pain in the lower extremities there are disturbances of locomotor function, which must be clinically diagnosed and which may cause pain by themselves, but which more often complicate pseudoradicular or true radicular syndromes.

One such lesion is a *blocked fibular head* (*see Figure 6.22,* page 211), which may cause pain at the fibular head and cramp in the calf; in the acute stage pain at flexion and extension of the knee may be felt, with negative findings at the knee joint.

Pain originating in the lower extremity

In a *painful knee* (not pain referred to the knee) it is most important not to overlook a *patella* that does not move easily and smoothly on the femoral and tibial articular surfaces. This has sometimes to be found by exerting gentle pressure on the patella from above, creating a grinding resistance. The technique described on page 212 is most effective in dealing with such lesions.

Most important of all is *movement restriction of the tarsal bones* and ankle joints, mainly affecting joint play. The joints most frequently affected are the ankle joint, the second, third and fourth tarsometatarsal joints, and the talocalcaneal joint. The most frequent symptoms are: pain in the foot, cramp which may also affect the calf and shin and dysaesthesia (which is also attributed to tunnel syndromes). For diagnostic and therapeutic techniques *see* Chapters 4 and 6.

There is one frequent complaint, however, which must be dealt with here: a painful *calcaneal spur.* In itself this is simply the insertion of the plantar aponeurosis. It becomes painful when there is increased tension in the aponeurosis, but the cause may be complex, as follows: (1) movement restriction between the tarsal bones, in particular between the calcaneus and the talus, navicular and cuboid; (2) movement restriction of the fibular head (!) or (3) frequently of the sacroiliac joints; and (4) increased tension in the muscles attached to the plantar aponeurosis. All these possibilities must be borne in mind for treatment to be successful.

For the *painful Achilles' tendon see Figure 6.105,* page 284.

Even such a condition as *meralgia paresthetica nocturna* is usually secondary to disturbed function of the lumbar spine and pelvis. It is usually explained as yet another entrapment or 'tunnel' syndrome, this nerve emerging from the lateral border of the psoas, crossing the iliacus, and passing under the inguinal ligament. It is reasonable to assume that increased pressure in that tunnel can result from spasm of the muscles that pass through it, i.e. principally the iliopsoas. Spasm or increased tension of the psoas and the iliacus is a very frequent condition indeed, caused by muscular imbalance in lesions of the thoracolumbar junction, the lumbosacral junction, the hip and even the coccyx. Hence if we normalize function of the lumbar and pelvic region and relax the iliopsoas, this condition usually clears up.

Pseudoradicular and other pain due to disturbed locomotor function of the upper extremities

In the upper extremity, too, pain frequently radiates from lesioned segments of the cervical spine, the cervicothoracic junction, and even from the upper ribs. Here, unlike the lower extremities, we do not as a rule see pain following a single dermatome exactly; the simple pseudoradicular pattern is usually hidden or distorted by what we would call a chain reaction of secondary lesions producing pain mainly in the shoulder, round the elbow and forearm, and at the wrist.

Shoulder pain

This is probably the most constant symptom of pain radiating into the upper extremity and constitutes a clinical problem as complex as that of low-back pain. This may be due to the fact that many structures refer pain to the dermatome C4, which covers the shoulder region and belongs to the same segment as the phrenic nerve.

Experience has shown that any type of pain originating in the cervical spine, even in its upper part to as far down as to the upper thoracic and the upper ribs – and even the viscera, the heart, lungs, liver, gall bladder and stomach – may be the origin of pain referred to the dermatome C4. (The dermatome chart of Hansen and Schliack (1962) used here differs from that of Keegan (1944) usually quoted in the American and British literature, where the shoulder region is covered by the dermatome C5.) The phrenic nerve, originating from the C4 segment, provides a much more credible explanation of this widespread irradiation than does the dermatome C5. This explains the somewhat vague term 'shoulder–arm syndrome'.

SHOULDER PAIN DUE TO DISTURBED MUSCLE FUNCTION

Here, too, muscular imbalance alone can be the cause of pain, producing symptoms as fatigue sets in. The muscle most susceptible to painful spasm (trigger points) is the trapezius, in its upper and middle sections, which produces shoulder pain. For clinical signs *see* 'upper crossed syndrome' (page 171).

Therapy
Immediate relief can be obtained by PR of the muscles with trigger points, but the underlying muscular imbalance should be treated by remedial exercise.

Pain radiating from the cervical and upper thoracic spine

Here pain is evoked by certain movements of – or positions of – the head. The most frequent cause is movement restriction, which is then the main object of treatment.

Pain originating in the upper ribs

The first four ribs produce pain radiating into the shoulder. In lesions of the second to fourth rib patients also feel pain in the shoulder-blade. In lesions of the first rib (*see Figure 4.18*, page 123) shoulder pain may be the only complaint. At examination there is usually tenderness at the vertebral margin of the scapula in lesions of the second to fourth rib, and tenderness of the (underlying) angle of the rib is found only after shoulder abduction. Tenderness of the first rib can be palpated at its attachment to the manubrium sterni below the clavicle. Here, too, movement restriction is the most frequent cause of pain and therefore the principal object of therapy.

The scapulohumeral joint

The clinical picture of involvement of this joint has been described in classic terms by Cyriax (1977). It corresponds to the 'frozen shoulder' which is unique in arthrology because it is caused by contracture of the joint capsule (Cyriax, 1977; De Sèze, 1960).

Symptoms

In patients of 45–65 years of age, more usually women, pain of severe intensity sets in, felt in the shoulder, radiating down the arm even to the forearm, and being worst at night (in bed), or when the arm hangs down, carrying a weight, or on moving the shoulder. At first there is only slight restriction of movement, but in the course of a few weeks this deteriorates. It is possible to distinguish three stages (as Cyriax points out), each lasting 3–4 months:during the first stage pain is intense and the symptoms exacerbate; during the second stage pain subsides although movement is still restricted; and during the third stage the frozen shoulder 'thaws', so that in about 1 year the patient is symptom free.

Clinical signs

At examination we find the typical capsular pattern (Cyriax, 1977; *see Figure 4.30,* page 133). It is worth noting that joint play (*see Figure 4.31,* page 134) remains unaffected as long as abduction of the arm is possible to about 90 degrees, which shows again that it is only the capsule that restricts mobility. The typical pain point is at the attachment of the deltoid muscle tendon and the subscapularis muscle. In severe cases there is muscle atrophy in the deltoid, the supra- and infraspinatus muscles, and there can be severe vasomotor disturbance in the whole of the upper extremity with cyanosis, oedema and even glossy skin on the fingers ('shoulder arm syndrome').

Therapy

In the acute stage we have to combat pain, using the classic analgesics but avoiding narcotics if possible. It is also important to combat pain indirectly, by treating all concomitant disturbances of the cervical spine and any muscle spasm in the shoulder. The usual mobilization and manipulation techniques are useless in dealing with the shoulder joint itself, but there is one technique that may give relief at any stage of the disease – traction using PR (*see Figure 6.10,* page 204). The most specific treatment, which should always be given a trial, is gravity induced PR or infiltration of the subscapularis. This is indicated whenever we diagnose a trigger point in this muscle (*see* Chapter 6, page 270, *Figure 6.87(b)*). Cortisone should be tried (or substances with similar effect – such as triamcinolone) as an intra-articular injection, but should be repeated only for a few times and only if it alleviates the pain. It is advisable for the patient to wear her arm in a sling during the acute stage and to perform only isometric exercises. More active exercise can be undertaken in the second stage, when pain has subsided, but it should never be such as to provoke the pain again.

Pain provoked by arm abduction

Pain during abduction of the arm is more common than the capsular pattern. It is caused by disturbance of the mechanism by which the head of the humerus slips through under the coracohumeral ligament during abduction. This movement is lubricated by the bursa subdeltoacromialis, and if the mechanism is impaired X-ray sometimes reveals calcifications.

Symptoms

There may be pain provoked by abduction of the arm, or even merely movement restriction, or there may even be severe spontaneous pain. There are two types of impaired movement that may be present:

1. The patient abducts the arm to the point at which the humeral head becomes engaged under the ligament and at this point the patient feels pain, but once he overcomes this 'obstacle', abduction may continue to 180 degrees without symptoms. This phenomenon is the 'painful arc' (Cyriax, 1977).
2. There may simply be restricted abduction.

Clinical findings
Restricted abduction, a painful arc, or both, with normal rotation in the shoulder joint; there is impairment of joint play at the humeroscapular joint (*see Figure 4.31*, page 134). There may be calcifications in the bursa subdeltoacromialis.

Therapy
Mobilization to restore joint play (*see Figure 6.11*, page 204); infiltration of the bursa subdeltoacromialis by injection of local anaesthetic under the acromion over the head of the humerus, or simply needling of the pain point.

Pain arising in the muscles of the rotator cuff and the long head of the biceps

In these cases symptoms occur mainly if the patient is forced to strain the painful muscle, pain being felt at the insertion point at the humeral head, with the exception of the long head of the biceps which is felt in the groove between the major and minor tubercles of the humerus. For clinical examination, *see Figure 4.29*, page 133).

Therapy
PR of each muscle found to give pain (*see Figures 6.85–6.87*, page 268). Needling or local anaesthetic can be applied to the attachment point of each muscle, or to the long biceps tendon in the groove between the tubercles.

Accessory shoulder joints

THE ACROMIOCLAVICULAR JOINT

This is a very frequent but rarely diagnosed cause of pain which the patient feels in the shoulder and fails to distinguish from pain in the shoulder joint. The pain is provoked by moving the raised arm in front of the chest. At examination passive adduction of the arm across the chest is painful and the joint is tender at palpation. Therapy consists mainly in mobilization (*see Figures 6.12* and *6.13*, page 205). Needling or the application of local anaesthetics is also helpful. Only in cases of true arthrosis, where this treatment has failed, should local application of cortisone be tried.

THE STERNOCLAVICULAR JOINT

Blockage of this joint, without arthrosis, is a much rarer condition. Symptoms are localized in the subclavicular region with much irradiation to the shoulder, sternum and neck; the pain is provoked by shoulder movements involving the scapula. It is important to point out that the frequently painful or tender medial end of the clavicle is not as a rule a sign of lesion of the sternoclavicular joint, but of tension in the sternocleidomastoid, and must be treated as such. True isolated arthrosis of this joint is not frequent either and is difficult to treat. In simple blockage mobilization is effective and can be combined with local anaesthetics or needling.

Pain in the elbow region

A very frequent complication of pain even of cervical origin is pain localized more often at the lateral than the medial epicondyle of the humerus. As the epicondyles are the attachment points of muscles, increased muscle tension plays an important role here and should be diagnosed and treated. Although the lateral epicondyle is palpated through the brachioradialis, the muscles producing increased tension at the epicondyle are the supinator, the extensor of the fingers and the hand, and the biceps brachii. Prehension causes pain, particularly if it is a cramped movement. It is no coincidence that tennis elbow and writers' cramp are forms of the same disease; pressure on the pen because the writer is tense and nervous and failure to relax the grip on the tennis racket in between strokes set up the same reaction.

Symptoms
Pain at the lateral aspect of the elbow, radiating up and down the arm, and more intense when the hand grasps something or holds firmly on to something. Patients often complain that things fall out of their hands.

Clinical signs
There is a very tender pain point at the lateral epicondyle. For diagnosis and treatment of increased tension in the pertinent muscles, *see Figures 6.81–6.83*, pages 266–267. In addition to increased muscle tension, there is resistance to springing the elbow joint in a lateral direction.

Therapy
The muscles in spasm must be relaxed, manipulation is effective, and local anaesthesia or needling can be used. The use of cortisone should be the exception. It is important to remember that the underlying cause of the condition is a cramped way of using the hands, and failure in treatment is due to inability to improve the patient's habits rather than to ineffective methods of treatment.

Medial epicondylar pain

Symptoms
Pain at the medial epicondyle.

Clinical signs
Tension in the flexors of the hand and fingers and impaired springing of the elbow in a medial direction.

Therapy
Relaxation of the finger and hand flexors, manipulation of the elbow in a medial direction, and if necessary local anaesthesia. Use of cortisone should be the exception.

Pain at the wrist

The structure most frequently found to be painful is the styloid process of the radius. This affection is closely linked with lateral epicondylalgia and lateral springing of the elbow joint is usually impaired (*see* page 135). Another structure that is frequently painful (with or without arthrosis) is the first carpometacarpal joint. In both these conditions the symptoms are local, generally getting worse with strain. The most significant sign in a painful styloid process, besides local tenderness, is restricted radial flexion of the hand. Therapy should be mainly directed to the underlying disturbance of function at the elbow. (De Quervain's tendovaginitis may be a secondary condition.) Joint mobilization is recommended, as for lesion of the first carpometacarpal joint; *see Figure 6.2* (page 198).

In rare cases there may be a painful os pisiforme, one cause being blockage against the underlying os triquetrum. This can easily be mobilized.

Entrapment syndromes

There are two important affections in the upper extremity which are quite often found in combination: the carpal-tunnel syndrome and the thoracic-outlet syndrome.

THE CARPAL-TUNNEL SYNDROME

This condition is attributed to compression of the median nerve in the tunnel formed by the carpal bones and crossed by the ligament carpi transversum, compression first affecting the vessels supplying the nerve.

Symptoms
The patient complains of numbness and tingling, or even pain, in the hand and fingers, at first when waking up in the morning and later such as to wake him up in the night. In the more advanced stage pins and needles and pain are felt even during the day, particularly on raising the arms. Relief is obtained when the arms hang loose, while shaking the hands improves the blood supply. Pain is also felt at the wrist and may radiate up the arm. Strain on the hands exacerbates the symptoms.

Clinical signs
In the initial stages we have to provoke the symptoms for examination; the simplest method is raising the arms while the patient is supine. Pressure on the median nerve above the wrist may elicit a sharp tingling pain (Tinel's sign). In the more advanced stage there is hypoaesthesia in the area supplied by the median nerve and weakness with atrophy of the abductor pollicis; this muscle must always be tested. One of the most significant findings is increased resistance to joint play between the carpal bones (*see* page 200).

Therapy
If joint play is impaired it must first be restored by mobilization (*see Figures 6.5* and *6.6,* pages 200–201) and the patient must be taught self-mobilization (*see Figure 6.71,* page 255). In the few cases in which joint play is not impaired, or if mobilization brings no relief, local anaesthetic should be applied in the carpal

tunnel. Only in exceptional cases should local application of cortisone be attempted. In the advanced stages, with thenar atrophy, when secondary changes hinder the success of this type of therapy, operation is indicated.

THE THORACIC-OUTLET SYNDROME ('SCALENUS SYNDROME')

This is attributed to compression of the bracchial plexus mainly at the gap between the anterior and middle scalenus and its attachment at the first (or cervical) rib, also between the clavicle and the first rib, causing numbness and tingling in the upper extremity, the pain being most intense in the hands and fingers. Thus it is not unlike the carpal-tunnel syndrome. In fact, at the time the syndrome was distinguished many cases at present diagnosed as carpal-tunnel syndromes were attributed to the scalenus syndrome.

The thoracic-outlet syndrome is apparently the result of a complex of lesions in structures forming the thoracic outlet, each requiring separate diagnosis and producing its specific symptoms. These are: increased tension of the scalenus (see Figure 6.76, page 261); increased tension of the other upper fixators of the shoulder girdle; movement restriction in the lower cervical and upper thoracic spine; and movement restriction of the upper ribs, in particular of the first rib. It is no wonder, in view of this complexity, that doctors unfamiliar with the diagnosis of these disturbances of function indicated operation, instead of conservative treatment of the underlying cause of the condition. This syndrome warrants operation only in exceptional cases where marked neurological signs are present.

Symptoms

Principally dysaesthesia – i.e. numbness and pins and needles – with pain in the upper extremity, including the hands, which gets worse when heavy carrying has to be done. The symptoms vary according to which structure (lesion) plays the principal role.

Clinical signs

The following tests are useful: Adson's manoeuvre, i.e. weakening (disappearing) pulse at the radial artery on bending the head back and turning it to the same side; raising the abducted arm bent at the elbow and observing the radial pulse; or pulling the arm down (as if carrying a heavy case) and observing the pulse. All these tests show concomitant compression of the subclavian artery. More important, however, is diagnosis of disturbance of the structures forming the thoracic outlet. Only in exceptional cases are true neurological signs found (atrophy of muscles of the hand); cervical myelopathy must then first be ruled out.

Therapy depends on the analysis of clinical findings and their relevance, and is less a technical question than one of pathogenic considerations.

Combined lesions

As with low-back pain, pain in the upper extremities is usually due not to one specific lesion but a combination of several. As we have seen in the thoracic-outlet syndrome, which is due to a complex of interconnected lesions, all the syndromes affecting the upper extremities form chains, as described on page 174. A key role is played by muscular imbalance at the shoulder girdle, producing tension of the upper fixators, and by faulty respiration with lifting of the thorax and increased tension in the scalenes. This increased tension is transmitted to the muscles of the upper arm and forearm and influences the epicondyles. Secondary movement restriction of the spinal and extremity joints soon follows, which increases muscle spasm. We can thus see combinations not only in space, so to speak, but also in time: pain radiating from the neck into the shoulders may be followed by pain in the epidondyles, the styloid process, and then by a carpal-tunnel syndrome followed by dysaesthesia due to blockage of the first rib. All this has to be considered and weighed up in order to indicate the proper place and the proper time for specific treatment, nor should the possibility of visceral involvement be forgotten.

The cervicocranial syndrome

This syndrome covers headache of cervical origin as well as other disturbances mainly of equilibrium, including minor neurological disorders like cervical nystagmus. The underlying disturbance of the cervical spine can be the same as in simple neck pain. It is of course true that the cause is more frequently a lesion in the upper cervical spine, in particular at the cervicocranial junction, just as the lower cervical spine is more likely to produce pain in the upper extremity, but there are frequent exceptions. This is understandable if we consider the musculature: long muscles like the sternocleidomastoid, the scalenes, trapezii, and levatores scapulae, with their frequent spasms and trigger points, cover all of the cervical region and may react to lesions at any segment of the cervical spine. Apparently, the reaction of the nervous system determines whether the patient will suffer only from pain in the neck, or in the shoulder or arm, or mainly from headache, although the same disturbance of function may underlie them all.

Headache of cervical origin

This is an extremely frequent condition and is in my opinion the commonest single type of headache. It includes 'tension headache' which was thought to be mainly psychological; increased muscle tension, as we have seen, is due to many factors, and in its classic description (Wolff, 1948) increased tension of the neck muscles is part of the clinical picture of tension headache. Increased muscle tension is the consequence of practically all disturbances of the cervical spine, from exogenic overstrain, faulty posture and muscular imbalance to movement restriction throughout the cervical spine. There is of course a close relationship between headache, increased tension and psychological problems (*see* page 40), but this does not alter the fact that increased muscle tension is a physiological phenomenon and that it should be treated by the most suitable physiological methods. Nor is 'vasomotor' headache incompatible with headache of cervical origin: the mere fact that a disturbance in the cervical region causes headache shows the presence of a factor of reflex origin. If we assume that disturbed function plays the role of a nociceptive stimulus, then a vasomotor reaction is part of the typical reaction, pain as a rule provoking vasoconstriction.

As this type of headache is very frequent, it should not be diagnosed only per exclusionem, i.e. only after any other origin has been ruled out, as most neurological textbooks teach. Admittedly, serious pathology must be excluded; but it should be remembered that headache of cervical origin has its own characteristic features, and as an important clinical entity it should be diagnosed as such.

Symptoms

All that is characteristic for vertebrogenic disorders (*see* page 103) is true for headache of cervical origin. I want to insist particularly on the position of the head, i.e. headache due to head anteflexion for long periods at work, and headache on waking, due to an unfavourable position of the head during sleep. Another feature of great importance is asymmetry, i.e. the fact that headache of cervical origin is usually one-sided or at least more intense on one side than on the other. It is also paroxysmal in character, i.e. there are either pain-free intervals or, if pain does not entirely disappear, there are at least paroxysms of intense pain. Summing up all of the features listed in Chapter 4 – including the role of psychological, endocrinological or even an allergic factor – we come to the conclusion that cervical headache has many features in common with migraine.

At this point the localization of cervical headache must be discussed. This diagnosis is certainly indicated if the patient complains of pain radiating from the neck into the occiput and from there towards the eyes and temples, more to one side than the other. However, this in itself is insufficient for a diagnosis. In young patients, particularly adolescents and children, headache is frequently the first sign of disturbed cervical function long before neck pain has been felt. In such cases the pain may be localized in the forehead or the temporal region. Even pain radiating into the face (but not typical trigeminal neuralgia!) can be of cervical origin. This is less surprising than it may seem: Travell (1981) has studied referred pain from trigger points in the sternocleidomastoid, which were frequently localized in the face.

Clinical signs

The most important are of course the signs of disturbed cervical function, which are common to neck pain, and include signs of muscular imbalance, spasm, faulty respiration and segmental lesions, particularly of the craniocervical junction. The most important pain points are on the lateral surface of the spinous process of the axis (more frequently on the right), at the posterior arch of the atlas (in the short extensors), at the transverse process of the atlas and in the sternocleidomastoid. The frequent pain points on the occiput itself are usually secondary, and there may sometimes be odd pain points of atypical localization on the skull. There is an important pain point at the temple in the temporalis muscle (not to be confused with a painful temporal artery!); other masticatory muscles may also cause headache, and should be examined for trigger points even through the open mouth. Even the pain point corresponding to the notch of the first division of the trigeminal nerve at the orbit can be of cervical origin.

Typical hyperalgesic skin zones are found medially below the mastoid processes, at the temples and eyebrows and at the forehead above the eyebrows and on both sides of the nose.

Therapy

This follows the same rules as for any other disturbance of the cervical region. It may be worth while stressing that here the significance of movement restriction at the craniocervical junction is so great that it is good policy to treat this first, since muscular imbalance cannot be improved until this obstacle has been removed. Movement restriction between atlas and occiput must be examined in all directions. If pain regularly begins on waking, we must enquire about the sleeping position of the patient. While trigger points in the muscles and at periosteal points of attachment are best treated by PR, pain points on the skull are better dealt with by needling. A tender temporalis muscle can be treated by PR (together with the masseter) or by local anaesthetic. The hyperalgesic zones on the forehead, temples and round the nose respond very well to skin stretching (*see* page 303).

ANTEFLEXION HEADACHE

This is of exceptional clinical importance because in present-day conditions large numbers of people work seated, with the head bent forward. Hypermobile subjects who are susceptible to ligament pain are particularly prone to this type of headache. Another group is made up of patients after injury. The largest group of sufferers, however, are schoolchildren; and according to Gutmann (1968), whose opinion I share, 'school headache' – originally considered to be psychological – is usually due to this mechanism.

Symptoms
The child is pain free on waking. Only after some time at school, perhaps several hours, and particularly when reading or writing, the child starts to fidget and change his position, until later headache is felt as such. During the holidays there are no symptoms. As the condition deteriorates, headache begins sooner and the child finds it increasingly difficult to concentrate so that his performance in school deteriorates. These same patients suffer from headache after jolting in public vehicles or on turning somersaults.

Clinical signs
The anteflexion test is positive, i.e. if the patient's head is held in maximum anteflexion without force but merely taking up the slack, pain sets in after 10–15 s. (Immediate pain is a sign of anteflexion blockage at C0/1.) There may be some movement restriction in the upper cervical spine. The typical pain point is the lateral edge of the spinous process of the axis. Typical signs of hypermobility may be visualized at X-ray (*see Figure 3.45*, page 97).

Therapy
If there is movement restriction it should be treated, as it aggravates the symptoms. The main therapeutic measure is to advise the patient to avoid head anteflexion – for instance, by using a sloping desk for reading and writing. One of the reasons why children suffer from this type of headache much more now than in the past is the introduction of flat school tables instead of the old-fashioned sloping desks. Further therapeutic and preventive measures are a supporting collar to be worn in jolting public vehicles, and the avoidance of PT exercises involving forced head anteflexion, such as somersaults.

Gutmann (1979) has recently described anteflexion headache as a consequence of stenosis of the vertebral canal at the craniocervical junction. In such cases he showed that pressure of the cerebrospinal fluid and headache increase during head anteflexion. In severe cases he had these patients operated by decompression, removing the posterior arch of the atlas and widening the foramen magnum.

TEMPOROMANDIBULAR JOINT

This is a type of headache not of cervical origin(!), which we should not miss: pain originating at the joint and/or the masticatory muscles. Palpation includes the TMJ, muscular trigger points (through the open mouth), tension of the digastricus and tenderness of the hyoid cornua with a possible shift of the hyoid.

RETROFLEXION HEADACHE

Another type of headache is aggravated during retroflexion. This is sometimes the case if there is very marked pain at the posterior arch of the atlas, if there is marked tenderness of the spinous processes below C2 and if there is involvement of the vertebral artery.

MIGRAINE

I have already pointed out that most of the characteristic symptoms of headache of cervical origin fit the clinical picture of migraine, and also that vasomotor disturbance is compatible with headache of cervical origin. Yet it would be wrong to suggest that migraine as such is just another 'vertebrogenic' disease, because there are cases of migraine with absolutely no involvement of the cervical spine. However, in the large majority of migraine patients (including children) we find some disturbance of locomotor function, including faulty respiration (Sachse *et al.*, 1982, in 22 cases of classic migraine). He found movement restriction in the cervical spine in all but three cases, and normal respiration patterns also only in three patients. Bakke *et al.* (1982) and Clifford *et al.* (1982) have found greatly increased EMG activity of head and neck muscles during attacks of migraine. Most migraine patients improve if disturbances of motor function are dealt with, perhaps because as in painful visceral affections the motor system reacts as a rule thus itself becoming a pathogenetic factor.

Differential diagnosis

I must again stress the importance of differential diagnosis. It cannot be the subject of this book, but just as headache due to serious pathological lesion will usually first be treated with analgesics before the true diagnosis is made, the same may happen – and does happen – with manipulation. With the latest manipulation techniques, however, the danger is less than rather than more than that presented by the mistaken use of analgesics or narcotics. The surest way to avoid diagnostic error, of course, is to see patients at intervals and to repeat or complete examination whenever anything unexpected appears during treatment.

Disturbances of equilibrium

The importance of the spinal column, particularly the craniocervical junction, for maintaining equilibrium was explained in Chapter 2. The most significant symptoms of disturbance are dizziness and vertigo, but in a great many patients we can determine disturbed equilibrium by the method shown in *Figure 4.33*, page 144. If as a routine measure patients are asked to stand with each foot on separate scales, putting equal weight on each, a difference of 5 kg or over will probably be accompanied by deviation in Hautant's test in some position of the head, usually in that corresponding to movement restriction. This type of clinically masked disturbance of equilibrium, which is far more frequent than dizziness, is almost invariably of cervical origin, showing the 'cervical pattern' which will be explained below, and which disappears after treatment of movement restriction. These patients are of the type with movement restriction in the craniocervical junction, in whom Norre *et al.* (1976) described cervical nystagmus.

Symptoms

These vary according to the type of vertigo or dizziness involved.

Classic vertigo (Menière's syndrome) – Typical attacks last for hours or even days; the patient suffers from rotational vertigo and is able to indicate the direction of rotation (clockwise or anti-clockwise); vertigo is accompanied by nausea *and* vomiting, usually coupled with tinnitus and disturbance of hearing. There are less severe cases, i.e. shorter, without disturbed audition and a rocking sensation (sea-sickness) may take the place of the typical rotation.

A polymorphous group of short attacks of dizziness provoked by certain head positions in relation to the trunk, the patient having the sensation of being pushed or pulled to one side, forwards or backwards, and apprehensive of falling. Nausea and tinnitus are usually absent, but headache is frequent. From its dependence on neck movement this type of disturbed equilibrium is widely recognized as 'cervical vertigo' or dizziness of cervical origin.

Positional vertigo – These patients suffer short attacks of true rotational vertigo on changing the position of the head in space, i.e. together with the rest of the body, and *not* necessarily changing the position of the head relative to the trunk. These attacks, though short, are very intense, and if the eyes remain open nystagmus of very short duration can be observed.

Severe attacks of short duration provoked by certain positions of the head relative to the trunk, during which the patient falls to the ground: drop attacks, cervical syncope with or without loss of consciousness.

Mixed and transitional forms – i.e. patients suffering from more than one type of attack, or border cases, the type of attack changing during the disease.

When questioning the patient, it is essential to make it quite clear what he or she means by 'dizziness', for the word is used to describe the feeling of fear of falling from a height, an attack of fainting or weakness due to circulatory disorder, or even for intoxication (cerebellar disturbance) and ataxia. When the patient complains of dizziness, then, cross-examination must first elicit more explicit information: does the world seem to be turning clockwise or anti-clockwise round his head? Does he feel pulled to one side, or to the other?

Clinical signs

Only if it is possible to examine the patient during a classic attack of true vertigo can we observe the typical signs of labyrinthine disorder, such as nystagmus to the right with deviation to the left, and deviation to the side of the weaker labyrinth – i.e. during Romberg's test, standing with eyes closed with the head in neutral position, there is deviation to the side; with the head turned to the side of the weaker labyrinth the trunk moves backwards, while it moves forward if the head is turned to the opposite side. If, however, we examine the patient in between attacks, and there are no pathological neurological findings, there is little to observe unless we carry out Hautant's test as described in Chapter 4 (page 144).

Using this as a routine examination method a characteristic pattern emerges if there is a cervical factor, regardless of the type of disturbance of equilibrium. In 72 examinations of 69 patients I found the most constant phenomenon was increased deviation of the forward-stretched arms at rotation of the head in the opposite direction to that of deviation, and at retroflexion of the head, and less or no deviation of the arms at head rotation in that direction, or at anteflexion. In 69 cases there were only two exceptions, and in neither of these did the cervical spine play any role. In what might be called 'typical cases', deviation increased if the 'pathogenic' head position coincided with the direction of movement restriction, as was the case in 50 examinations (70 per cent). In many cases side deviation is provoked only if the head is rotated and/or bent back, but deviation of the arms is in the opposite direction to that of head rotation. It is also significant that deviation disappears after treatment of movement restriction, or at least becomes much less marked, the effect being visible a few minutes after treatment.

It is important to stress here that a cervical factor may be present in all forms of vertigo and dizziness; this was as true in a group of typical vertigo (54 patients) as in 70 patients with cervical and mixed-type vertigo, the results of treatment showing little difference (the figure for improvement in both was 90 per cent). The type of vertigo that reacts least to treatment of the cervical spine appears to be positional vertigo; this is a much less frequent form. Disturbed audition, too, is affected by manipulation only in a few cases. Disturbed cervical function is usually found in all forms, most frequently in the craniocervical junction, including C2/3.

In Chapter 2 I set out some of the theoretical reasons for the importance of the spinal column and in particular of the craniocervical junction. Clinical evidence corroborates this: the pattern described above, in which moving the head in the direction of movement restriction aggravates deviation, and the fact that the direction of cervical nystagmus changes in the rhythm of neck rotation (Norre *et al.*, 1976) provide additional evidence of the role of receptors in joints and muscles in the maintenance or disturbance of equilibrium. In two of my cases there was only spasm of the short extensors at the craniocervical junction, and by simple PR of these muscles deviation was abolished.

It is not only afferent stimuli from joints and muscles by which the cervical spine may cause disturbance of equilibrium, however; it can affect intracranial structures, including the labyrinth, by impinging on the vertebral artery. In fact there is a tendency to ascribe most disturbances of equilibrium of cervical origin to some involvement of this artery, which in my view is a gross exaggeration.

It is therefore important to know in which cases of disturbed equilibrium involvement of the vertebral artery should be suspected:

1. In patients of advanced age, particularly if there are other signs of arteriosclerosis.
2. If there are drop attacks (cervical syncope).
3. If back bending of the head coupled with rotation has a marked effect on dizziness, particularly in the absence of movement restriction, or if dizziness persists after manipulation; a positive De Kleyn's test is also suggestive.
4. Certain X-ray findings: retrolisthesis, in particular if oblique pictures of the cervical spine in head retroflexion show a narrowed intervertebral foramen (*see Figure 3.23*, page 102), a difference in the obliquity of the intervertebral apophyseal joints at one segment (*see Figure 3.52*, page 102) or marked arthrosis of the neurocentral joint.

All of these clinical criteria are indirect signs, the only proof being provided by arteriography.

Cervical syncopes (drop attacks) are certainly proof of ischaemia and are most frequently provoked by sustained head retroflexion during work. If cerebral ischaemia is marked, even epileptic seizures can occur. The importance of cervical syncope is unfortunately largely underrated, as it is certainly much more frequent than the Adams–Stokes syndrome.

So far it might seem only a question of differential diagnosis, which in itself is a difficult matter in disturbances of the equilibrium. However, in the large majority of cases with involvement of the vertebral artery there is also involvement of the cervical spine. This is not just coincidence: there is not only a close anatomical relationship, while the average age of patients suggests a degree of arteriosclerosis, but a sclerotic artery is itself much more susceptible to mechanical irritation than is a normal vessel. For the same reason complications at arteriography are more frequent in cases with arteriosclerosis than, for instance, in tumour patients. A disturbance of the cervical spine will therefore be much more harmful in a patient with a sclerotic vertebral artery than in a patient with normal arteries.

The great majority of patients with vertebral artery involvement also suffer from disturbances of the cervical spine, as is borne out by clinical experience and by the literature (Barré, 1926; Bärtschi-Rochaix, 1949). Both authors describe a combination of cervical headache and disturbance of equilibrium due to vertebral artery involvement even with possible minor neurological symptoms. Vítek (1970) made the point that headache in patients with cerebral arteriosclerosis is as a rule caused by simultaneous involvement of the cervical spine.

It is necessary to stress these relationships because of the significant therapeutic consequences involved. Realization of the deleterious effect of mechanical irritation of a sclerotic vertebral artery by disturbance of the cervical spine makes adequate treatment of the spinal lesion mandatory. Nevertheless this is the subject of considerable controversy because of possible complications due to damage to the vertebral artery by manipulation (*see* page 180).

Clearly, such complications are not the result of manipulation as such, but of grave technical mistakes. Leaving disturbed function untreated is tantamount to leaving mechanical irritation free to endanger the vertebral artery unchecked. Again, in the great majority of cases the disturbance is at the craniocervical junction. This is important because this is the site of treatment that most regularly gives relief, probably because (1) in normal functioning of the craniocervical junction the loops of the vertebral artery in this region allow for head rotation without increasing tension in the artery; and (2) if head rotation is impaired here, it has to take place below C2, i.e. where the vertebral artery runs through its canal, exposed to shearing forces if rotation takes place.

This is borne out by clinical practice. In a recent group of 70 patients with dizziness, vertigo or both, 21 showed the signs given above as indicating vertebral artery involvement; whereas in the patients without arterial involvement treatment failed in only 10 per cent (the results were similar to those in the larger group already quoted), in the group with involvement of the vertebral artery there were 28.5 per cent failures, but 38 per cent excellent and 33.5 per cent good results. The lesion treated was, for the most part, at the craniocervical junction.

These results are also significant for diagnosis. If no improvement of the condition follows on normalization of the function of the cervical spine, it can be surmised that there is serious involvement of the vertebral artery either by arteriosclerosis or by gross deformity in the lower cervical spine, which may require surgical treatment (Jung and Kehr, 1972). Adequate manipulative treatment thus not only gives satisfactory results in cases where no other non-surgical methods are effective, but enables us to single out those patients in whom arteriography is indicated with a view to possible surgical treatment.

I must close this section by pointing out the importance but also the difficulty of differential diagnosis. This complex problem touches on neurology, otorhinolaryngology and ophthalmology; if there is involvement of the vertebral artery minor neurological signs due to ischaemia are not uncommon, so that other pathological conditions have to be excluded. I must stress again, here, that (as I know from experience) improvement after manipulation does not rule out posterior fossa tumour. In fact, if correct techniques are used, the danger of manipulation lies not in any immediate harm to the patient, but in possible neglect of the true diagnosis if manipulation is (temporarily) successful. This should not discourage us, however, for in no field is manipulation more effective than in the treatment of disturbances of equilibrium.

The syndrome of 'the upper quarter'

The different clinical pictures of disturbance to the cervical spine have been presented so far as they affect the upper extremity, the head, the neck, or the upper thorax. As can be expected, however, we find patients suffering from symptoms all over the area connected with the cervical spine, at least on one side, in the 'upper quarter' of the body. As infiltration of the ganglion stellare can affect the whole area, this syndrome has been attributed to involvement of this ganglion, but this is a quite unfounded assumption. However, not only is the cervical spine a functional unit, but it presents typical chain reactions (*see* pages 173–174) which explain why, even if patients fortunately do not suffer from all possible symptoms of cervical origin at one and the same time, they may nevertheless experience quite a few of them if the disease takes its typical chronic intermittent course. It is muscle tension in particular, involving the long muscles of the neck, which is likely to produce symptoms over a large area. There is also an interesting phenomenon often observed during treatment of cervical lesions: their tendency to 'descend'. For instance, we frequently find that after treating the craniocervical junction in a patient with cervical headache, he will arrive at the next session with movement restriction in the mid-cervical region, complaining of neck pain; at the third session he will be suffering in the lower cervical region, with symptoms in the shoulder, until we finally get him symptom free after treating the upper thoracic spine or ribs for pain round the shoulder-blade or in the upper thorax.

Basilar impression and a narrow cervical spinal canal

These two anomalies have in common the ability to cause compression, the former of the medulla, the latter of the cervical cord and particularly of the intumescence. They also share a tendency for symptoms to appear in the higher age groups, although the anomalies causing them are congenital. A process of decompensation in which disturbed function is involved therefore probably plays a role. In both conditions, so long as surgery is not proposed, I have found manipulative treatment very useful. In basilar impression there are frequently no signs of structural neurological damage, the only symptoms being headache, dizziness or both, and in such cases the treatment is the same as for patients who do not present the anomaly. Even patients with some signs of compression, however, may improve after manipulation, or even after traction. The same is true particularly of pain in the upper extremities in patients with cervical myelopathy with a narrow spinal canal (and spondylosis!), and there may even be some improvement in locomotor function. For similar reasons pain in syringomyelia improves after manipulative treatment of the cervical spine. This is not without importance for the patient, as surgery is not always successful and any improvement achieved by non-surgical methods is to be valued.

Root syndromes

In discussing compression of the vertebral artery, of the medulla or of the cervical cord by basilar impression or a narrow spinal canal, not only disturbance of function but also a clearly defined pathological condition was considered, where the disturbance of function plays a part in the pathogenesis of the clinical manifestations.

The same can be said of root compression: in root syndromes of the lower extremity the most important pathological change is disc herniation; in the upper extremity there may be a complex of changes producing a narrow foramen intervertebrale where root compression takes place, disc herniation being only one of the possible mechanisms. There are other pathological conditions of significance both in the cervical and in the lumbar region, like a narrow spinal canal and, of course, expanding lesions which may also cause root compression.

However, with the exception of expanding lesions, most of the pathological conditions listed here are not an absolute indication for operation; most cases of radicular syndrome recover without operation, thanks to compensation, in which function plays an important role. This is why conservative treatment is so often successful – i.e. traction, manipulation, various types of reflex therapy and remedial exercise; serious cases require systematic rehabilitation. Indeed, surgery *alone* fails, more often than not, if it is not followed by rehabilitation, i.e. if we do not help the patient to normalize function. This is why root syndromes and disc herniation should be dealt with in this book. The interplay of changes in structure and function constitutes an intricate and complex problem of diagnosis and therapy.

The clinical differences between root syndromes in the upper and lower extremities, respectively, are considerable and so the two will be dealt with separately, but first I shall summarize what was said about root syndromes in Chapter 2 (page 41ff.).

Root syndromes in the lower extremities

CASE HISTORY

Although root syndromes share many features with other vertebrogenic disturbances (*see* page 103ff.) there are specific important features. The first is that in most cases pain radiating into the lower extremity is preceded by low-back pain. This is why disc herniation is thought to be the main cause not only of root pain, but also of low-back pain. Since, however, the latter is a much more frequent condition, the correct interpretation is that only those cases of low-back pain that are caused by disc herniation (*see* page 309) are likely to produce root syndromes at some stage of the disease. There are, however, cases in which root pain, for example in the calf, is the first complaint in patients who have never suffered from low-back pain, which appears only later during the disease, if at all. Pain felt in the buttocks is certainly a prominent feature in many cases, hence the old term 'sciatica'. Much like low-back pain, root pain may have a sudden onset after some awkward movement, when getting out of bed in the morning, lifting a heavy object, etc., or it may begin so stealthily that the patient cannot readily remember or describe the first symptoms. For correct management in individual cases we have to elicit from the patient all the attendant circumstances that aggravate symptoms, and, equally important, those in which there is (relative) freedom from pain.

Symptoms
Pain radiating into the legs, in typical cases as far as to the toes; pain exacerbating on coughing or sneezing (a violent sneeze or attack of coughing may even precipitate a root syndrome!). Pain is frequently combined with dysaesthesia (numbness, tingling, or pins and needles). There may be symptoms due to locomotor impairment, such as weakness, clumsiness, or the patient feeling unable to support himself on the affected leg.

Clinical signs
In the acute stage we often find the typical antalgesic posture described in acute lumbago due to disc herniation (*see Figure 7.1*, page 310). Like every rule this also has its exceptions, however, and there are acute cases in which the patient holds the trunk and lumbar spine erect in lordosis, unable to bend forward. The most frequent antalgesic posture, that of kyphosis with scoliosis of the *low* lumbar spine to the side of the lesion, is easily explained as the position that keeps the intervertebral foramen as wide as possible. Other, less typical antalgesic positions, including lordosis, have been ingeniously explained by De Sèze (1957) in diagram form, by the varying positions of the disc prolapse in relation to the root inside the spinal canal. The kyphotic–scoliotic position goes together with movement restriction, particularly of movements that would cause narrowing of the intervertebral foramen, i.e. back bending and lateral flexion to the side of the lesion. If straight leg raising is impaired stooping with straight legs will also be affected. In patients who hold themselves erect, trunk anteflexion will often be impaired, even when the patient is seated with knees bent. In the less acute stage posture may be more or less normal, but stooping with straight legs will be reduced so long as straight leg raising is impaired. In some cases there will be a painful arc as in lumbago due to disc herniation (*see* page 115).

It is important to point out that movement restriction and antalgesic posture in root syndromes are not due to blockage in individual mobile segments, and that indeed such blockage may be absent when the patient is examined (*see Figures 4.10 and 4.11*, page 118). Another feature of root syndromes is the positive straight leg raising test, which in typical cases may be very marked. There can be atypical straight leg raising tests: (1) a painful arc (Cyriax, 1977), pain felt early on in the test but passing at further raising; (2) although pain is felt from a certain point, it is still possible to raise the patient's leg further.

Of major significance are neurological signs of root involvement, such as motor deficit and hypoaesthesia, without which the diagnosis of true root syndrome is inconclusive because of the alternative possible diagnosis of pseudoradicular radiating pain. For this reason the slightest indication of motor or sensory deficit is highly significant. The specific signs and symptoms will now be given for each relevant root. Only three are important: L4, L5 and S1.

L4 root syndrome – Pain radiates over the ventral aspect of the thigh to the knee and can radiate further on the anteromedial aspect of the leg down to the medial ankle and even to the medial aspect of the big toe; in this syndrome a positive femoral nerve stretch test is very marked. There is weakness of the quadriceps and of the hip flexors (often neglected at examination!). The patellar reflex is weakened or absent. There is hypoaesthesia mainly on the anterior aspect of the thigh in the L4 dermatome. Owing to weakness of the knee extensors and hip flexors, walking may be difficult.

L5 root syndrome – Pain radiates on the lateral aspect of the thigh and leg to the lateral ankle and over the instep to the big toe and to the second and third toes. There is weakness of the foot and toe extensors, the muscles most affected being the extensors of the big toe and the extensor digitorum brevis. Very slight impairment in the L5 root can therefore be detected by comparing the force of extension of the big toe on each foot, and by palpation of the digitorum brevis muscle above and in front of the lateral ankle, and testing the tonus of the extensors at the shin, parallel to the tibia. If there is marked weakness the patient cannot walk on his heels and in the most severe cases there is typical drop foot. It is important to remember that drop foot is only exceptionally due to paresis of the peroneal nerve, and far more often to severe L5 nerve root compression. Tendon reflexes are usually little affected by this syndrome. Hypoaesthesia is found in the L5 dermatome.

S1 root syndrome – Pain radiates on the dorsal aspect of the thigh and leg, towards the heel and over the lateral aspect of the foot to the 4th and 5th toes. Muscle weakness may be found in the gluteal muscles, particularly in the gluteus maximus, and in the triceps surae and the flexors of the toes. In very slight root lesion the first sign of motor impairment is that when the patient is told to lean forward without lifting his heels from the ground there is no toe flexion on the side of the lesion. If motor impairment is marked the patient cannot walk on his toes on the affected side. The Achilles' tendon reflex is weakened or abolished. There is hypoaesthesia at the dorsal aspect of the thigh and leg, the lateral aspect of the foot and the fourth and fifth toe.

Therapy

In the acute stage the most important single measure is absolute rest in bed, if possible in a position that gives maximum relief; it is essential to improvise pillows to support the patient in this position. If traction can be carried out in the relief position (*see Figure 6.28,* page 218) it should be attempted. If there is blockage and some of the gentle mobilization techniques are practicable, they can give substantial relief. Treatment of lesions in the craniocervical and thoracolumbar junctions, if found, can also be helpful. If relief cannot be obtained either by positioning of the patient or by traction, and manipulation is ruled out because of acute pain, then root infiltration or an epidural application of local anaesthetics is the treatment of choice. If there is a very tender pain point – for example at the fibular head, in the proximity of the ankle, or a very tender interdigital fold – needling or infiltration may give relief. The same goes for a tender scar, in particular on the lower abdomen, the hips or legs, especially if the pain during needling is felt *very intensely*. Analgesics play an important supporting role, but are often insufficient in themselves. If, however, complete rest *alone* brings relief, little else is needed during the acute stage, the essential point being not to discontinue it too soon.

During the chronic stage, or after the acute stage has been passed, it is necessary to restore function according to the principles laid down in this book: we restore joint mobility by manipulative techniques wherever it has been lost, we train weak muscles, restore movement patterns and so on. However, care must be taken to avoid for a long time any movements that cause pain, and similarly to avoid positions that are painful. It is notoriously common that sitting is tolerated badly in kyphosis, for example. It is particularly important to teach the patient how to stoop correctly. Once walking is painless short walks should be encouraged. If pain becomes chronic although blockages have been treated, and traction no longer relieves it, reflex therapy is very important. Pain points and hyperalgesic zones must be sought, particularly in the periphery (the interdigital folds are very important), and pathogenic scars must be diagnosed. These are treated by the most adequate methods: attachment points of tendons by PR, or by needling if there is no increased muscle tension; hyperalgesic zones by skin stretching or by other methods of 'reflex massage'; the same methods may be applied to scars, which react very well to simple skin stretching.

It is important to remember that during the chronic stage other lesions in the lower extremity may complicate recovery: cramp may occur, due to blockage at the fibular head or of tarsal bones; there may be coxalgia without coxarthrosis, pain at the tuber ossis ischii simulating 'sciatica', or pain of the piriformis. Each of these lesions is easily treated. Vasomotor disturbances such as cold feet should be treated with physiotherapy; a simple and effective method is to roll a cold water-bottle and a hot water-bottle with the feet, giving training in mobilization at the same time.

Despite the effective therapeutic measures described, there remain cases of root syndrome in which conservative therapy fails and surgery is indicated; because conservative therapy is effective it is easier to detect the type of case in which conservative therapy is ineffective, for this is after all the main reason for indicating surgery. The problem is: at what point do we consider our conservative therapy to have failed? Naturally opinions vary, partly because the course of the disease varies from one case to the next. If it were simply a case of *absolutely no* improvement, one might say that 4–6 weeks is long enough if pain is severe, and even a shorter time if pain is excessive. However, in most cases we do achieve *some* improvement, which may turn out to be merely temporary – and it is this course that makes our decision more difficult.

Although the failure of conservative treatment is the main reason for indicating surgery, it is not sufficient in itself. We must satisfy ourselves that the underlying cause of the condition warrants surgery; this is not infrequently disc herniation, but the diagnosis must be clearly established.

There are some specific questions of importance here: is muscle weakness with typical signs of lower motor neurone lesion in itself an indication for operation if the diagnosis of disc herniation, for example, is established? The answer here is that by our definition, neurological deficit is one of the principal characteristics of a true root syndrome; experience has shown that even patients with marked weakness with atrophy and loss of reflexes usually recover after pain has improved. There is nevertheless one exception, which fortunately is not frequent, but which must be borne in mind: sudden onset of weakness or paralysis. In typical cases the patient described excruciating pain, after which he fell asleep; on waking he felt no pain, but found he could not lift his foot or toes. We confirm the signs of drop foot, and if in such cases no improvement takes place within 24 hours operation must be performed immediately; otherwise it is too late and permanent paralysis results.

Another exception is disturbance of sphincter function and impending caudal lesion. Signs of caudal involvement are among the most urgent indications for surgery. This is mentioned here because doctors practising manipulative therapy may miss these signs, because unless sphincter disturbance is very serious or complete the patient may not mention it. On the one hand they suffer much more from their severe pain symptoms, so that some difficulty in passing water seems of little importance; on the other hand they may feel embarrassed, and not see the connection. It is therefore essential for the examining doctor to know *when* to ask patients with spinal disorders about their control of micturition and bowel action. The answer is clear: this question is relevant when during an attack of acute root pain or lumbago *the Achilles' tendon reflex is absent on both sides*.

In addition to disc herniation, which is certainly the most frequent cause of operation, in recent years the importance of a narrowed spinal canal has also been stressed. Combined with degenerative changes this may be the cause of root compression,or it may be the reason why disc herniation takes a very unfavourable course. Its most characteristic clinical feature is radicular claudication, a condition in which the patient (with hardly any other clinical signs) has to stop walking after some distance, because of pain shooting down the leg, and has to crouch; after a few moments he can walk on, but the episode is soon repeated.

In exceptional cases pathological hypermobility in one segment may be an indication for surgery. This is the case in spondylolisthesis particularly in adolescents or young adults; this hypermobility can be proved by X-ray in ante- and retro-flexion.

Finally, operation cannot do more than remove a local mechanical lesion that constitutes an obstacle to conservative treatment. It does not and cannot automatically restore the function of the locomotor system. Operation is one episode in the treatment of a disturbance that affects the whole of locomotor function and which must be dealt with by the appropriate methods of locomotor rehabilitation which include manipulative therapy. Gentle mobilization can be used a few weeks after the operation, if indicated; at sites further from the operated segment it can be applied even earlier.

Root syndromes in the upper extremities

GENERAL SYMPTOMS

Patients complain of pain radiating down the arm to the fingers, coming either from the neck, or 'from under the shoulder-blade', or both. Pain is frequently worst in bed, exacerbating on bending the head back; the patient requires a high pillow. Pain is typically accompanied by dysaesthesia and a feeling of weakness.

GENERAL CLINICAL SIGNS

There are two typical pain points: Erb's point above the clavicle and a point between the medial angle of the upper border of the scapula and the spinous process of T2 or T3. The former is in the mass of the scalenes, the latter in the interscapular part of the trapezius, both responding well to PR (*see Figures 6.76* (page 261) and *6.93* (page 275), respectively). Pain usually worsens at head retroflexion and at side-bending or rotation to the side of the lesion, i.e. movements that cause narrowing of the intervertebral foramina, even if there is no segmental blockage, i.e. even after manipulation. There are also cases, however, in which head and neck anteflexion is painful (Frykholm, 1969). This depends on whether the root involved has a descending course inside the spinal canal: such roots stretch at head anteflexion, causing pain (Adams and Logue, 1971) whereas the movement otherwise tends rather to give relief, as it facilitates widening of the intervertebral foramina.

Individual root syndromes
C6, C7 and C8 are of practical importance.

C6 root syndrome – Pain radiates over the radial (lateral) aspect of the arm to the thumb and forefinger, and here hypoaesthesia may be found. There is weakness of pronation and in some cases an alar scapula can be observed. This is best tested by the patient stretching both arms forward, while seated, and maintaining this position for a while. Vitek (1950) has described a reflex that is specific: with the patient's arm flexed at the elbow in semi-pronation, the examiner taps the radius above the wrist, from the palmar aspect, and obtains a pronatory jerk. (The usual tapping on the styloid process produces flexion at the elbow, corresponding more to segment C5.)

C7 root syndrome – Pain radiates over the posterior aspect of the arm towards the second to fourth fingers, with dysaesthesia; hypoaesthesia may also be found in this area. There is typical weakness and even wasting of the triceps and the triceps reflex is weak or absent. (Thenar atrophy is sometimes given as a sign of C7 involvement; this can be misleading, as thenar atrophy is mainly a sign of the carpal-tunnel syndrome.)

C8 root syndrome – Pain radiates over the ulnar (medial) aspect of the arm to the fourth and fifth fingers, with dysaesthesia; hypoaesthesia may be found in this area. There is weakness of finger flexion and the flexor reflex is impaired. (This is elicited by tapping on the tendons of the finger flexors just proximal to the carpal tunnel, with the fingers in a semi-flexed position.) There can be wasting of interosseal muscles and of the hypothenar, with weakness of abduction of the little finger, but care must be taken to differentiate this from paresis of the ulnar nerve and from cervical myelopathy.

GENERAL THERAPY

Although in the upper extremity true root syndromes present a more serious disturbance than pseudoradicular pain, treatment follows the same principles; greater emphasis is laid, however, on traction and reflex therapy. I have already mentioned the treatment of Erb's point and the frequent pain point medial to the upper border of the scapula by PR. Whatever the interpretation, infiltration of the stellate ganglion by local anaesthetic can be useful. In the upper extremity, as in the lower, failure of conservative therapy is an indication for surgery; however, this is rare.

Vertebrovisceral relations

The possible correlation of structures belonging to the same segment, the possibility of referred pain and some of the consequences have already been discussed (*see* page 42). Here we shall consider the practical clinical aspects.

The following possibilities should be envisaged:

1. The vertebral column (locomotor system) is causing symptoms that are mistaken for visceral disease.
2. Visceral disturbance is causing symptoms simulating affection of some part of the locomotor system.
3. Visceral disease is causing a reflex (pseudoradicular) reaction in the segment, including blockage in the corresponding mobile segment of the vertebral column.
4. Visceral disease that has caused segmental movement restriction has subsided, but blockage remains, causing symptoms simulating visceral disease (as in (1)).
5. (Conjectural.) Disturbance of the locomotor segment is causing visceral disease.

The first two points show that our first concern is differential diagnosis. The spinal column with its mobile segments can produce symptoms in each body segment that may imitate those arising in the viscera and are frequently ascribed to them both by laymen and by medical practitioners, as we shall see below. This explains why lay manipulators are believed to have 'cured' visceral disease (and believe it themselves). Another reason is that some doctors ignore this field of differential diagnosis and use the term 'functional' for disturbances in which no pathological changes are found in the visceral organs, 'functional' being used as a euphemism for psychological trouble, if not for malingering. When a doctor treats a patient for symptoms thought to be of visceral origin and finds no pathological changes to correspond to them, before opting for a 'psychological' origin he or she should first look for changes in the segment (*see* page 40). The pejorative use of the word 'functional' is characteristic of the underestimation of the significance of disturbed function, in particular of the locomotor system. It is this underestimation, combined with ignorance, that gives the unqualified manipulator the opportunity to claim 'miracle' cures.

The other side of the problem, as it is put in point (2), is a fair warning to every therapist concerned with pain in the locomotor system: that there may be organic disease lurking behind this pain. Particularly when pain and the typical signs of segmental disturbance show a tendency to relapse, the cause may be a visceral affection in the corresponding segment. Error in point (1) is common; error in point (2) can be fraught with danger.

Point (3) is of great theoretical significance, explaining why one of the possible causes of segmental movement restriction is visceral disease (*see* page 22). In fact, clinical experience has taught us that disease of individual organs produces a specific pattern of reactions in various segments; these patterns are of considerable diagnostic importance and will be described here. The regularity is so striking that if after treatment of segmental disorders (blockage, muscle spasm, pain points, etc.) we find a tendency to relapse, we have to conclude that visceral disease is either still active, or has also relapsed. This shows that we have an important pointer not only for diagnosis but also for prognosis.

Point (4) follows on from this; if visceral disease has been cured and we treat the changes in the segment caused by it, we obtain most satisfactory results and can thus confirm the success of the internal treatment. Here patients and therapists tend to draw a wrong conclusion: because secondary changes still caused symptoms in the segment, after internal therapy, all credit is given to the therapist who treated them. On the other hand, relapse of disturbed function in the segment is often the first sign of recurring internal disease.

Point (5) is one most cherished by lay manipulators, in the past, and it is still controversial today. It would seem to be fairly well established that lesions in the mobile segment of the vertebral column affect some functions of internal organs; this is borne out by vasoconstriction in the whole segment affected by a pseudo-radicular syndrome. In such cases we can see the disorder clearing up as soon as we treat the mobile segment. Other such conditions have been described in connection with the craniocervical syndrome, including disturbance of equilibrium; still others will be dealt with in some disturbances of heart rhythm without organic changes, and in menstrual pain. I will now discuss our experience in treating individual conditions.

Tonsillitis

Taking the case history in patients with vertebrogenic disturbances I was so struck by the high incidence of chronic relapsing tonsillitis that I took a random sample of 100 cases from my files and found that 56 had a history of chronic relapsing tonsillitis or tonsillectomy for that reason, while only 44 had no or only incidental tonsillitis.

This led to a systematic study of a group of 76 children with chronic tonsillitis under the care of an otorhinolaryngologist (Lewit and Abrahamovič, 1976). The most striking and constant clinical finding was movement restriction at the craniocervical junction, in the great majority between occiput and atlas (70 cases, or 92 per cent). Twenty-eight patients underwent operation, without having been manipulated; 25 suffered from movement restriction, and in 19 of these cases blockage was unaffected by tonsillectomy and was treated later, 3–6 months after operation.

Thirty-seven children were given manipulative treatment and followed up for 5 years; in 18 cases tonsillitis never recurred after manipulation, but in seven of them movement restriction did recur and had to be treated. Two patients had a few relapses of tonsillitis without recurrence of blockage; in three there were frequent relapses and blockage, and nine had to be operated on for recurring tonsillitis.

In addition to blockage mainly between C0 and C1, with spasm of the short neck extensors, we frequently find increased tension in the muscles below the mandible in the vicinity of the tonsils.

It can be seen from this study that tonsillitis goes hand in hand with movement restriction in the craniocervical junction, mainly between occiput and atlas, with little tendency to spontaneous recovery, i.e. with the danger of permanently disturbed function in one of the most sensitive regions of the locomotor system. In addition, our experience suggests that blockage at this level increases the susceptibility to recurrent tonsillitis.

Lungs and pleura

As our attention was drawn to the role of respiration in correct functioning of the locomotor system, the relation between the lungs and the function of the thorax became clearer. Pain due to rib lesions must be differentiated from pleural pain.

Severe incoordination of respiratory movement may produce dyspnoea, while chronic asthma with emphysema will produce rigidity of the thorax. The respiratory disease in which involvement of the thorax has been studied most is obstructive respiratory disease (Bergsmann, 1974; Köberle, 1975; Sachse, 1970; Steglich, 1972). There are two obvious mechanisms by which disturbed thorax function influences respiration in asthmatics: rigidity of the thorax wall further increases resistance during respiration and the inspiratory position of the thorax in asthmatics is worsened by further lifting of the thorax during inspiration, which is typical for that disease.

In addition to rigidity of the ribs Köberle (1975) found blockage mainly of the segments T7–T10. In a group of 30 asthmatics Sachse (1970) found a taut trapezius in 23 patients, a taut pectoralis in 15 and a weak lower trapezius in 15. Increased tension in the scalene muscle is the most constant change in muscular activity directly connected with lifting of the thorax during inspiration.

The mobilization of the ribs and of blocked segments of the thoracic spine, and training of correct breathing patterns, will thus be the logical treatment for patients with respiratory disorders, particularly those with obstructive respiratory disease.

The heart

Of all vertebrovisceral relations, that between the heart and the spinal column (thorax) has received most attention. This is due not only to the importance of the problem, but also to the role of pain in the largest group of patients, i.e. in those with ischaemic heart disease, pain being of course the principal manifestation of disturbance of spinal and thoracic function. Pain of cardiac origin is localized mainly in the structures of the locomotor system, including the (left) shoulder and the arm.

The following pattern of disturbance of the locomotor system seems characteristic of ischaemic heart disease: blockage affecting the thoracic spine from T3 to T5, most frequently between T4 and T5 and at the cervicothoracic junction, and of the 3rd to 5th rib on the left side; there is muscular spasm (increased tension) of the erector spinae between T4 and T8 on *both* sides, more on the left; spasm of the pectoralis mainly on the left, with pain points in the mammary and axillary line on the third to fifth rib; and increased tension with trigger points in the upper part of the trapezius. Increased tension in the scalenus is connected with pain points at the sternocostal joints on both sides, and is linked to faulty respiration producing the feeling of oppression which is also characteristic of angina. Tension in the scaleni is frequently linked with a lesion of the first rib, producing a pain point on the lateral aspect of the manubrium sterni. If it is on the left side it may easily be interpreted by the patient as coming from the heart.

It is obviously most important to distinguish between ischaemic heart disease producing this pattern and primary disturbance of the locomotor system of a similar pattern (the vertebrocardial syndrome). Rychliková (1975) showed that the more complete this pattern, i.e. the more severe the (reflex) changes in the locomotor system, the more likely it is to be *secondary* to heart disease. Important clinical criteria are: the effect of physical effort like climbing stairs and susceptibility to nitroglycerine treatment – both characteristic of true ischaemia. On the other hand, pain provoked by certain positions of the body is more characteristic of locomotor disturbance. The painful attacks are shorter in true angina than in the vertebrocardial syndrome. The course of the disease is significant: if despite specific treatment of locomotor lesions these relapse or are aggravated, the cause must be primary heart disease. The role of the locomotor system in the pathogenesis of pain is borne out by the fact that in a group of patients with myocardial infarction *without pain* Rychlíková (1975) did not find any signs of disturbance of the locomotor system.

Since the pattern of locomotor disturbance described above will present symptoms closely similar to those of ischaemic heart disease, they have to be treated according to the principles laid down here, whether they are primary or secondary. More often than not mobilization of movement restriction and muscle relaxation will have to be followed by the training of correct breathing patterns and correct posture if the results achieved are to be more than temporary. It is important here to warn readers of the complexity of this problem, and the many pitfalls to be met with; constant supervision of these patients by a cardiologist is essential.

Taking the role of ischaemic heart disease in causing characteristic locomotor disturbance as established, the question of the role of locomotor disturbance as a factor in heart disease remains open. There is one condition, however, where the latter presumption seems well founded: paroxysmal tachycardia with no organic heart lesion. Here the changes found in the spinal column are linked with tachycardia in such a way that when we normalize the function of the spinal column, heart rhythm also becomes normal and remains so as long as there is no relapse in the spinal column. Although direct evidence of disturbed motor function causing organic heart disease is lacking, it would seem reasonable to grant it the role of a possible risk factor.

The prime significance of the treatment of locomotor disturbance in heart disease lies in the relief of pain, which greatly enhances the rehabilitation of these patients.

Stomach and duodenum

As in heart disease, painful conditions in these organs are most likely to produce reflex changes in the locomotor system, for this reason clinical experience of vertebrovisceral correlation is greatest in these conditions. The data given below are based on a group of 79 adolescents suffering from duodenal and/or gastric ulcer (Lewit, 1975, 1976; Rychlíková, 1975, 1976).

The following pattern was characteristic of disturbance in the locomotor system: blockage of thoracic segments between T4 and T7 with a clear maximum occurrence at T5/6; compared with a control group there was increased incidence of blockage in the craniocervical junction; but the most striking change was pelvic distortion (87 per cent as compared with 44.4 per cent in the healthy controls). There was increased muscle tension in the thoracic erector spinae in the segments T4–T9, again with the maximum at T5/6, and the same was true of hyperalgesic skin zones, the incidence of the latter being about half that of increased muscle tension. It is interesting that these changes were almost symmetrical, with a slight preponderance on the right; there was hardly any difference between the cases of gastric and of duodenal ulcer. Increased tension of the abdominal muscles, however, was more marked on the right.

In this group the intensity of reflex changes was clearly correlated to pain; where there was no pain, as in some cases after operation, the pattern did not present itself. It must be added that this pattern was found in young patients (15–22 years old); in older patients suffering from ulcers the incidence of pelvic distortion is much lower.

For clinical practice it is useful to remember that reflex changes are a useful criterion of the severity of the disease, and if we find this pattern in patients who do not complain of abdominal symptoms, the stomach and duodenum should be examined.

Liver and gall bladder

Since pain plays a prominent role in affections of the liver and especially of the gall bladder, reflex changes must be expected. According to Rychlíková (1974) the segments most frequently affected are T6–8. Frequent radiation of pain into the shoulder is borne out by HSZ in the C4 dermatome and increased tension in the upper part of the trapezius on the right. There is also increased tension in the thoracic erector spinae, more on the right than on the left. For differential diagnosis with psoas spasm, see below. On the other hand, Tilscher, Bogner and Landsiedl (1977), studying 30 patients with hepatitis, found movement restriction in the segments T8–T10 in 20 cases and (interestingly) restricted rotation of the right hip in 15.

The kidneys

Apart from the pain directly associated with a diseased kidney, pain in the lumbar region (back pain) is also found in this condition. A thorough analysis of reflex changes in the locomotor system in kidney disease has been made by Metz *et al.* (1980); in 206 cases of chronic kidney disease (pyelonephritis, glomerulonephritis) he found the following pattern: movement restriction at the thoracolumbar junction (T10–L1), and at the lowest ribs; pelvic distortion; increased tension in the thoracolumbar erector spinae, the psoas quadratus, the thigh adductors, the piriformis; and flabbiness of the abdominal muscles and the glutei. There was accompanying ligament pain and disturbed statics. These changes were not very susceptible to therapy so long as the underlying kidney disease was still active.

In a group of 40 (mainly women) patients with nephroptosis and another 40 patients after nephropexy, there was marked hypermobility, in particular at the L5/S1 segment which showed a high promontory; the reflex changes were similar, with marked muscular imbalance, faulty statics and ligament pain. In these cases, however, disturbance of the locomotor function proved to be the decisive cause of the symptoms; treatment of disturbed locomotor function brought relief while nephropexy proved ineffective.

The psoas and the abdominal muscles

As the psoas is located in the abdominal cavity, in many ways it behaves like an internal organ; differential diagnosis is therefore very important. As we have seen, tension in the psoas may be secondary to kidney disease; it is most frequently associated with movement restriction at the thoracolumbar junction; but it can also be a sign of motor imbalance, very often as a result of faulty athletic training. For examination, *see Figure 4.42*, page 153. Palpation may be difficult if pain is intense, because tension in the muscles of the abdominal wall will also be increased, as in any other painful abdominal condition. In such cases the abdominal wall softens after proper treatment of the psoas. Psoas spasm is usually associated with spasm of the thoracolumbar erector spinae, and relaxation of one muscle induces relaxation of the other.

Tension in the abdominal muscles, which may be due to any intra-abdominal pain, as we have seen, can however produce trigger points in the abdominal muscles, especially in the rectus abdominis. In turn these points may simulate abdominal disease. Palpation is not easy; it can best be performed by a pincer movement of the two hands, avoiding pressure from above. The most reliable signs are painful insertions at the upper aspect of the pubic symphysis and at the xiphoid process.

The most frequent clinical manifestation of psoas spasm is the 'post-cholecystectomy syndrome', or pain simulating gall-bladder disease after the organ has been removed; treatment of a blocked thoracolumbar junction is usually very effective. It is interesting to note that the pattern of true gall-bladder disease does not regularly include psoas spasm. Because of its size and site, the psoas can imitate almost any visceral disturbance: duodenum, appendix, pancreas or kidneys. Not only is the pain imitated, but so are the concomitant disorders of the autonomic nervous system such as loss of appetite, the feeling of indigestion, etc. In diagnosis of 'functional disturbance' of an abdominal organ, therefore, examination of the psoas should never be omitted, as very few conditions can be more effectively relieved than those due to psoas spasm.

Gynaecological disorders and low-back pain

Gynaecological disorders have always been traditionally associated with low-back pain, and this is certainly no mere coincidence. There are significant clinical correlations. The usual pattern includes lesions of the lumbosacral junction, the sacroiliac joint (in young women frequently pelvic distortion), a tender coccyx, spasm of the iliacus, muscular imbalance of the pelvic muscles, and ligament pain.

Novotný and Dvořák (1972) made a survey of almost 600 patients, showing the vertebrogynaecological relations. There was menstrual pain (algomenorrhoea) with regular gynaecological findings, felt also in the low back, and with typical onset at the menarche; this condition rarely deteriorates and very often improves after childbirth. Another important group developed symptoms during pregnancy and after delivery, i.e. at a period of increased strain and susceptibility of the lumbar spine and increased disturbance of pelvic function; in another group, low-back pain followed upon or deteriorated after gynaecological affections, minor surgery or both. The largest group of patients were women suffering from low-back pain due to disturbed function of the spinal column, in whom gynaecological examination was carried out as a routine diagnostic procedure, with negative findings.

In a group of 150 healthy pregnant women (Lewit, Knobloch, Faktorová, 1970) there was anamnestic menstrual pain in 48; in 38 there was either pelvic distortion or lumbosacral movement restriction. Findings in the lumbosacral spinal column and the pelvis were normal only in 10. Moreover, menstrual pain without lesion at the lumbosacral spine or pelvis was felt mainly in the hypogastric region, while in cases with disturbed function of the lumbosacral region pain was usually felt also in the low back.

In another group of 70 women with menstrual pain and negative gynaecological findings, treatment of the spine mainly by manipulation gave excellent results in 43 cases, favourable in 13, and no change in 14. At delivery women with disturbed function of the lumbosacral spine and pelvis frequently feel labour pains in the low back, even if delivery is normal in other respects.

From these data we may conclude that:

1. Low-back pain may be precipitated by gynaecological conditions such as pregnancy, parturition, gynaecological disease or operation.
2. In a very large number of patients low-back pain of locomotor origin is mistakenly ascribed to gynaecological disturbances. One reason for this may be spasm of the iliacus which is palpated as a site of tender resistance in the hypogastric region.
3. Menstruation pain with otherwise normal gynaecological findings, especially when localized in the low back, is usually of vertebrogenic origin and often the first clinical manifestation of disturbance in the lumbosacral region. Labour pains felt in the low back in an otherwise normal delivery can be a similar pointer.

Since the findings of Head (1893/4) and later McKenzie (1920) and Hansen and Schliack (1962), quite an important body of literature has built up about segmental changes in the skin, the subcutaneous tissues and muscle spasm in visceral disease. Little has been written about segmental movement restriction and changes in muscular pattern in these conditions, however, and for this reason I have included important data on these significant changes in locomotor function, and their clinical relevance in vertebrovisceral correlations.

8

Prophylaxis

Importance of the problem

Since the decisive role of impaired function has been demonstrated in the theoretical part of this book, it would be inconsistent not to discuss prophylaxis. Not only do we apply some preventive principles in our therapy (*see* page 182), but the very principles of rehabilitation are to a large extent identical with those of prophylaxis; indeed it is one of the main goals of rehabilitation to prevent relapses and complications.

Before going into detail, let us consider for a moment the importance and at the same time the enormity of the task, bearing in mind that patients with disturbed function of the locomotor system form the vast majority of those suffering from back pain and associated problems. The statistical data illustrating this are necessarily inexact, the true incidence of these conditions being much higher. The reason is that a large number of our patients are registered under quite different headings, such as headache, vertigo, pain in the chest or pelvic region, etc. Not all patients who suffer from these symptoms go to see a doctor, since they have found out by experience that conventional treatment is ineffective: they learn to live with their symptoms, in this way escaping registration. Even so, the figures are impressive.

Mindful of all these difficulties, Wood and Badly (1980) give the following figures for morbidity per 1000 persons in the USA and Great Britain (the latter in brackets): arthritis and rheumatism, 79 (30 'arthropathies'); back or spine problems, 52 (34); heart trouble, 29; high blood pressure, 47.

The total visits per year for back troubles, in Great Britain, amounted to 3 401 000 to general practitioners, 1 819 000 to orthopaedic surgeons, 637 000 to osteopaths and 361 000 to chiropractors.

Table 8.1 gives official data from Czechoslovakia. These give a clear picture and are significant economically. They cover only patients who missed work because of their symptoms.

Obviously among the cases headed 'soft-tissue rheumatism' there will be many patients suffering mainly from disturbed locomotor function. It is certainly striking that only the common respiratory infections are a more frequent cause of absenteeism than locomotor disturbances or vertebrogenic disease. If we take into account vertebrogenic disease alone we come almost to the figure of 15 000 000 lost

TABLE 8.1. Number of cases of conditions causing absenteeism; per 100 000 inhabitants of Czechoslovakia

Complaint	Year				Average duration of working incapacity (days)
	1968	1973	1979	1984	
Disease of the locomotor system	7897		9451	10 432	22.5
Soft-tissue rheumatism	2138		1975	1622	20.4
Vertebrogenic disease	3763	4623	4895	6406	20.8
Circulatory disease			3114	3324	42.4
Psychiatric disease			1403	1276	32.8
Neurological disease			1087	961	29.1
Respiratory infections			36 538	44 652	9.7

working days in a total population of 15 000 000. With 98 fresh applications for invalidity pensions per 100 000 inhibitants annually, diseases of the locomotor system (15.5 per cent of applications) take first place with ischaemic heart disease.

However impressive these figures, they are far from reflecting the true incidence of these conditions, for working incapacity can be a misleading criterion; it is mainly low-back pain and pain in the lower extremities that cause working incapacity, and here the type of work plays an important role. There are, however, data that show the incidence of symptoms due to disturbed locomotor function more directly.

In his classic 'Munkfors Investigation', covering 1200 workers in various trades, Hult (1954) found symptoms due to cervical lesion in 51 per cent and symptoms due to lumbosacral lesion in 60 per cent, either in the patient's history or at examination. In a country district near Prague, Uttl (1964) found that 61 of a representative sample of 100 subjects had suffered from vertebrogenic symptoms.

To this it must be added that back pain and associated complaints affect patients at the age of maximum work capacity, and that treatment is frequently time consuming and costly (e.g. spa treatment and physical therapy). As the most frequent symptom is pain, there is immeasurable suffering and frustration as well. Even if loss of working capacity can be registered, the factors of reduced efficiency and psychological implications cannot be.

Principles of prophylaxis

As disturbed locomotor function plays a highly important role in the pathogenesis of back pain, prevention must be concerned with the conditions under which this most frequently occurs. We find on analysis that imbalance of muscle function due to faulty movement patterns plays a prominent part. This is largely due to environmental factors: modern industrialized civilization not only greatly changes our eating habits, pollutes the air and water and endangers us with toxic materials or even radiation; it changes our locomotor habits most radically. To put it briefly: while reducing movement it increases static overstrain, hence producing the typical imbalance between mainly postural and mainly phasic muscles (Janda, 1975). This is also the main reason why the incidence of disturbed function shows a constant tendency to rise.

Instead of walking, or even riding, we sit or stand in vehicles in which we are jolted or slumped; most work in offices and even in factories is carried out in a more or less fixed (static) position, frequently stooping. As agriculture becomes more mechanized work in the fields is not much better in this respect than work in mines or offices. Indeed the unfavourable trend begins as soon as the child first goes to school and is forced to *sit* most of the day. Young and healthy, he rebels at times, and rushes about wildly (if he gets the chance); as he grows he soon learns to prefer the motor bike and the TV.

This must be emphasized, because public attention is so narrowly focused on environmental pollution that the harm done to man himself by changes in locomotor behaviour is easily overlooked. There are two logical approaches to prevention under modern conditions: one is to avoid static overstrain as far as possible; the other is to seek to compensate it.

As most of our work is done seated, a correct sitting position is of great importance (*see Figures 4.58* and *4.59,* page 164). This, however, depends on the chair used: the height of the chair is correct if the thighs are horizontal and the whole of the foot rests on the floor, even if the knees are bent at slightly more than right angles. The back should be supported at the summit of the kyphotic arch, which is more often in the lumbar than in the thoracic region of the back. If the subject does not lean against the chair-back but can prop his elbows on the work-table or the arms of the chair, the height of the table should be such that by letting the upper arm hang naturally, the subject can lie his elbows on the table (sitting erect). If neither chair nor table offer support, the seat should slope upwards towards the back, tilting the pelvis forward and preventing lumbar kyphosis. Another way of avoiding the unfavourable effects of kyphotic sitting posture of long duration is for the patient to learn Brügger's relief position (*see Figure 6.119,* page 295).

A special problem is posed by the prevention of head and neck anteflexion (*see* anteflexion headache, page 324). Because the plane of the visual field must correspond to the plane of the object we are looking at, inclination of that object is what matters. If the book we are reading or the paper on which we are writing lies on a horizontal desk, raising or lowering the desk will not prevent us having to bend head and neck forward. What is needed is a tilted surface; a book can of course be held or supported on a book-rest at the correct angle.

The unfavourable effect of sitting is further enhanced by jolting in vehicles, the worst being lorries or tractors travelling over uneven ground. The importance of good springs and shock absorption must be stressed.

If work is performed standing, it is important that the subject should stand erect, if possible, since a stooping position held for any length of time is always a strain. At this point I must stress that a slight stooping movement, such as bending over a wash-basin while shaving, may be more dangerous than maximum stooping, because it is in the former position that the erector spinae contracts most, exerting maximum pressure on the discs (*see* the 'painful arc', page 115).

If lifting weights causes symptoms (or relapses), correct lifting must be taught, like correct stooping. Only very heavy weights are lifted with the spinal column erect, by bending and straightening the knees. Otherwise we have to insist on the harmonious synergism of leg and trunk flexion and use the technique of 'uncurling' with the aid of the abdominal muscles, as described in Chapter 4 (*see* page 164 and *Figure 4.60*). If stooping we should always put one leg forward, slightly bent.

It would be ideal if everyone obliged to work in a fixed static position were encouraged to change this position occasionally, or given a short break in which to do so.

Just as important as the position held during the day is the way the body lies at night, in bed. In fact, there are few more effective ways of avoiding relapse than correcting an unsuitable sleeping position. The patient is usually asked about the type of bed he sleeps on, and advised to have a soft thick mattress over a firm hard bed. This is the wrong approach. The patient should first describe the position in which he usually sleeps, and only then should we advise improvements. For this we have to distinguish whether his symptoms are mainly in the lumbar or sacral region, or are mainly cervical.

If symptoms are mainly in the low back we need to know whether the patient lies on his side, supine or prone. If the answer is supine or prone, and symptoms occur during the night, or if the patient is wakeful, the trouble is usually due to lordosis. We may then advise him either to lie on his side, or – if he lies supine – to put a pillow or even a low padded stool beneath his legs. If he lies prone, it is usually best to advise a different position, but here, too, the pelvis can be raised by a pillow, thus flattening lordosis. If lying on the side produces symptoms this may be due to scoliosis, and then a pillow under the waist will help to straighten the lumbar and low thoracic spine.

Sleeping in the right position may be even more important for the cervical spine; this is in part borne out by our experience that acute wry neck most frequently occurs after rest in bed, cervical headache is frequently worse in the morning, and even radicular pain in the upper extremity has a tendency to be worst at night. Only too frequently the well-meant advice is given to patients to lie flat, with no pillow or a very small one; this may be good for a young person with a flat back, *lying supine*. However, a small soft pillow, or no pillow at all, means that if the patient lies on his side the head and neck are bent, and probably also rotated towards the mattress, because the head is narrower than the shoulders. To keep the cervical spine in the neutral position the *head must be supported*. The correct height for this support will of course vary from patient to patient, according to the width of the shoulders and also according to how the patient lies – which we must first inquire. He may lie exactly on his side, or slightly rotated, the shoulder pushed slightly forward or slightly back, all of which affects the height of the support needed. It is therefore best to let the patient demonstrate his favoured sleeping position, and then to determine the height of the support. There are patients who place one arm under the head, which simply means that they feel the need for such a support, for nobody can lie on his own arm for any length of time. The support should be square and not too big; it must never be put under the shoulders, and should be firm enough to give constant support. It should not be wedge shaped.

If the patient has the unfortunate habit of lying prone, this should be discouraged, because it is a position that forces the cervical spine into maximum rotation. Again, a firm pillow giving him the necessary support to lie comfortably on his side will both encourage him to do so and prove an obstacle should he turn to lie prone. There are specially constructed pillows with a hole for the nose, enabling the patient to lie prone with his neck straight. Using such a support, however, he must take care not to lift the head into retroflexion. The most suitable compromise for those who cannot drop this habit is to place a pillow under the shoulder on the side to which the head is turned, thus lessening head and neck rotation. The habit of lying prone usually dates from early childhood, when the position has much to recommend it; later in life, unfortunately, it becomes less and less well tolerated.

Even when lying supine, most older people need a head support; many become round shouldered and stiff, and if the head is not supported it falls into retroflexion. This is not only unfavourable for the cervical spine but can be positively dangerous in subjects with some degree of cerebral arteriosclerosis, since it favours ischaemia, particularly of structures supplied by the vertebral arteries.

To conclude: it is most important to find out which conditions precipitate symptoms, and to detect faults in the patient's daily habits that should be avoided or corrected in order to prevent relapse. In fact, there is probably no more effective way of helping these patients than by judicious advice about their habits of working, sitting or sleeping. And, which comes to the same thing, our best therapeutic measures will fail if we do not discover the faulty position a typist maintains at her work, an unsuitable driver's seat, a wrong position during sleep. It is therefore a grave omission on our part if, after learning that symptoms occur in the morning, we do not ask the patient what position he usually sleeps in – or if we learn that symptoms are precipitated by lifting objects and do not investigate the way the patient stoops to lift things. Indeed, one of the main purposes of taking a case history is to investigate these matters exactly. This shows that prophylaxis and correct management of patients cannot be separated.

The other approach to prevention of disturbed locomotor function, as I pointed out at the beginning of this chapter, is to seek ways to compensate for civilization's ills during our leisure time. If we have too little movement at work, for instance, we may make up for it in our free time. This, as everyone knows, ought to be the main reason for taking up gymnastics and sports, and we are often asked by patients which sport or other physical activity we would recommend them to take up for prophylactic reasons. The question seems straightforward, but we are instantly aware that the answer is not simple. Not only do the various forms of sport affect our bodies in very different ways, but they can even be positively harmful. It is essential to analyse each type of sport carefully, bearing in mind the constitution of the person asking our professional advice. Then there is the question of competitive sports: in view of the extreme and ever-increasing demands made by competitive sports on their devotees, their usefulness for prevention of disturbances, or for the maintenance of normal good health, is most questionable. In fact, as I shall be showing later, most of those who compete in sports must be considered among the most threatened population groups.

It cannot fall within the scope of this book to give a comprehensive picture of the effect of various types of sport on the locomotor system. It may be useful, however, to give a few examples of how to approach the question. Take swimming, for example, considered by most people to be a particularly 'healthy' sport: all the muscles are brought into play, the body weight does not act on the spinal column and there is very little risk of injury. On further analysis, however, we find that the breast stroke and even the crawl make the pectoralis muscle overactive and taut, so that most swimmers become round-shouldered. On the other hand, the breast stroke and even more so the 'butterfly' produce lumbar hyperlordosis and hypermobility. In the older age groups most people hold their head out of the water while swimming, keeping the cervical spine in hyperlordosis. This having been said, I do not want to suggest that swimming is altogether harmful; advising a round-shouldered patient or one with a hypermobile low back, I would suggest that he swims on his back, and I would explain that the crawl is better than the breast stroke for a hypermobile low back.

Doctors should be aware of the dangers of volley-ball for the locomotor system: those who play at the net must, as they leap up and drop back to the ground, keep the lumbar spine in hyperlordosis so as not to touch the net; this is most unphysiological and a danger to the low lumbar discs. Diving is a dangerous sport by the operation of a similar mechanism, spondylolisthesis being significantly more frequent among divers than in the rest of the population. Gymnastics as usually taught make muscular imbalance even worse, particularly in exercises in which the trunk and legs are held straight and at right angles to each other. In order to achieve this the action of the abdominal muscles naturally approaching the sternum to the pubic symphysis must be overcompensated and inhibited by the erector spinae and the iliopsoas – the best way to provoke the 'lower crossed syndrome' (*see* pages 170–171). The important mechanism of curling up the lumbar spine is discarded and instead there is leverage at the lumbosacral junction, with deleterious effect on the discs. Gymnastics on apparatus tend to make the upper fixators of the shoulder girdle overactive. The emphasis on swift movement in gymnastics makes safe control of the body difficult, and it is not easy to avoid a movement that may be harmful. For this reason some types of Yoga exercise (but not those resembling acrobatics!) and Tai-chi are probably more suitable for prophylactic purposes than traditional European gymnastics.

A leisure activity to be recommended is regular walking, preferably on soft paths or wearing crêpe-rubber soles; it is without risk, since it is the most physiological form of locomotion. Similarly, cross-country skiing has much in its favour; it also makes use of all four limbs, and the snow provides a soft terrain.

We should not forget that dancing is among the oldest forms of movement that people have enjoyed. Since, unlike gymnastics, it can be carried on for hours at a time it is as effective as exercise; with few exceptions it is harmless, and it can also be recommended to combat obesity.

These examples should suffice to show the need for a judicious approach to sport as a preventive of locomotor disturbance, and to warn against oversimplifying the question.

Clothing

Although posture and movement, and their correction, naturally play the principal role in preventing disturbed locomotor function and its sequelae, there are other important factors such as food and clothing. It is notoriously well known that regions highly susceptible to pain, like the neck and the low back, are sensitive to cold and draughts, and those who suffer from pain in these areas will try to protect them. This is fully justified by experience, but we should not forget the antinomy of necessary protection and desirable resistance, or hardening. Thus although we should protect regions that we know are apt to cause symptoms, we should try to harden the body as a whole. Nor should we forget that the susceptibility to cold of a region like the low back is usually due to a latent lesion, and that after successful treatment cautious hardening may be undertaken. One of the main purposes of wearing clothes is to protect the body from the cold, but this should be judicious to maintain thermoregulation or resistance to heat and cold at an optimum. Besides clothing, this also applies to the question of when and to what extent we should expose our bodies to the air, water and the sun.

There is yet another side to the question, what might be called the mechanical side; tight corseting is no longer a menace to the modern woman, but there are other hazards – hair and cap styles that force a forward and upward tilt of the head, bags slung from one shoulder and, of course, shoes. High heels not only change the gait but also the body statics: they produce forward pelvic tilt with its unfavourable effect on muscle function (imbalance), affecting spinal curvature and even the position of the head, as well as the breathing. There should be no need to emphasize here how important the shape of the shoe is for the development and proper functioning of the foot.

Another important point concerns the abdominal muscles; the modern fashion of pantihose is harmless for slim young women with strong muscles, but for the obese or older woman with weak abdominal muscles – especially after operation or several pregnancies – a firm belt is most desirable. Obese elderly men, too, with poor abdominal muscles, should wear a broad belt. On the other hand care must be taken to see that the belt does not cut into the abdomen. A suitable brassiere is also extremely important for women with heavy breasts. Only too often do we see women patients lifting their breasts with brassieres that are too small, with narrow ribbons that cut deep into the flesh of the shoulders. This constant drag on the shoulders is enough to foil any attempt to treat the cervical spine, or to correct body statics. It is a grave mistake not to point out the patient's lack of wisdom in this respect; women with very heavy breasts should be advised most emphatically to wear a corset.

It is only too obvious that the campaign against obesity common to many fields of medicine is very relevant for the correct functioning of the locomotor system. A vicious circle is easily set up, in which obesity causing overstrain with faulty statics manifests itself in low-back pain; the patient is reluctant to move because of the pain and gets even fatter. I cannot deal here with ways of combating obesity, but it is important to decide whether obesity is a relevant factor in any given case of locomotor disturbance. We should remember that increased weight will seriously affect the lower extremities, the pelvis and the lumbar spine but is of only slight relevance to the cervical spine. There are subjects with very little fat on the trunk but obese buttocks and thighs; this may be practically irrelevant for the spinal column and body statics. The physical type of the patient is important; the pyknic tolerates obesity much better than the asthenic. A heavily built subject who weighs about 80 kg at 20 years and 90 or even 100 kg at 50 years may suffer very little, whereas an asthenic subject who weighs 50 or 60 kg at 20 years and 80 or 90 kg at 50 years will be decompensated. When advising weight reduction we must have good reason to think that obesity is a potential cause of the symptoms.

Having discussed some of the basic principles of prevention, we now come to the question of preventive correction of specific disturbances. As I pointed out on page 182, we not only indicate treatment of those lesions that manifest themselves by causing pain, but we also treat lesions in key positions although they may still be latent, because we are convinced that they are a potential source of trouble. We are therefore justified in asking whether, and under what conditions, we should treat clinically latent lesions in persons without symptoms. This is particularly to the point in joint or segmental movement restriction (blockage) which is potentially harmful, and at the same time can be quickly and safely diagnosed as well as treated.

Manipulation as a prophylactic measure

Having discussed the usefulness of manipulation as prophylaxis we must now turn to its practical possibilities. It is certainly not possible, and probably not even useful, to suggest prophylactic manipulative treatment for the whole population, but it may be reasonable to envisage such medical supervision for pre-school and schoolchildren. Our experience suggests that a check-up once a year or even every other year would be sufficient, and carried out by experts this would not even be time consuming, as it is usually the craniocervical junction and the pelvis that are affected. This would present an effective way of dealing with disturbed locomotor function at the very outset.

There are some groups of patients for whom preventive manipulation is of great importance. The first are patients recovering from injury; trauma was listed among the chief causes of blockage in Chapter 2, and indeed after any type of mechanical injury there is likely to be movement restriction which can complicate recovery. This is particularly true of the spinal column.

Head injury, including concussion, is a significant example. It stands to reason that any force acting on the head must also affect the cervical spine, while it is obvious that the big, firm skull is less fragile than the seven vertebrae and (vital) soft parts of the mobile cervical spine. In fact what is called the post-concussion syndrome with headache and vertigo can scarcely be distinguished from the cervicocranial syndrome. Indeed Bärtschi-Rochaix (1949) describing 'migraine cervicale' found that most of his patients had suffered head injury. Torres and Shapiro (1961) compared 45 cases after concussion with 45 cases after whiplash injury to the cervical spine; they found little difference in symptoms or neurological findings, or even EEG, the only significant observation being a higher incidence of neck and upper extremity pain in whiplash injury. Junghanns wrote as early as 1952 that recent experience suggested that symptoms usually attributed to concussion were in reality due to contusion of the cervical spine. This is also borne out by autopsy findings; in all 20 cases of death after head injury Leichsenring (1964) found serious damage to the cervical spine.

In a group of 65 of my patients after concussion (with loss of consciousness), clinical findings in the cervical spine were normal only in six. The results of manipulative treatment were similar to those in other cases of headache and vertigo of cervical origin (37 'excellent', 18 'fair' and 10 failures). Failure was most frequently due to ligament pain and anteflexion headache; the most frequent site of blockage was between atlas and axis.

In the light of this experience manipulative treatment given (in hospital) for preventive purposes, during the first days after concussion, seemed justified; all of the patients were fully conscious, with no suspicion of intracranial haemorrhage, and negative X-ray findings in the skull and cervical spine. In 24 out of 32 cases any pain they felt ceased immediately after treatment. Bartel (1980) has published almost identical results: in 50 cases examined immediately after head injury there was blockage in all but two, the lesion most frequently located at C1/2. In 40 cases one treatment was sufficient (for the most part this was mobilization), while in six cases treatment was repeated once. Forty of the cases were then symptom free; six were improved; there were two failures.

In the light of this experience, the high incidence of traumatic neurosis must be put down mainly to mismanagement; in the vast majority of cases without gross neurological findings doctors not trained in the manual diagnosis of movement restriction and segmental reflex change come to the disastrous conclusion that there are 'no organic findings' and hence dismiss the trouble as 'functional', i.e. psychological disturbance. The patient thus has insult added to injury, receives no adequate treatment and is forced into a neurotic reaction which is taken to confirm the mistaken original diagnosis. There can hardly be a better illustration of the identity of prophylaxis and the correct management of the patient.

What is true for head injury is equally valid for other parts of the locomotor system: a patient who falls on a hand may suffer from indirect injury to the cervical spine in addition to fracturing his radius, while a patient who falls on to his feet or buttocks may also injure his lumbar spine.

There are typical lesions in the extremity joints after injury. A patient who falls on his hand, whether the radius is fractured or not, pushes it upward at the elbow, resulting in blockage at the elbow joint. The clinical consequence is pain at the styloid process after the removal of the plaster, with impaired radial flexion due to blockage at the *elbow* and absence of radial springing (as in a painful radial epicondyle, *see Figure 6.8,* page 202). In such cases treatment of the elbow gives immediate relief. If pain does not subside after a fall on the shoulder, the cause is frequently a blocked *acromioclavicular joint* or a *first rib,* or again a cervical lesion. After foot injury with or without fracture we usually find blocked tarsometatarsal or tarsal joints, or both, as well as blockage at the ankle joint in many cases; after knee injury there is often a blocked fibular head. Treatment of these joints invariably gives immediate relief, which is often permanent. Again the question arises as to whether we should treat these lesions immediately after injury or not. This is purely a question of diagnosis: *if we can rule out fracture and haematoma or hypermobility,* the sooner treatment is given the better, to prevent late sequelae.

Another important group comprises patients who have suffered from internal disease giving rise to segmental movement restriction (*see* page 336ff., vertebrovisceral correlations). This is particularly important where surgical treatment has been needed, because then operation trauma has been added to the internal lesion. It is indeed rather the exception if such patients do *not* suffer from complications owing to disturbed locomotor function (e.g. after gall bladder or gynaecological operations). General anaesthetic with intubation frequently causes cervical lesions which it is imperative to treat.

Whether preventive manipulation could be envisaged for those engaged in some particularly demanding professions is doubtful; in fact, as we have seen, most occupations in modern society are carried on in conditions that are harmful. However, there is one group that is at such risk that manipulative treatment for preventive purposes is justified, and even to some extent carried out: professional sportsmen and sportswomen, a fact which throws light on the effects of competitive sport.

There is another possible approach to the prevention of locomotor disturbance in particularly demanding professions: the choice of employment, taking into account the individual's constitution. Here we are most concerned with hypermobility; it is the hypermobile subject who suffers most from static overstrain and is most susceptible to the consequences of a confined sitting position, stooping, head anteflexion and jolting.

It would of course be very misleading to give the impression that the only therapeutic measure to be applied for prevention was manipulation. The importance of this method, and its possible application, have been dwelt upon because it is the subject of this book, and has proved both effective and practicable in prevention.

The classic therapeutic measure is, of course, remedial exercise, and this has been given its due importance in Chapter 6. I should add that it is effective only if the principles laid down in that chapter are consistently followed, i.e. if the type of muscular imbalance and faulty locomotor pattern is accurately analysed and the therapeutic plan worked out accordingly. It can readily be seen, however, that remedial exercise is much more demanding as a form of prevention than is manipulation, and it is therefore not easy to determine its practicability.

Remedial exercise has always been used for children with bad posture, but there are few children who can really profit from it. A more effective approach would be to introduce elements of remedial exercise into normal physical training in schools: teaching correct respiration, stooping, weight carrying, standing and sitting. It would be possible to devise different types of exercise for hypermobile children and for stiff and very muscular children. I have pointed out the great shortcomings of traditional European physical training on page 348, but the greatest misfortune is the attitude of many if not most physical training instructors. Like sports trainers they are primarily interested in those children who shine in sports and gymnastics, those who are 'promising' as future competitive sportsmen (to their own detriment). The 'awkward' child, the child who really needs more of the teacher's attention, is put into a quiet corner in preparation for a sedentary life and obesity.

There are two groups of adults who ought to be given remedial exercise as a first priority: women after childbirth and, for the same reason, patients with weak abdominal muscles after abdominal operation. Not to indicate remedial exercise in such cases is gross negligence.

9

Problems of expertise

Expertise poses considerable problems in patients suffering from pain originating in the locomotor system, among whom those with back pain form the most numerous group. Although their lives are not endangered, they may nevertheless not be fit for the work they are expected to perform, temporarily or permanently, and in some cases they are even threatened with invalidity. In addition, the question of damage traceable to the type of work they do, and particularly to occupational injury, has often to be settled by litigation requiring expert opinion.

Any decision taken in so complex and responsible a matter must be the outcome of scientifically based assessment of pathogenesis and prognosis, as well as management of the patient. From all that has been written here, it is evident that opinions differ widely, yet if disturbed function is accepted as one of the most significant factors in pain deriving from the locomotor system, this must necessarily find expression in our expertise. The difficulties are obvious.

In the first place, in most of the cases where our expertise is called for, the patient has received neither adequate therapy nor rehabilitation. An even greater obstacle is that most doctors are not taught detailed diagnosis and analysis of locomotor function and its disturbance, so that even significant lesions pass unnoticed. This is particularly serious in view of the principal symptom, i.e. pain: the doctor who does not recognize changes in muscle and tissue tension brought about by pain will have to rely (reluctantly) on what he is told by the patient, or else simply refuse to believe him. The unfortunate consequence is that the expert, in order to find 'objective' criteria, feels bound to base his decision on the morphological findings, i.e. mainly on X-rays. This is also easier to 'prove'; changes in function are far more difficult to show. There are psychological factors at work, too, something like public opinion working to the same end: the patient himself is informed, more often than not, of the changes found in his X-rays and presented to him as the cause of his pain, with the inevitable psychological consequences. It is the patient so 'informed' who becomes a hopeless problem for further management, and invalidity is then not the consequence of the disease but of misguided 'expert opinion'. On the other hand, young patients with serious symptoms including true disc herniation are considered malingerers because their X-rays show 'no changes', i.e. no degenerative changes.

It is thus important to give some indication here of how expert opinion can and should be expressed with regard to disturbed function. We cannot deal with all types of pain caused by locomotor disturbance; back pain and root syndromes will be discussed. To present a problem for expertise, pain must have had a chronic course; we shall therefore exclude acute cases. It has to be assumed, too, that such pathological conditions as ankylosing spondylitis, tuberculosis, osteoporosis etc., have been ruled out.

In chronic cases without pathological findings there is decompensation as a consequence of articular lesions, faulty statics and muscular imbalance. Our chief concern will be to correct these, so as to achieve compensation, but at the same time we have to assess to what extent the work the patient is expected to perform contributes to decompensation or even causes relapses. This has to be assessed specifically for each case, in view of the effect of different types of work on the locomotor system.

For instance, if the patient gets backache whenever he has to sit for a longer period we shall have to forbid him to do sedentary work but may encourage him to walk, if he reacts favourably. First, however, we must make sure that the bad effect of sitting is not due to an unsuitable chair, a table at the wrong height, etc. Similarly, if lifting and stooping or weight carrying causes symptoms, we must first find out whether the patient's movement patterns are not at fault – in which case he must be taught correct techniques – but not allow him to return to this type of work before making sure it will not cause relapse. Since one of the frequent factors involved is movement restriction, we should be reluctant to forbid movement as long as it is well tolerated; it is one of the principles of the management and rehabilitation of such patients to improve locomotor function by appropriate movement – despite public opinion shocked by the sight of a patient not fit for work enjoying country walks or even moving about on skis! Sometimes the trouble lies not in the work performed by the patient, but in how he gets to and from work, particularly if jolting in public vehicles is not well tolerated.

Here again there is an important distinction between back pain with or without pseudoradicular (i.e. radiating) pain in the lower extremities, and true radicular syndromes. In the former, movement is usually well tolerated and should be encouraged, while in the latter it is harmful so long as the radicular signs are acute – which may be for a considerable time. Another condition in which walking is not well tolerated and where we must be cautious about allowing it is pain due to articular involvement of the lower extremities. Here walking on hard ground (paved streets) is particularly harmful.

There is a specific problem in the case of patients who have been unfit for work for a long period, such as several months; this is often the case with radicular syndromes of the lower extremities, particularly where operation has been necessary. These people are out of training. If a young footballer, for example, has to lie in bed for several weeks, nobody expects him to play in a match the day he recovers his health. Working people, however physically demanding their job, do not enjoy the same consideration, although it should be obvious that some readaptation is necessary. If we do not want to risk relapse, the patient should work for a time under somewhat easier conditions, i.e. either not full time, or omitting some of the more demanding operations involved, until he fully recovers his former strength. There is sometimes an attempt in this direction, giving the patient 'easier work'; alas, this usually means transfer to office work or to that of a doorman, which has nothing to do with his real job and gives him no chance to readapt to it.

Pain in the low back and the lower extremities is certainly a more frequent cause of working incapacity than pain in the neck, shoulders and upper extremities, even if the pain is equally intense, because the latter type of pain does not have the same effect on movement. If pain in the low back and lower limbs is sufficiently severe, the patient cannot get to his feet, whereas pain in the shoulder or headache are often the same whether he goes to work or stays at home. Indeed, unless the pain interferes directly with his work, as shoulder pain may do, the patient may suffer less at work than left to his own resources at home.

Before turning to the much discussed question of trauma, it may be appropriate to say a few words about occupational 'damage'. In the preceding chapter we saw that Western civilization has altered living conditions in such a way as to make the large majority of professions unfavourable to a healthy locomotor system. There are occupations that are particularly undesirable from this point of view: drivers, particularly those exposed to severe jolting like in a tractor, and jobs involving extreme static overstrain, like that of the dentist or the seamstress. Yet it seems exaggerated to regard back pain as an occupational disease in such cases. Frequently, patients get worse at a job for which they are clearly physically unsuited; this is due to a lack of medical expertise in eliminating individuals from work detrimental to their physical constitution. This is most marked when workers are forced to change jobs at an age when adaptation is no longer easy. They then rightly claim that symptoms appeared or got much worse because of their new job – but the real fault lies in lack of prevention.

The role of trauma

As injury, and particularly injury at work, gives the patient the right to claim compensation, it is a frequent subject of litigation requiring expert opinion. The questions put to the doctor in such cases are (1) whether there was trauma at all, and (2) whether and to what degree trauma is responsible for the patient's condition. The answers to both these questions may cause considerable controversy, particularly if the injury has affected the spinal column. I shall therefore deal mainly with that issue here.

The infliction of trauma

If a heavy object falls on a toe and causes fracture, nobody would question that the fracture was due to injury. When stooping to lift a heavy object, the force of contraction of the erector spinae may amount to several hundred kilograms. If in such a situation a man's foot slips, or if two men are lifting a weight and one of them unexpectedly drops it, a sudden force of several hundred kilograms is brought to bear on the lumbosacral junction. It would be illogical not to regard the sudden, unexpected effect of such a force as an injury. This does not mean that the lifting of a heavy object, in itself, constitutes an injury, even if the force deployed by the muscles is indeed considerable; lifting quite heavy objects is an activity that within limits is quite physiological. It is the unforeseen, incoordinated, jerky movement that should be recognized as traumatic.

A further point is that injury to the spinal column is more often than not indirect, as I pointed out in the preceding chapter (*see* pages 350–351). Therefore, if symptoms pointing to spinal involvement occur after a fall on the extremities, buttocks or shoulders, they should be considered as caused or exacerbated by the trauma even if the patient himself does not realize the connection. The greater the damage to the structure directly injured, the more easily spinal involvement is overlooked. Immediately after fracture of the arm or pelvis, local pain is such that it draws all attention to the major trauma, while the insidious injury to the spinal column is barely noticed. (In the cervical region, this is often of the whiplash type.) As the fracture heals and the cast is removed, symptoms due to that apparently minor and therefore unrecognized injury get worse instead of clearing up, and should be clearly diagnosed as such. Finally, although by now whiplash injury is a familiar traumatic entity, its seriousness and the relatively unfavourable prognosis are not sufficiently admitted. The fact that whiplash injury need not be caused exclusively by rear-end collisions but also by similar mechanisms brought into play – e.g. by a fall (Berger, Gerstenbrand, 1981) – is still not sufficiently recognized.

The most serious aspect, as I have pointed out in Chapter 8, is that the patient's symptoms after trauma are frequently due to disturbed function, while only relatively few doctors have the ability to recognize and assess them as such. Even more difficult than the diagnosis of movement restriction can be that of hypermobility, as in fresh whiplash injury, resulting later in ligament pain with or without blockage.

This situation only too frequently ends with patients who have suffered injury – whose pain typically persists because of disturbed function – being diagnosed as having no objective signs of illness; they are then treated as 'psychological' cases or as malingerers. The inevitable result is that the patient feels wronged and a typical conflict ensues, leading to neurosis which in the end justifies the diagnosis which began as a grave error and which could have been avoided.

The effect of trauma

Where trauma has been admitted as such, the question to be answered is whether the patient's symptoms are indeed the result of that trauma. This is a difficult question in some circumstances, e.g. if symptoms do not follow immediately upon injury and if there is a symptom-free interval of days, weeks or even months. We know, fundamentally, that injury may cause disturbed function, as it may cause movement restriction; this may be clinically latent for some time and may become apparent only as the result of additional strain, the influence of cold, or of infection. Another significant aspect is whether the trauma affects a structure that was completely intact, or whether the structure now affected has previously been injured. This question is frequently put in cases of elderly patients in whom degenerative changes are no surprise. At first glance it would seem logical to assume that trauma that does not (yet) cause serious morphological damage such as fracture or torn ligaments, but only disturbs function in the form of blockage or hypermobility in an intact terrain, will have much less serious consequences than if the structure has suffered before. In the first case there is 'only' disturbed function, which if treated adequately should recover in time without sequelae. In the second case, we may assume that even if our patient was without symptoms previous to injury, he was in fact in a state of compensation and that trauma has now brought about decompensation, which may be (and frequently is) a much more serious condition.

What usually happens is that expert opinion arrives at more or less the opposite conclusion: the usual argument is that in view of the changes (i.e. degenerative, morphological) that can be proved, the patient would sooner or later have suffered from the same symptoms, and therefore the trauma did not cause the symptoms but merely precipitated what would have happened anyway. As this type of argument is dealt with below, I will not discuss it here.

The question of whether trauma is or is not the cause of symptoms is also often put in cases of disc herniation producing radicular syndromes. Again the argument runs like this: if trauma affects an intact spinal column, fracture of the vertebra is more likely to result than disc prolapse. If, however, disc degeneration is already present, prolapse with its clinical consequences would have occurred anyway, so that again the trauma would have been no more than the precipitating factor.

Taking this line of argument point by point, it is important to stress the following:

1. There are conditions under which a disc may rupture even if intact; this occurs in lordosis or hyperlordosis and is known from those tragic cases in which a diver strikes his head on the bottom of a pool and sudden quadriplegia results. There may be no vertebral fracture at all, because what happened was due to an acutely prolapsed disc causing cervical-cord compression.
2. Disc degeneration is a very frequent condition; routine examination of the population over 50 years of age showed that it exists in the majority. Yet relatively few suffer from clinical manifestations, let alone from (true!) root syndromes.
3. Even if a disc is prolapsed, it may be asymptomatic – at autopsy it is often found in subjects who never suffered root syndromes (McRae, 1956). Even if a patient with disc prolapse recovers without operation, the prolapse is still there, although without clinical manifestations.

To sum up: it is an untenable argument that in view of certain morphological (mainly degenerative) changes we must expect a certain type of syndrome, either as a direct consequence of these changes or, indirectly, as a direct consequence of 'inevitable' disc prolapse which necessarily or even probably produced this syndrome. This attitude is also unjustifiable, because the young victim of injury with a perfectly intact locomotor system would then be given maximum compensation after injury, while the victim who showed no symptoms because his changes were well compensated but who becomes decompensated would get next to nothing, although he will have much greater difficulty in recovering from his injury than his younger colleague.

The crucial question now is: by what criteria can we give expertise in the matter of changes in function? The basis is a thorough clinical examination establishing (1) the changes in function and (2) the reflex changes that are the direct sign or clinical manifestation of pain (nociceptive stimulation). The role played by the trauma can be decided only on the basis of the anamnesic data. If it can be proved that (1) according to the given criteria trauma really occurred and (2) the patient was symptom free before the incriminated trauma, then the trauma must be recognized as having caused the symptoms. On the other hand, if the patient has had symptoms previously that took the typical course of pain-free intervals alternating with relapses then the trauma was at best a precipitating cause, or even irrelevant. Since most employed persons are registered with a doctor who has to confirm sick leave, it is not usually difficult to establish the true state of affairs.

10

The place of manipulative therapy and its future

There are two aspects to manipulation. First, it causes marked reflex effects in many types of pain, a feature that it shares with many other methods of physical therapy such as massage, electric stimulation and local anaesthesia. The other aspect is that it is a specific form of treatment of impaired locomotor function, i.e. of reversible joint movement restriction or blockage. This aspect became crucial for further clinical development and application.

It soon became clear that treatment of restricted joint movement had its limits and that passive mobility in itself involves not only joints but also muscles. This close relationship between joints and muscles became the starting point for further advances; the logical step was to turn our attention to active muscle function and its typical impairment in patients with pain due to disturbed function of the locomotor system, in particular in vertebrogenic lesions. This was locomotor imbalance due to faulty motor patterns.

No less important than movement is posture, or statics, owing to contemporary conditions of static strain and overstrain. Integration of various aspects of disturbed function of the locomotor system shed some light on the no man's land between neurology, orthopaedics and rheumatology which is the home of the vast majority of patients with pain deriving from the locomotor system, in whom no definite pathomorphological changes can be found. We suggest 'functional pathology of the locomotor system' as the name for this no man's land. The most frequent symptom of impaired locomotor function is pain, reflected clinically by reflex changes such as muscle spasm trigger points, hyperalgesic skin zones, or periosteal points.

Manipulation owes its pioneeering role in this field not only to the two aspects already discussed, but also to the fact that it has furnished the necessary diagnostic tools. Manipulation, rightly compared to surgery in this respect, requires absolutely accurate diagnosis. The criteria necessary for manipulation have since been consistently applied to movement patterns, statics, and reflex changes. It thus became possible to obtain the necessary diagnostic data for a judicious analysis of the clinical picture, and to plan rational therapy, i.e. to choose (1) the structure where treatment is most urgent and promising, and (2) the most adequate method of treatment.

Preoccupation with active, i.e. muscular, function was not without consequences for the development of manipulative techniques. In recent years we have tended to make use of the patient's own muscles to restore impaired joint movement, i.e. we have learned increasingly how to make use of the patient's inherent forces, rather than those of the therapist. Indeed, by involving muscular physiology we have increasingly engaged the patient's own activity; originally passive manipulative techniques became semi-active, until finally the patient began to learn self-treatment independent of the therapist. Since these techniques are very effective in producing muscular relaxation, they can also be used to treat muscular spasm, trigger points and even referred pain. In this way these semi-active and ultimately active methods of self-treatment take an increasingly evident share in remedial gymnastics and in rehabilitation medicine.

This is understandable, for since the locomotor system is the organ of voluntary movement, it should be efficiently controlled by the patient. It is then no coincidence that the aims of rehabilitation (to restore lost function) using active co-operation on the part of the patient converge with those of modern manipulative techniques which use muscular facilitation and inhibition. Rehabilitation medicine is not only interested in the locomotor system but also makes use of voluntary movement in dealing with other systems. Here again we have the same problem as that presented by viscerovertebral correlations, particularly in the field of correlation between the locomotor system and respiration, which is under direct motor control.

It is this combination of methods from modern techniques of rehabilitation and manipulative medicine that gives scope for an almost unlimited array of combinations and variations, with the final aim: to make correction of locomotor function almost automatic, i.e. using the minimum of conscious control of movement, but such physiological factors as inspiration, expiration, eye movements and even the force of gravity. This flexibility and variability in method opens up further as yet unforeseen possibilities of combination and progress.

Conscious, active co-operation by the patient is another important feature shared with rehabilitation medicine. In most other fields of medicine, the attitude of the doctor is only too often that of the ancient shaman: the patient comes *to be cured,* whether by drugs, surgery, or miracle. The patient (as the word implies) patiently does nothing about it; he is only the *object* of medicine. In rehabilitation, on the contrary, the patient is the *subject,* and as doctors we merely advise him how to deal with his predicament. This involves overcoming the comfortably passive role of the patient and dealing with the difficult problem of psychological motivation. The close relationship between psychological motives and locomotor function is very clear, since the locomotor system is controlled by the will. This is also borne out by the importance of the human factor in manipulation as well as in locomotor rehabilitation. In this field of medicine we have to rely mainly on our eyes and hands, and to learn (re-learn!) the skills modern medicine so sadly neglects in favour of sophisticated equipment. Only the skilled hand can adapt as promptly as is required to the patient's reactions, keeping fully in contact with his requirements both physical as well as psychological. In this field of medicine a personal relationship between doctor and patient is vital.

The logical conclusion to be drawn is that manipulation has its place within the framework of physical medicine and rehabilitation, all of which serve the aim of restoring function by the most adequate means.

The realization of this task requires teamwork, the three members of the team being the doctor, the physiotherapist and the patient. The role of the doctor is to form the diagnosis and analyse the locomotor disturbance; he should also start treatment, for in straightforward cases one or two treatments suffice. In more serious cases he should be aware – if not after the first, then after the second or third examination and treatment – how the case should be treated further by the physiotherapist. This is not only a question of remedial exercise, massage, electrotherapy and so forth, but also of repeated mobilization and relaxation techniques taught to the patient for self-treatment. As this combination of self-treatment and physiotherapy proceeds, the doctor has to assess the results and see the patient again whenever treatment seems ineffectual; it is of course the doctor who decides when to terminate treatment.

There is much to be said for reserving thrust techniques for the doctor alone. The physiotherapist is by her training best fitted to use her hands and must understand the increasingly sophisticated methods of remedial exercise; restoring muscular balance and correcting locomotor patterns, she will use mobilization techniques and teach them to her patients. This manner of proceeding entails a reasonable partnership between doctors and physiotherapists, so that they divide their roles judiciously.

Tuition plays a crucial part in realizing this ideal, for the complex subject of locomotor function and the truly difficult skills of diagnostic and therapeutic techniques are rarely taught in medical schools, even with specialization in those fields of medicine dealing with the locomotor system. In some countries a first step has already been taken, in the shape of postgraduate training of a certain number of doctors (as yet inadequate to the dimensions of the task); they will be the pioneers and initiators. Many will have to overcome too narrow an interest in one particular approach, such as manipulation, in order to be able to handle efficiently a team whose aim is to combat disturbances of the locomotor system.

The next step is the specialized training of physiotherapists to make effective partnership possible. It will then be necessary to introduce the basic principles of manipulation and locomotor rehabilitation to the university curriculum, so that medical students become aware of the importance, possibilities and attractiveness of this field of medicine. This is closely linked with the final step, which is as yet no more than a pious hope. Since disturbances of the locomotor system are the most frequent cause of painful disorders, every general practitioner comes up against them daily; at present he can only prescribe analgesics and hope for the best. He should be given the opportunity to learn how to deal with simple cases, to acquire a limited number of techniques that are both easily learned and safe. This goal is now attainable, thanks to the mobilization techniques that use muscular facilitation and inhibition.

This brings us back to the question of ultimate goals. The vast number of painful disorders designated as 'functional', in reality due to disturbed function of internal organs and the locomotor system, constitute the majority of minor ailments afflicting our fellow humans. It is here that manipulative and other techniques of physical medicine are the adequate method to deal with disturbed function and the ensuing reflex changes, treating them in the most specific and physiological way. It would indeed be a significant contribution to modern medicine if these methods, judiciously used, were to be brought into play where the heavy and often only too effective armament of drug therapy, with all of its side-effects, is sometimes called upon in the 'front line' of 'minor every day troubles' – the heavier weapons could then be saved for the right moment.

The locomotor system which appears to play the major part in these disorders is the principal object of the diagnostic and therapeutic techniques described in this book. They should teach us how to make ever-increasing use of this most intricate and perfect instrument at our disposal, our own locomotor system, at a time when we are learning to use increasingly sophisticated mechanical systems but are losing intelligent control of our own bodies.

References

ABRAMS, A. (1912) *Spondylotherapy*. San Francisco: Philopolis Press

ADAMS, C. B. T. and LOGUE, V. (1971) Studies in cervical myelopathy. I. Movement of the cervical roots, dura on cord and their relation on the course of the extrathecal roots. *Brain*, **94**, 557

ANDERSON, B. (1980) *Stretching*, Bolinas, California: Shelter

ANDERSON, J. A. D. (1980) Back pain and occupation. In *The Lumbar Spine and Back Pain*, 2nd edn, p. 57. Ed. Jayson, M.I.V. London: Pitman Medical

ANGRIST, A. A. (1973) The inevitable decline of chiropractic. *N.Y. State Journal of Medicine*, **73**, 324

ANKERMANN, K. J. (1982) Die iliosakrale Diskordanz, eine funktionell reversible Fehlstellung der Iliosakralgelenke. *Zeitschrift für Physiotherapie*, **34**, 377

BABIN, E and MAITROT, D. (1977) Signes radiologiques osseux des varietées morphologiques des canaux lombaires étroits. *Annales Radiologiques*, **20**, 491

BAJER, A., BOHRN, K. and KAMENÍK, M. (1959) Funkční zkouška poruch pruchodnosti cév kmene mozkového pomocí De Kleynova testu. (Examination of brain stem circulation with the aid of De Kleyn's test.) *Československá Otolaryngologie*, **8**, 55

BAKKE, M., TFELT-HANSE, P., OLESEN, J. and MØLLER, H. (1982) Action of some pericranial muscles during provoked attacks of common migraine. *Pain*, **14**, 121

BAKKE, S. N. (1931) Röntgenologische Beobachtungen über die Beweglichkeit der Wirbelsäule. *Acta Radiologica (Stockholm)*, Suppl. XIII

BALMER, H. (1972) Die Bewegungsachsen der Lumbalwirbelsäule bei Flexion und Extension. *Zeitschrift für Unfall-Medizin und Berufskrankheiten*, **63**, 11

BARBOR, R. (1964) A treatment for chronic low back pain. In *Proceedings of the 4th International Congress of Physical Medicine, Paris, September 6–11*. International Congress Series, No.107. Amsterdam: Excerpta Medica

BARBOR, R. (1972) Das Schultergelenk. *Manuelle Medizin*, **10**, 25

BARON, J. B., BESSINETON, J. C., BIZZO, G., NOTO, R., TÉVANIAN, G and PACIFICI, M. (1973) Correlation entre le fonctionnement des systèmes sensorimoteurs labyrinthiques et oculomoteur ajustant les déplacements du centre de gravité du corps de l'homme en orthostatisme. *Agressologie*, **6 (14) B**, 79

BARR, J. (1937) Sciatica caused by intervertebral disc lesion. *Journal of Bone and Joint Surgery*, **19**, 323

BARRÉ, J. A. (1926) Le syndrome sympathique cervical postérieur. *Revue Oto-Neuro-Ophthalmologique*, **4**, 65

BARRÉ, J. A. (1926) Sur un syndrome sympathique cervical postérieur et sa cause fréquente, l'arthrite cervicale. *Revue neurologique*, **33**, 1246

BARRÉ, J. A. (1952) Troubles neuro-ophthalmologiques d'origine cervicale. *Revue Oto-Neuro-Ophthalmologique*, **24**, 18

BARTEL, W. (1980) Die Häufigkeit und Behandlung von Blockierungen im Bereich der Kopfgelenke nach Schädel-Hirntrauma. In *Manuelle Medizin, Tagungsbericht, Potsdam, 28 – 31.1.1980*, p. 92. Eds Metz, E. G. and Badtke, G. Wissenschaftlich-Technisches Zentrum der Pädagogischen Hochschule. Potsdam: K. Liebknecht

BARTEL, W. (1980) Die Wirksamkeit der Manuellen Therapie bei der Nachbehandlung von Sprunggelenksverletzungen. In *Manuelle Medizin, Tagungsbericht, Potsdam, 28 – 31.1.1980*, p. 118. Eds Metz, E. G. and Badtke, G. Wissenschaftlich-Technisches Zentrum der Pädagogischen Hochschule. Potsdam: K. Liebknecht

BÄRTSCHI-ROCHAIX, W. (1949) *Migraine Cervicale.* Bern: Huber

BASMAJIAN, J. V. (1978) *Muscles Alive,* 4th edn. Baltimore: Williams and Wilkins

BEAL, M. C. (1979) Grundlagen der Osteopathie. In *Theoretische Fortschritte und praktische Erfahrungen der Manuellen Medizin,* p. 32. Eds Neumann, H. D. and Wolff, H. D. Bühl: Konkordia

BECKER, F. (1978) Über Schwindelerscheinungen besonders aus der Sicht der Manuellen Therapie. *Manuelle Medizin,* **16,** 95

BENN, R. T. and WOOD, P. H. N. (1975) Pain in the back. An attempt to estimate the size of the problem. *Rheumatology and Rehabilitation,* **14,** 121

BERGER, M. (1982) Differentialdiagnose des Schulter-Nackenschmerzes aus neuroorthopädischer Sicht. *Wiener medizinische Wochenschrift,* **23–24,** 583

BERGER, M. (1984) Neuroorthopädische Diagnostik und Therapieeffekte bei cervikalen Rotationsstörungen. In *Schmerzstudien 6. Schmertz und Bewegungssystem,* p. 163. Eds. Berger, M., Gerstenbrand, F., Lewit, K. Stuttgart, New York, Gustav Fischer

BERGER, M. and GERSTENBRAND, F. (1981) Kopfschmerzen als Spätsymptom nach Peitschenschlagtrauma der Halswirbelsäule, neuroorthopädische Aspekte. In *Schmerzstudien 5, Kopfschmerz,* p. 264. Eds Gross, D. and Frey, R. Stuttgart and New York: Gustav Fischer

BERGER, M., GERSTENBRAND, F. and LEWIT, K. (1984) *Schmerzstudien 6. Schmerz und Bewegungssystem,* Stuttgart and New York, Gustav Fischer

BERGER, M. and LEWIT, K. (1984) Der antalgetische Effekt der postisometrischen Muskelrelaxation. In *Schmerzstudien 6. Schmerz und Bewegungssystem,* p. 214. Eds Berger, M., Gerstenbrand, F., Lewit, K. Stuttgart, New York, Gustav Fischer

BERGSMAN, O. (1974) Das mechanisch-dyspnoische Syndrom – thorakale Störung der Atembewegung. *Manuelle Medizin,* **12,** 79

BIEDERMANN, F. (1954) *Grundsätzliches zur Chiropraktik.* Ulm: Haug

BIEDERMANN, F. and EDINGER, A. (1957) Kurzes Bain, schiefes Becken. *Fortschritte auf dem Gebiete der Rontgenstrahlen,* **86,** 754

BISCHKO, J. (1984) Die Akupunturtherapie beim Bewegungssystem. In *Schmerzstudien 6. Scherz und Bewegungssystem,* p. 261. Eds Berger, M., Gerstenbrand, F., Lewit, K. Stuttgart, New York, Gustav Fischer

BITTERLI, J., GRAF, R., ROBERT, F., ADLER, R. and MUMENTHALER, M. (1977) Zur Objektivierung der manualtherapeutischen Beeinflussbarkeit des spondylogenen Kopfschmerzes. *Nervenarzt,* **48,** 259

BITTERLI, J., SCHLAPBACH, P. and FELLMANN, N. (1978) Traitement de l'arthrose fémoropatellaire par pollissage manuel. *Cinésiologie,* **69,** 55

BJELINSKIJ, V. E. (1973) Vliyanie vesa tyeli i myshetshnyck sil na formirovanie fisiologitsheskich izgibov pozvonotschnika. (Influence of body weight and muscle forces on the formation of spinal curvature.) *Ortopedia, traumatologia i protezirovanie,* **34,** 45

BOUDIN, G., BARBIZET, J. and MASSON, S. (1959) Vertige et perte de connaissance. *Revue Neurologique,* **101,** 747

BOURDILLON, J. F. (1982) *Spinal Manipulation,* 3rd edn. London: Heinemann Medical; New York: Appleton-Century-Crofts

BREIG, A. (1964) Dehnungsverschiebungen von Dura und Rückenmark im Spinalkanal. *Fortschritte in der Neurologie und Psychiatrie,* **32,** 195

BRENA, S. F., WOLF, S. L., CHAPMAN, S. L. and HAMMONDS, W. D. (1980) Chronic back pain: electromyographic, motion and behavioral assessment following sympathetic nerve blocks and placebos. *Pain,* **8,** 1

BROCHER, J. E. W. (1966) *Die Wirbelsäulenleiden und ihre Differentialdiagnose,* 4th edn. Stuttgart: Thieme

BRODIN, H. (1979) Principles of examination and treatment in manual medicine. *Scandinavian Journal of Rehabilitation Medicine,* **11,** 181

BRODIN, H. (1982) Cervical pain and mobilisation. *Manuelle Medizin,* **20,** 90

BRODIN, H. (1982) Inhibition–facilitation technique for lumbar pain. *Manuelle Medizin,* **20,** 95

BRÜCKMANN, W. (1956) Osteochondrose der Halwirbelsäle und Koronarinfarkt. *Deutsche Medizinische Wochenschrift,* **81,** 1740

BRÜGGER, A. (1960, 1962) Uber vertebrale radikuläre und pseudoradikuläre Syndrome. *Acta Rheumatologica,* Documenta Geigy, No. 18, No. 19

BRÜGGER, A. (1977) *Die Erkrankungen des Bewegungsapparates und seines Nervensystems.* Stuttgart and New York: G. Fischer

BRÜGGER, A. (1984) Neurologische und morphologische Grundlagen der sogenannten rheumatischen Schmerzen – ein Beitrag zum Verständnis der Funktionskrankheiten. In *Schmerzstudien 6. Schmerz und Bewegungssystem,* p. 56. Eds Berger, M., Gerstenbrand, F., Lewit, K. Stuttgart, New York, Gustav Fischer

BRUNSTRÖM, A. A. (1962) *Clinical Kinesiology.* Philadelphia: F. A. Davis

BUCHMANN, J. (1980) Motorische Entwicklung und Wirbelsäulenfunktionsstörung. *Manuelle Medizin*, **18,** 37

BUCHMANN, J. and BÜLOW, B. (1983) Funktionelle Kopfgelenksstörungen bei Neugeborenen im Zusammenhang mit Lagereaktionsverhalten und Tonusassymetrie. *Manuelle Medizin*, **21,** 59

BUERGER, A. A. (1977) Clinical trials of manipulation therapy. In *Approaches to the Validation of Manipulative Therapy*, p.313. Eds Buerger, A. A. and Tobis, J. S. Springfield: Charles C. Thomas

BUERGER, A. A. (1980) A controlled trial of rotational manipulation in low back pain. *Manuelle Medizin*, **18,** 17

BUETTI–BÄUML, C. (1954) *Funktionelle Röntgendiagnostik der Halswirbelsäule*. Stuttgart: Thieme

BURAN, I., NOVÁK, J. (1984) Der Psychische Faktor bei schmerzhaften vertebragenen Syndromen, seine klinische und elektromyographischen Erscheinungsforman. *Manuelle Medizin*, **22,** 5.

BURTON, C. V. (1981) Conservative management of low back pain. *Postgraduate Medicine*, **70,** 168

CAMPBELL, E. J. M., AGOSTONI, A. and NEWSOM DAVIS, J. (1970) *The Respiratory Muscles. Mechanics and Neural Control*. London: Lloyd-Luke

CAVIEZEL, H. (1974) Entwicklung der theoretischen Grundlagen der manuellen Medizin. *Schweizer Rundschau für Medizin (Praxis)*, **63,** 829

ČERNÝ, R. (1948) Autodermografie bolesti a čití. (Autodermography of pain and sensibility.) *Sborník lékařský*, **50,** 315

CHRÁST, B. and KORBIČKA, J. (1962) Die Beeinflussung der Strömungsverhältnisse in der Arteria vertebralis durch verschiedene Kopf – und Halsstellungen. *Deutsche Zeitschrift für Nervenheilkunde*, **183,** 426

ČIHÁK, R. (1970) Variations of lumbosacral joints and their morphogenisis. *Acta Universitatis Carolinae Medica*, **16,** 145

CLIFFORD, T., LAURITZEN, M., BAKKE, M., OLESEN, J. and MØLLER, E. (1982) Electromyography of pericranial muscles during treatment of spontaneous common migraine attacks. *Pain*, **14,** 137

COLACHIS, S. C., WORDEN, R. E., BOCHTAL, C. O. and STROHM, B. R. (1963) Movement of the sacroiliac joint in the adult male: a preliminary report. *Archives of Physical Medicine and Rehabilitation*, **44,** 490

CRAMER, A. (1958) Funktionelle Merkmale der Wirbelsäulenstatik. In *Wirbelsäule in Forschung und Praxis*, vol.5, p.84. Ed Biedermann, F. Stuttgart: Hippokrates

CRAMER, A. (1965) Iliosakralmechanik. *Asklepios*, **6,** 261

CYRIAX, J. (1977) *Textbook of Orthopaedic Medicine*, Vol. 1. London: Cassel.

CYRIAX, J. (1978) *Textbook of Orthopaedic Medicine*, Vol. 2. London: Baillière

CYRIAX, J. and CYRIAX, P. J. (1983) *Illustrated Manual of Orthopaedic Medicine*. London, Butterworth

CYRIAX, J. and SCHIÖTZ, E. H. (1975) *Manipulation Past and Present*. London: Heinemann

DALSETH, I. (1974) Anatomic studies of the osseous craniovertebral joints. *Manuelle Medizin*, **12,** 130

DANZ, J. (1982) Gelenkspielbefunde an der Hand bei Patienten mit Rheumatoid-Arthritis. *Manuelle Medizin*, **20,** 70

DECHER, H. (1969) *Die zervikalen Syndrome in der Hals-Nasen-Ohren-heilkunde*. Stuttgart: Thieme

DECHER, H. (1976) Morbus Meniere und zervikale Syndrome. *Archives of Oto-Rhino-Laryngology*, **212,** 369

DÉJÉRINE, J. (1901) Sémiologie du système nerveux. *Pathologie générale* 5, p.359. Paris: Bouchard

DERBOLOWSKI, U. (1956) Beckenmechanik-chiropraktisch gesehen. *Hippokrates*, **27,** 310

DOLTO, B. J. (1976) *Le Corps entre les Mains*. Paris: Hermann

DORAN, D. M. L. and NEWELL, D. J. (1975) Manipulation in treatment of low back pain: a multicentre study. *British Medical Journal*, **2,** 161

DOVE, C. I. (1982) The occipito-atlanto-axial complex. *Manuelle Medizin*, **20,** 11

DRECHSLER, B. (1970) Spinale Muskelsteuerung und Wurzelkompression. In *Manuelle Medizin und ihre wissenschaftlichen Grundlagen*, p.92. Ed. Wolff, H. D. Heidelberg: Physikalische Medizin

DUCKWORTH, J. W. A. (1970) The anatomy and movements of the sacroiliac joints. In *Manuelle Medizin und ihre wissenschaftlichen Grundlagen*, p.56. Ed. Wolff, H. D. Heidelberg: Physikalische Medizin

DUL, J., SNIJDERS, C. J. and TIMMERMAN, P. (1982) Bewegungen und Kräfte im oberen Kopfgelenk beim Vorbeugen der Halswirbelsäule. *Manuelle Medizin*, **20,** 51

DUUS, P., KAHLAU, G. and KRÜCKE, W. (1951) Allgemeinbetrachtungen über die Einengung der Foramina intervertebralia. *Langenbecks Archiv und Deutsche Zeitschrift für Chirurgie*, **268,** 341

DVOŘÁK, J. (1982) Manuelle Medizin in den USA im Jahre 1981. *Manuelle Medizin*, **20,** 1

DVOŘÁK, J. and DVOŘÁK, V. (1983) *Manuelle Medizin, Diagnostik*. Stuttgart: Thieme

DVOŘÁK, J. and ORELLI, F. (1982) Wie gefährlich ist die Manipulation der Halswirbelsäule? *Manuelle Medizin*, **20,** 44

EBBETTS, J. (1971) Manipulation of the foot. *Physiotherapy*, 194

EBBETTS, J. (1975) Manipulation in treatment of low back pain. *British Medical Journal*, **2,** 393

EDER, M. (1984) Indikationen und Erfolgsaussichten der Manualtherapie lumbaler Syndrome. In *Neuroorthopädie 2, Lendenwirbelsäulenerkrankungen mit Beteiligung des Nervesystems*, p. 454. Eds Hohmann, D., Kügelgen, B., Liebig, K. and Schirmer, M. Berlin, Heidelberg, New York, Tokyo, Springer

EDMEALS, J. (1978) Headache and head pains associated with diseases of the cervical spine. *Medical Clinics of North America*, **62**, 533

EMMINGER, E. (1967) Die Anatomie und Pathologie des blockierten Wirbelgelenks. *Therapie über das Nervensystem*, vol.7, *Chirotherapie-Manuelle Therapie*, p.117. Ed. Gross, D. Stuttgart: Hippokrates

EPSTEIN, B. S., EPSTEIN, J. A. and LAVINA, L. (1964) The effect of anatomic variation in lumbar vertebrae and spinal canal on cauda equina and nerve root syndromes. *American Journal of Roentgenology*, **91**, 1055

ERDMANN, H. (1956) Die Verspannung des Wirbelsockels im Beckenring. In *Wirbelsäule in Forschung und Praxis*, vol.1, p.51. Ed. Junghams, H. Stuttgart: Hippokrates

ERDMANN, H. (1960) Zur Statik des symmetrischen Assimilationsbeckens. In *Wirbelsäule in Forschung und Praxis*, vol.15, p.103. Ed. Junghanns, H. Stuttgart: Hippokrates

ERDMANN, H. (1965) Vergleichend anatomische Untersuchungen zum Verständnis der Statik und Dynamik von Becken und Lendenwirbelsäule bei verschiedenen Beckentypen. *Asklepios*, **6**, 1

ERKRATH, F. A. and STRAUCH, W. (1968) Kreuzschmerzen und Leistungsminderung bei weiblichen Beschäftigten. *Deutsches Gesundheitswesen*, **23**, 1125

EVANS, D. P., BURKE, M. S., LLOYD, K. N., ROBERTS, E. E. and ROBERTS, G. M. (1978) Lumbar spinal manipulation on trial. Part I – clinical assessment. *Rheumatology and Rehabilitation*, **17**, 46

EVJENTH, O. and HAMBERG, J. (1981) *Muskeldehnung*. Zug, Schweiz: Remed

FAHLSTRÖM, G. (1978) On specific mobility 0–C2 and specific treatment of the cervical spine. *Manuelle Medizin*, **16**, 92

FALKENAU, H. A. (1977) Pathogenese und Chirotherapie des pharyngoösophagealen zervikalen Syndroms. *Laryngologie, Rhinologie, Otologie*, **56**, 466

FARELL, J. P. and TWOMEY, L. T. (1982) Acute low back pain. Comparison of two conservative treatment approaches. *Medical Journal of Australia*, **1**, 160

FARFAN, H. F. (1973) *Mechanical Disorders of the Low Back*. Philadelphia: Lea and Febiger

FARFAN, H. F. (1980) The scientific bases of manipulative procedures. In *Low Back Pain*, p.159. Ed. Grahame, R. Clinics in Rheumatic Diseases. Philadelphia: W. B. Saunders

FEINSTEIN, B., LONGTON, J. N. K., JAMESON, R. M. and SCHILLER, F. (1954) Experiments on pain referred from deep somatic structures. *Journal of Bone and Joint Surgery*, **36A**, 981

FELD, M. (1954) Subluxations et entorse sousoccipitales. Leurs syndrome fonctionel consécutif aux traumatismes craniens. *Semaine des Hôpitaux*, **30**, 1952

FIGAR, Š. (1970) Objektivierung der Reflextherapiewirking auf Grund der Gefässreaktivitätsregistratur. In *Manuelle Medizin und ihre wissenschaftlichen Grundlagen*, p.89. Ed. Wolff, H. D., Heidelberg: Physikalische Medizin

FIGAR, Š. and KRAUSOVÁ, L. (1975) Measurement of degree of resistance in vertebral segments. In *Functional Pathology of the Motor System, Rehabilitácia*. Suppl. 10–11, p.60. Eds. Lewit, K. and Gutmann, G. Bratislava: Obzor

FINEMAN, S. F., BORELLI, F. J., RUBINSTEIN, B. M., EPSTEIN, H. and JACOBSON, H. G. (1963) The cervical spine. Transformation of the normal lordotic pattern into a linear pattern in neutral posture. *Journal of Bone and Joint Surgery*, **45A**, 1179

FISK, J. W. (1977) *The Practical Guide to Management of the Painful Neck and Back; Diagnosis, Manipulation, Exercises, Prevention*. Springfield: Charles C. Thomas

FISCHER, A. A. and CHANG, C. (1981) EMG evidence of paraspinal muscle spasm during sleep in patients with low back pain. *Pain*, Suppl. 1, 225

FORD, F. R. and CLARK, D. (1956) Thrombosis of the basilar artery with softening in the cerebellum and brain stem due to manipulation of the neck. *Bulletin of the Johns Hopkins Hospital*, **1**, 57

FORESTIER, J. and LAGIER, R. (1971) Hyperostoses vertébrales ankylosantes. *Médicine et Hygiene*, **29**, 668

FOX, E. J. and MELZACK, R. (1976) Transcutaneous electrical stimulation and acupuncture: comparison of treatment for low back pain. *Pain*, **2**, 141

FRANK, G. (1971) Der Lagerungsschwindel und seine diagnostische Bedeutung. *Deutsches Gesundheitswesen*, **26**, 2122

FRANKSHTEIN, S. I. (1951) *Reflexi Patologitsheski Izmyenyenyck Organov*. (Reflex changes in visceral disease.) Moscow: Medgiz

FREDERICKSON, J. M., SCHWARZ, D. and KORNHUBER, H. H. (1976) Convergence and interaction of vestibular and deep somatic afferents upon neurons in the vestibular nuclei of the cat. *Acta Otolaryngologica (Stockholm)*, **61**, 169

FRIED, K. (1966) Die zervikale juvenile Osteochondrose. *Fortschritte auf dem Gebiet der Röntgenstrahlen*, **105**, 69

FRISCH, H. (1973) Die theoretischen Grundlagen der Manuellen Medizin. *Zeitschrift für Orthopädie und ihre Grenzgebiete*, **111**, 573

FRISCH, H. (1983) *Programmierte Untersuchung des Bewegungsapparates*. Berlin, Heidelberg, New York, Tokyo, Springer

FROST, F. A., JESSE, B. and SIGGAARD-ANDERSSEN, J. (1980) A controlled double blind comparison of Mevipacain injection versus saline injection for myofascial pain. *Lancet*, **ii**, 499

FRYETTE, H. H. (1954) *Principles of Osteopathic Technique*. Carmel: Academy of Applied Osteopathy

FRYKHOLM, R. (1969) Die zervikalen Bandscheibenschaden. In: *Handbuch der Neurochirurgie*, vol.VII/I, p.73. Eds. Olivecrona, H. and Tonnis, W. Heidelberg: Springer

FULLENLOVE, T. M. and JUSTIN WILLIAMS, A. (1957) Comparative Roentgen findings in symptomatic and asymptomatic backs. *Radiology*, **68**, 572

GAGEY, P. M., BARON, J. B., LESPARGOT, J. and POLI, J. P. (1973) Variations de l'activité tonique posturale et activité des muscles oculocéphalogyres en cathédrostatisme. *Aggressologie*, **6(14)B**, 87

GAIZLER, G. (1965) Die Beurteilung der Ruhehaltung der Halswirbelsäule – eine erledigte Frage? *Fortschritte auf dem Gebiet der Röntenstrahlen*, **103**, 566

GAIZLER, G. (1970) Eidogram. Neue, die Gravitationsrichtung berücksichtigende radiologische Messmethode der Wirbelsäule. *Zeitschrift für Orthopädie und ihre Grenzgebiete*, **107**, 197

GAIZLER, G. (1973) Die Aufrichtungs – und Erschlaffungsprobe. *Der Radiologe*, **13**, 247

GAIZLER, G. and MADARÁSZ, J. (1979) Funktionelle Röntgendiagnostik der Halswirbelsäule. *Manuelle Medizin*, **17**, 82

GAY, J. R. and ABBOTT, K. H. (1953) Common whiplash injuries of the neck. *Journal of the American Medical Association*, **152**, 1698

GAYMANS, F. (1971) Die Messung der Körperrotation und ihre Bedeutung für die Diagnose und Therapie vertebragener Störungen. *Manuelle Medizin*, **9**, 31

GAYMANS, F. (1980) Die Bedeutung der Atemtypen für Mobilisation der Wirbelsäule. *Manuelle Medizin*, **18**, 96

GAYMANS, F. (1982) Mobilisation of the spinal column by stimulation of reflex points. Communication at the International Symposium 'Spine and Muscles' Prague, 6 May

GAYMANS, F. and LEWIT, K. (1975) Mobilisation techniques using pressure (pull) and muscular facilitation and inhibition. In *Functional Pathology of the Motor System. Rehabilitácia Supplementum, 10–11*, p.47. Eds Lewit, K. and Gutmann, G. Bratislava: Obzor

GEERINCKX, P. (1979) Vorlaugphänomen der Rippen. *Manuelle Medizin*, **18**, 76

GEIGER, Th. and GROSS, D. (Eds) (1967) *Chirotherapie, Manuelle Therapie. Therapie über das Nervensystem*, vol.7 Stuttgart: Hippokrates

GEIGER, W. (1952) Zur zervikalen Migräne. *Deutsche Medizinische Wochenschrift*, **77**, 198

GEISER, M. (1972) Rückenuntersuchungen in einer Infanterie-Rekrutenschule. *Schweizer Medizinische Wochenschrift*, **102**, 1301

GERSTENBRAND, F., TILSCHER, H. and BERGER, M. (1980) Radikuläre und pseudoradikuläre Symptome der mittleren und unteren Halswirbelsäule. In *Nacken-Schulter-Armsyndrom, Schmerzstudien 3*, p.82. Eds Kocher, R., Gross, D. and Kaeser, H. E. Stuttgart and New York: G. Fischer

GHIA, J. N., MAO, W., TOOMEY, T. C. and GREGG, J. M. (1976) Acupuncture and chronic pain mechanisms. *Pain*, **2**, 285

GITELMAN, R. (1980) A chiropractic approach to biomechanical disorders of the lumbar spine. In *Modern Developments in Principles and Practice of Chiropractic*, Ed. Haldemann, S. New York: Appleton-Century-Crofts

GLÄSER, O. and DALICHO, A. W. (1962) *Segmentmassage*. Leipzig: Thieme

GLOVER, J. R., MORRIS, J. G. and KHOSLA, T. (1974) Back pain: a randomized clinical trial of rotational manipulation of the trunk. *British Journal of Industrial Medicine*, **31**, 59

GOOD, A. B. (1979) Spinal joint blocking. *The British Osteopathic Journal*, **11**, 4

GOODRIDGE, J. P. (1981) Muscle energy technique: definition, explanation, methods of procedure. *Journal of the American Osteopathic Association*, **81**, 249

GORDON, I. B. (1973) O znatshenii shejnovo osteochondrosa v praktike terapevta kardiologa. (Importance of cervical osteochondrosis in cardiological practice.) *Novokuznetsk: Osteochondroz pozvonotshnika*, **1**, 213

GORMAN, R. F. (1978) Cardiac arrest after cervical spine mobilisation. *Medical Journal of Australia*, **2**, 169

GRABER-DUVERNAY, J. (1972) Coxarthroses mineurs et réactions ostéophytiques. *Rheumatologie*, **24**, 123

GRAHAME, R. (1980) Clinical trials in low back pain. In *Low Back Pain*. Clinics in Rheumatic Diseases, vol.6, p. 143. Ed. Grahame, R. London and Philadelphia: W. B. Saunders

GREENMAN, P. E. (1978) Manipulative therapy in relation to total health care. In *The Neurobiologic Mechanisms in Manipulative Therapy*, p.43. Ed. Korr, I. M. New York and London: Plenum Press

GREENMAN, P. E. (1979) Verkürzungsausgleich – Nutz und Unnutz. In *Theoretische Fortschritte und praktische Erfahrungen der Manuellen Medizin*, p.333. Eds Neumann, H. D. and Wolff, H. D. Bühl: Konkordia GmbH für Druck und Verlag

GREENMAN, P. E. (1979) Manuelle Therapie am Brustkorb. *Manuelle Medizin*, **17,** 17

GREENMAN, P. E. (1984) Wirbelbewegung. *Manuelle Medizin*, **22,** 13

GREENMAN, P. E. (1984) Eingeschränkte Wirbelbewegung. *Manuelle Medizin*, **22,** 15

GREENMAN, P. E. (1984) Schichtweise Palpation. *Manuelle Medizin*, **22,** 46

GREINER, G. F., CONRAUX, C. and THIEBAUT, M. D. (1967) Le nystagmus d'origine cervical. *Revue Neurologique*, **117,** 677

GRIEVE, G. P. (1976) The sacro-iliac joint. *Physiotherapy*, 62

GRIEVE, G. P. (1978) *Mobilisation of the Spine*. Edinburgh: Churchill Livingstone

GRIEVE, G. P. (1981) *Common Vertebral Joint Problems*. Edinburgh: Churchill Livingstone

GROENEVELD, H. B. (1976) *Metrische Erfassung und Definition von Rückenform*. *Wirbelsäule in Forschung und Praxis*, vol.66. Stuttgart: Hippokrates

GROH, H. (1972) Wirbelsäule und Leistungssport. *Selecta*, **14,** 324

GROSS, D. (1972) *Therapeutische Lokalanästhesie*. Stuttgart: Hippokrates

GROSS, D. (1979) Sympathalgien des Nacken-Schulter-Arm-Bereiches. *Münchner Medizinische Wochenschrift*, **121,** 1167

GROSS, D. (1982) Contralateral local anaesthesia in the treatment of phantom limb and stump pain. *Pain*, **13,** 313

GROSS, D. and KOBSA, K. (1981) Motor coordination – polymyographic functional testing of the support and locomotor system. *Folia rheumatologica, Documenta Geigy*, pp. 1–8 Basel, Ciba-Geigy Ltd.

GROSSIORD, A. (1966) Les accidents neurologiques des manipulations cervicales. *Annales de Médicine Physique*, **9,** 283

GUNN, C. C. and MILDBRANDT, W. E. (1976) Tennis elbow and the cervical spine. *Canadian Medical Association Journal*, **114,** 803

GUNN, C. C., DITCHBURN, F. G., KING, M. H. and RENWICK, G. (1976) Acupuncture loci: a proposal for their classification according to known neural structures. *American Journal of Chinese Medicine*, **4,** 183

GURFINKEL, V. S., KOC, Ya. M. and SHIK, M. L. (1965) *Regulaciya Pozi Tsheloveka*. (Control of posture in man.) Moscow: Nauka

GUSTAVSON, R. (1981) *Trainingstherapie*, Stuttgart, New York, Thieme

GUTMANN, G. (1955) Schädeltrauma und Kopfgelenke. *Deutsche Medizinische Wochenschrift*, **80,** 1503

GUTMANN, G. (1956) Einführung in die statisch-funktionelle Röntgendiagnostik der Wirbelsäule unter besondrer Berücksichtigung der Kopfgelenke und Halswirbelsäule. In *Wirbelsäule in Forschung und Praxis*, vol.1, p.70. Ed. Junghanns, H. Stuttgart: Hippokrates

GUTMANN, G. (1960) Die Wirbelblockierung und ihr röntgenologischer Nachweis. *Wirbelsäule in Forschung und Praxis*, **15,** 83

GUTMANN, G. (1963) Das cervico-diencephale Syndrom mit synkopaler Tendenz und seine Behandlung. *Wirbelsäule in Forschung und Praxis*, **26,** 112

GUTMANN, G. (1965) Zur Frage der konstruktionsgerechten Beanspruchung von Lendenwirbelsäule und Becken beim Menschen. *Asklepios*, **6,** 263

GUTMANN, G. (1965) Das schmerzhaft gehemmte und das schmerhaft gelockerte Kreuz. *Asklepios*, **6,** 305

GUTMANN, G. (1968) Schulkopfschmerz und Kopfhaltung. Ein Beitrag zur Pathogenese des Anteflexions-Kopfschmerzes und zur Mechanik der Kopfgelenke. *Zeitschrift für Orthopädie und ihre Grenzgebiete*, **105,** 497

GUTMANN, G. (1970) X-ray diagnosis of spinal dysfunction. *Manuelle Medizin*, **8,** 73

GUTMANN, G. (1970) Klinisch-röntgenolotische Untersuchungen zur Statik der Wirbelsäule. In *Manuelle Medizin und ihre wissenschaftlichen Grundlagen*, p.109. Ed. Wolff, H. D. Heidelberg: Verlag für Physikalische Medizin

GUTMANN, G. (1975) Die pathogenetische Aktualitäts-Diagnostik. In *Functional Pathology of the Motor System. Rehabilitácia supplementum 10–11*, p.15. Eds. Lewit, K. and Gutmann, G. Bratislava: Obzor

GUTMANN, G. (1979) The subforaminal stenosis headache. *Acta Neurochirurgica*, **50,** 201

GUTMANN, G. (1981) Die funktionsanalytische Röntgendiagnostik der Halswirbelsäule und der Kopfgelenke. In *Funktionelle Pathologie und Klinik der Wirbelsäule*, vol.1. *Die Halswirbelsäule*, Teil 1. Ed. Gutmann, G. Stuttgart and New York: G. Fischer

GUTMANN, G. (1983) Verletzungen der Arteria vertebralis durch manuelle Therapie. *Manuelle Medizin*, **21,** 2

GUTMANN, G. and BIEDERMANN, H. (1984) Allgemeine funktionelle Pathologie und klinische Syndrome. In *Funktionelle Pathologie und Klinik der Wirbelsäule Vol. 1, die Halswirbelsäuue Teil 2*. Ed Gutmann, G. Stuttgart and New York, Gustav Fischer

GUTMANN, G. and TIWISINA, T. (1959) Zum Problem der Iriitation der Arteria vertebralis. *Hippokrates*, **30,** 545

GUTMANN, G. and VÉLE, F. (1978) *Das aufrechte Stehen.* Westdeutscher Verlag, Forschungsberichte des Landes Nordrhein-Westfahlen No. 2796, Fachgruppe Medizin

GUTMANN, G. and WOLFF, H. D. (1959) Die Wirbelsäule als volkswirtschaftlicher Faktor. *Hippokrates,* **30,** 207

GUTZEIT, K. (1951) Wirbelsäule als Krankbeitsfaktor. *Deutsche Medizinische Wochenschrift,* **76,** 112

GUTZEIT, K. (1953) Wirbelsäule und innere Krankheiten. *Münchner Medizinische Wochenschrift,* **100,** 47

GUTZEIT, K. (1981) Der vertebrale Faktor im Krankheitsgeschehen. *Manuelle Medizin,* **19,** 66

HACKETT, G. S. (1956) *Joint Ligament Relaxation Treated by Fibro-osseous Proliferation.* Springfield: Charles C Thomas

HADLEY, L. A. (1957) The uncovertebral articulations and cervical foramen encroachment. *Journal of Bone and Joint Surgery,* **39A,** 911

HALDEMANN, S. (1980) *Modern Developments in the Principles and Practice of Chiropractic.* New York: Appleton Century Crofts

HAMBERG, J. and EVJENTH, O. (1979) Untersuchung und Behandlung der Hypermobilität an der Lendenwirbelsäule. In *Theoretische Fortschritte und praktische Erfahrungen der Manuellen Medizin,* p.187. Eds Neumann, H. D. and Wolff, H. D. Bühl: Konkordia GmbH für Druck und Verlag

HANÁK, L., MORÁVEK, V. and SCHRÖDER, R. (1970) Elektromyografie v předoperační diagnostice u bederních diskopatií. (Electromyography in preoperational diagnosis of the nerve root in disc lesions.) *Československá Neurologie,* **33,** 6

HANRAETS, P. R. M. G. (1959) *The Degenerative Back and its Differential Diagnosis.* London, New York, Amsterdam: Elsevier

HANSEN, K. and SCHLIACK, H. (1962) *Segmentale Innervation, ihre Bedeutung für Klinik und Praxis.* Stuttgart: Thieme

HARGRAVE-WILSON, W. and SHERREY, J. H. (1966) Cervical spondylosis and vertigo. *Lancet,* **ii,** 1262

HARTMAN, L. S. (1983) *Handbook of osteopathic Technique,* Headley Wood, N.M.K. Publishers

HARZER, K. and TÖNDURY, G. (1968) Zum Verhalten der Arteria vertebralis in der alternden Halswirbel-säule. *Fortschritte auf dem Gebiete der Röntgenstrahlen,* **104,** 687

HASNER, E., SCHALIMZEK, M. and SNORASSON, E. (1952) Roentgenological examination of the function of the lumbar spine. *Acta Radiologica,* **37,** 141

HAUSAMANN, E. (1970) Grenzfälle zwischen Chirurgie und manueller Medizin. *Manuelle Medizin,* **8,** 49

HAUSAMANN, E. (1971) Hüftschmerz und Iliosakralgelenk. *Manuelle Medizin,* **9,** 73

HEAD, H. (1893, 1894) On disturbances of sensation with especial reference to the pain of visceral disease. *Brain,* **16,** 1; **17,** 339

HEILIG, D. (1981) The thrust technique. *Journal of the American Osteopathic Association,* **81,** 244

HEITHOFF, K. B. (1981) High-resolution computed tomography of the lumbar spine. *Postgraduate Medicine,* **70,** 193

HELLPAPP, W. (1959) Zur Geschichte und Entwicklung manipulativer Heilmethoden. *Wirbelsäule in Forschung und Praxis,* **13,** 69

HELLSTEN, W. (1969) Epikondyläre Schmerzen. *Manuelle Medizin,* **7,** 59

HENRY, M. J., GRIMES, H. A. and LANE, J. W. (1967) Intervertebral disc calcification in childhood. *Radiology,* **89,** 81

HENSELL, V. (1976) Neurologische Schäden nach Repositionsmassnahmen an der Wirbelsäule. *Medizinische Welt,* **27,** 656

HERRSCHMANN, H. (1976) Ein Beitrag zur Behandlung des Sudeck-Syndroms. *Zeitschrift für Physiotherapie,* **28,** 143

HETTINGER, T. (1983) *Isometrisches Muskeltraining,* 5th Edn., Stuttgart, New York, Thieme

HINZ, B. and ERDMANN, H. (1967) Zur manuellen Untersuchung der Halswirbelsäule in der Gutachterpraxis. *Zeitschrift für Orthopädie und ihre Grenzgebiete,* **104,** 28

HIRSCH, C. (1959) Studies on the pathology of low back pain. *Journal of Joint and Bone Surgery,* **41B,** 237

HIRSCHFELD, P. (1962) Die konservative Behandlung des lumbalen Bandscheibenvorfalls nach der Methode von Cyriax. *Deutsche Medizinische Wochenschrift,* **87,** 299

HIRSCHKOFF, S. (1966) La palpation dynamique. *Rheumatologie,* **18,** 47

HOAG, J. M., COLE, W. V. and BRADFORD, S. G. (1969) *Osteopathic Medicine.* New York: McGraw-Hill

HOCKADAY, J. M. and WHITTY, C. W. M. (1967) Patterns of referred pain in the normal subject. *Brain,* **90,** 481

HOEHLER, F. K., TOBIS, J. S. and BUERGER, A. A. (1981) Spinal manipulation for low back pain. *Journal of the American Medical Association,* **245,** 1835

HOHL, M. and BAKER, H. R. (1964) The atlanto-axial joint. *Journal of Bone and Joint Surgery,* **46A,** 1739

HOHL, M., BAKER, H. R. and HILLS, B. (1964) Normal motion of the upper portion of the cervical spine. *Journal of Bone and Joint Surgery,* **46A,** 1777

HOWE, J. F., LOESER, J. D. and CALVIN, W. H. (1977) Mechanosensitivity of dorsal root ganglia and chronically injured axons: a physiological basis for radicular pain of nerve root compression. *Pain*, **3**, 25

HOWELL, J. F., ALLEN, T. W. and KAPPLER, R. E. (1975) The influence of osteopathic manipulative therapy in the management of patients with chronic obstructive lung disease. *Journal of the American Osteopathic Association*, **74**, 757

HUBER, E. H., GINZEL, H. and TILSCHER, H. (1977) Die Belastung des Skeletts von Kindern und Jugendlichen durch Ausübung verschiedener Sportarten. *Pädiatrie und Pädologie*, **12**, 272

HUGUENIN, F. (1976) Das Iliosakralgelenk. *Manuelle Medizin*, **14**, 61

HUGUENIN, F. (1984) Der intrakanalikuläre Bandapparat des zerviko-okzi-pitalen Überganges. Eine klinische und diagnostische Studie seiner Funktion und Verletzungen. *Manuelle Medizin*, **22**, 25

HÜLSE, M. (1981) Die Gleichgewichtsstörungen bei der funktionellen Kopfgelenksstörung. *Manuelle Medizin*, **19**, 92

HÜLSE, M. (1983) *Die zervikalen Gleichgewichtsstörungen*. Berlin, Heidelberg, New York, Tokyo, Springer

HULT, J. (1954) The Munkfors Investigation. *Acta Orthopaedica Scandinavica*, Suppl. 16

HULT, J. (1954) Cervical, dorsal and lumbar spinal syndromes. *Acta Orthopaedica Scandinavica*, Suppl. 17

HULT, L. (1972) Freqeuency of symptoms for different age groups and professions. In *Cervical Pain*, Eds Hirsch, C. and Zotterman, Y. Oxford: Pergamon Press

HUNEKE, F. (1947) *Krankheit und Heilung anders gesehen*. Köln: Staufen

HUNEKE, W. (1953) *Impletholtherapie*. Stuttgart: Hippokrates

ILLI, F. (1954) *Wirbelsäule, Becken und Chiropraxis*. Ulm: Haug

IVANICHEV, G. A. (1983) Funkcionalnoye sostoyanie sheynikh segmentov spinovo mazga u bolnykh s lokalnoi gypertonii myshc (The state of function of spinal segments of the spinal cord in patients with localised muscular hypertonus.) *Zhurnal Nevropatologia i Psichiatria*, **83**, 646

IVANICHEV, G. A. and POPELYANSKI A.Ya. (1983) Manualnya terapia spondylogennych porazhenii perifericheskoi nervnoi sistemy (Manipulative therapy in vertebrogenic lesions of the peripheral nervous system). *Zhurnal Nevropatologia i Psichiatria*, **83**, 523

JACOBSON, G. and ADLER, D. C. (1953) An evaluation of lateral atlantoaxial displacement in injuries of the cervical spine. *Radiology*, **61**, 355

JACOBSON, G. and ADLER, D. C. (1956) Examination of the atlantoaxial joint following injury with particular emphasis on rotational subluxation. *American Journal of Roentgenology*, **76**, 1081

JACOBSON, G., ADLER, D. C. and BLEECHER, A. A. (1959) Pseudosubluxation of the axis in children. *American Journal of Roentgenology*, **82**, 472

JAKOUBEK, B. and ROHLIČEK, V. (1982) Changes of electrodermal properties in the acupuncture points in men and rats. *Physiologia bohemicoslovaca*, **31**, 143

JANDA, V. (1967) Einige Bemerkungen zur Entwicklung der Motorik in der Pathogenese der Fehlhaltung und vertebragener Störungen. *Physikalische Medizin und Rehabilitation*, **8**, 260

JANDA, V. (1967) Die Motorik als reflektorisches Geschehen und ihre Bedeutung in der Pathogenese vertebragener Störungen. *Manuelle Medizin*, **5**, 1

JANDA, V. (1972) *Vyšetřování Hybnosti*. (Examination of Mobility.) Praha: Avicenum – Zdravotnické nakladatelství

JANDA, V. (1975) Muscle and joint correlations. In *Functional Pathology of the Motor System, Rehabilitácia*, Suppl. 10–11, p.154. Eds Lewit, K. and Gutmann, G. Bratislava: Obzor

JANDA, V. (1978) Muscles, central nervous regulation and back problems. In *Neurobiologic Mechanisms in Manipulative Therapy*, p.27. Ed. Korr, I. M. New York and London: Plenum Press

JANDA, V. (1979) Die muskulären Hauptsyndrome bei vertebragenen Beschwerden. In *Theoretische Fortschritte und Praktische Erfahrungen der Manuellen Medizin*, p.61. Eds. Neumann, H. D. and Wolff, H. D. Bühl: Konkordia

JANDA, V. (1983) On the concept of postural muscles and posture. *The Australian Journal of Physiotherapy*, **29**, 83

JAYSON, M. I. V. (1970) The problem of backache. *Practitioner, Symposium on The Rheumatic Diseases*, **205**, 615

JAYSON, M. I. V. (1981) *The Lumbar Spine and Back Pain*, 2nd edn. London: Pitman Medical

JENKER, F. L. and DOSSI, A. (1977) Zusammenhänge und Diskrepanzen zwischen klinischer Symptomatologie und röntgenologischen Veränderungen an der Halswirbelsäule beim Zervikalsyndrom und beim Arm-Schulter-Syndrom. *Manuelle Medizin*, **15**, 115

JIROUT, J. (1956) Studies on the dynamics of the spine. *Acta Radiologica*, **46**, 55

JIROUT, J. (1957) The normal mobility of the lumbosacral spine. *Acta Radiologica*, **47**, 345

JIROUT, J. (1967) Studien der Dynamik der Halswirbelsäule in der frontalen und horizontalen Ebene. *Fortschritte auf dem Gebiet der Röntgenstrahlen*, **106**, 236

JIROUT, J. (1968) Die Rolle der Axis bei der Seitneigung der Halswirbelsäule und die 'latente Skoliose'. *Fortschritte auf dem Gebiet der Röntgenstrahlen*, **109**, 74

JIROUT, J. (1969) Röntgendiagnostik der Halswirbelsäule und der Kopfgelenke. *Manuelle Medizin*, **7**, 121

JIROUT, J. (1970) Die Kippung der Halswirbelsäule in der sagittalen Ebene der Halswirbelsäule. *Fortschritte auf dem Gebiet der Röntgenstrahlen*, **112**, 793

JIROUT, J. (1971) Patterns of changes in the cervical spine on lateroflexion. *Neuroradiology*, **2**, 164

JIROUT, J. (1972) The effect of mobilisation of the segmental blockade on the sagittal component of the reaction on lateroflexion of the cervical spine. *Neuroradiology*, **3**, 210

JIROUT, J. (1972) The influence of postural factors on the dynamics of the cervical spine. *Neuroradiology*, **4**, 239

JIROUT, J. (1973) Changes in the atlas–axis relations on lateral flexion of the head and neck. *Neuroradiology*, **6**, 215

JIROUT, J. (1974) The dynamic dependence of the lower cervical vertebrae on the atlanto-occipital joints. *Neuroradiology*, **7**, 249

JIROUT, J. (1976) Bedeutung der Synkinesen für die Entstehung der Wirbelblockierungen. *Manuelle Medizin*, **14**, 43

JIROUT, J. (1978) Veränderungen der Beweglichkeit der Halswirbel in der frontalen und horizontalen Ebene nach manueller Beseitigung der Segmentblockierung. *Manuelle Medizin*, **16**, 2

JIROUT, J. (1979) The rotational component in the dynamics of the C2–3 spinal segment. *Neuroradiology*, **17**, 177

JIROUT, J. (1979) Persistence of synkinetic patterns of the cervical spine. *Neuroradiology*, **18**, 167

JIROUT, J. (1980) Einfluss der einseitigen Grosshirndominanz auf das Röntgenbild der Halswibelsäule. *Radiologe*, **20**, 466

JIROUT, J. (1981) Rotational synkinesis of occiput and atlas on lateral inclination. *Neuroradiology*, **21**, 1

JIROUT, J. (1981) Die Beziehung zwischen dem klinischen und röntgenologischen Befund der synkinetischen Rotation der Axis bei Seitneigung. *Manuelle Medizin*, **19**, 58

JIROUT, J. (1983) Röntgenstudien der Dynamik der 1. Rippe. *Manuelle Medizin*, **21**, 20

JIROUT, J. (1984) Röntgenologische Symptome der Überlastung. In *Schmerzstudien 6. Schmerz und Bewegungssystem* p. 107. Eds Berger, M., Gerstenbrand, F. and Lewit, K. Stuttgart, New York, Gustav Fischer

JONES, L. H. (1963) Spontaneous release by positioning. *Clinical Osteopathy: Manipulative Therapy*, September, 128

JONES, L. H. (1981) Foot treatment without hand trauma. *Journal of the American Osteopathic Association*, **72**, 481

JONES, A. and WOLF, S. L. (1980) Treating chronic low back pain. EMG biofeedback training during movement. *Journal of the American Physical Therapy Association*, **60**, 58

JÖNSSON, M. (1966) Einstellungsuntersuchungen bei Berglehrlingen unter besonderer Berücksichtigung der Wirbelsäule. *Deutsches Gesundheitswesen*, **21**, 1809

JUNG, A. and KEHR, P. (1972) Das zerviko-enzephale Syndrom bei Arthrosen und nach Trauma der Halswirbelsäule. *Manuelle Medizin*, **10**, 97, 127

JUNG, A., KEHR, P. and JUNG, F. M. (1976) Das posttraumatische Zervikalsyndrom. *Manuelle Medizin*, **14**, 101

JUNGHANNS, H. (1930) Spondylolisthesen ohne Spalt im Zwischengelenksstück. *Archiv der Orthopädischen Chirurgie*, **29**, 118

JUNGHANNS, H. (1952) Die funktionelle Röntgenuntersuchung der Halswirbelsäule. *Fortschritte auf dem Gebiete der Röntgenstrahlen*, **76**, 591

JUNGHANNS, H. (1955) Ergebnisse der Wirbelsäulenpathologie und ihrer Auswirkung auf Röntgenologie und praktische Medizin. *Die Medizinische*, **15**, 513

JUNGHANNS, H. (1957) Leistungsfähigkeit und Grenzen chiropraktischer Massnahmen. *Deutsches Medizinisches Journal*, **8**, 194

JUNGHANNS, H. (1974) Die Bedeutung der Insufficientia intervertebralis für die Wirbelsäulenforschung. *Manuelle Medizin*, **12**, 93

JUNGHANNS, H. (1979) *Die Wirbelsäule in der Arbeitsmedizin. Wirbelsäule in Forschung und Praxis*, vols. 78 and 79. Stuttgart: Hippokrates

KABAT, H. (1965) Proprioceptive facilitation in therapeutic exercise. In *Therapeutic Exercise*, 2nd edn., p.301. Ed. Licht, S. New Haven: E. Licht

KABÁTNÍKOVÁ, Z. and KABÁTNÍK, Z. (1966) Význam chrbtice pri bolestiach hlavy v detskom veku. (The role of the spinal column in children's headache.) *Lékařský Obzor*, **15**, 361

KALCHER, B. (1979) Die Beeinflussung der körperlichen Leistungsfähigkeit durch skelettbedingte Störungen der Atemtechnik. In *Theoretische Fortschritte und praktische Erfahrungen der Manuellen Medizin*, p.134. Eds Neumann, H. D. and Wolff, H. D. Bühl: Konkordia

KALTENBORN, F. M. (1966) *Frigjøring av Ryggraden*. Oslo: F. M. Kaltenborn

KALTENBORN, F. M. (1976) *Manuelle Therapie der Extremitätengelenke*. Oslo: Olaf Norlis Bokhandel

KAMIETH, H. (1958) Das Syndrom der Beckenringlockerung. *Die Medizinische*, **25**, 1014

KAMIETH, H. (1983) Röntgenbefunde von normalen Bewegungen in den Kopfgelenken. In *Wirbelsäule in Forschung und Praxis*, Vol. 101, Ed Schulitz, K. P., Stuttgart, Hippokrates

KANE, R. L., LEYMASTER, C., OLSED, D., WOOLLEY, F. R. and FISHER, F. D. (1974) Manipulating the patient. A comparison of the effectiveness of physician and chiropractor care. *Lancet*, **i**, 1333

KAPANDJI, I. A. (1970) *The Physiology of Joints*. Edinburgh: Churchill Livingstone

KAPPLER, R. E. (1981) Postural balance and motor pattern. *Journal of the American Osteopathic Association*, **81**, 239/53

KEEGAN, J. (1944) Neurosurgical interpretation of dermatome hypalgesia with herniation of lumbar intervertebral disc. *Journal of Bone and Joint Surgery*, **24**, 236

KEEGAN, J. (1947) Relations of nerve roots to abnormalities of lumbar and cervical portions of the spine. *Archives of Surgery*, **55**, 246

KELLGREN, J. H. (1938) Observation of referred pain arising from muscles. *Clinical Science*, **3**, 15

KELLGREN, J. H. (1939) On the distribution of pain arising from deep somatic structures with charts of segmental pain areas. *Clinical Science*, **4**, 35

KELLY, M. (1956) Is pain due to pressure on nerves? *Neurology*, **6**, 32

KELTON, I. and WRIGHT, W. (1949) The mechanism of easy standing in man. *Australian Journal of Experimental Biology and Medical Science*, **27**, 505

KENDALL, H. O., KENDALL, F. P. and WADSWORTH, G. E. (1971) *Muscle Testing and Function*. Baltimore: Williams and Williams

KIBLER, M. (1958) *Das Störungsfeld bei Gelenkerkrankungen und inneren Krankheiten*. Stuttgart: Hippokrates

KIM, J. H. and PARTRIDGE, L. D. (1969) Observations on types of response to combination of neck, vestibular and muscular stretch signals. *Journal of Neurophysiology*, **32**, 239

KIMBERLEY, P. E. (1980) Bewegung – Bewegungseinschränkung und Anschlag. *Manuelle Medizin*, **18**, 53

KIRITSHINSKI, A. R. (1959) *Reflektornaya Fisikoterapia*. (Reflex Physical Therapy.) Kiev: Gosudarstvennoye Medicinskoye Izdatelstvo

KITZINGER, G. (1978) Skoliose und Beckenverwringung. *Manuelle Medizin*, **16**, 35

KLASMEIER, H. (1961) Bandscheibenprolaps und Konstitutionstyp der Wirbelsäule. *Fortschritte auf dem Gebiete der Röntgenstrahlen*, **94**, 479

KLAWUNDE, G. and ZELLER, H. J. (1974) Über den Zusammenhang zwischen reversibler Gelenksblockierung an der Wirbelsäule, subjektiven Beschwerden und beruflichen Tätigkeitsmerkmalen. *Zeitschrift für Physiotherapie*, **26**, 167

KLAWUNDE, G. and ZELLER, H. J. (1975) Elektromyographische Untersuchungen des M.iliacus (Sagittale Blockierung im lumbo-iliosakralen Bereich). *Beiträge zur Orthopädie und Traumatologie*, **22**, 420

KLAWUNDE, G. and ZELLER, H. J. (1979) Klinische, elektromyographische and reflexographische Untersuchungen über den Einfluss von iliolumbosakralen Blockierungen auf die Steuerung zugeordneter Muskelaktivitäten. *Manuelle Medizin*, **17**, 74

KLAWUNDE, G. and ZELLER, H. J. (1980) Über die Verwendbarkeit verschiedener Parameter der Nervenleitfähigkeit zur Objektivierung manualmedizinischer Befunde und Therapieeffekte. *Manuelle Medizin*, **18**, 56

KLEIN, K. and BUCKLEY, J. C. (1967) Asymmetries of growth in the pelvis and legs of growing children. *Journal of the Association of Physical and Mental Rehabilitation*, **21**, 40

KNOTT, M. and VOSS, D. E. (1968) *Proprioceptive Neuromuscular Facilitation*, 2nd edn. New York: Harper and Row

KNUTSSON, F. (1944) The instability associated with disc degeneration in the lumbar spine. *Acta Radiologica*, **25**, 593

KÖBERLE, G. (1976) Neue Aspekte in der Behandlung des akuten Schiefhalses. *Zeitschrif für Physiotherapie*, **28**, 135

KÖBERLE, G. (1975) Arthrologische Stömuster bei chronisch-obstruktiven Atemwegserkrankungen. In *Functional Pathology of the Motor System. Rehabilitácia*, Suppl. 10–11, p.96. Eds. Lewit, K. and Gutmann, G. Bratislava: Obzor

KOGAN, O. G. *et al.* (1981) *Klassifikacia nevrologicheskikh proyavlenii osteokhoncroza pozvonochnika i principy formulirovania diagnoza* (Classification of neurological manifestations of spinal osteochondrosis and the principles of how to formulate a diagnosis) Novokuznetsk, Polygrafkombinat

KOMENDANTOV, G. L. (1945) Proprioceptivyne reflexi glaza i golovy u krolikov. (Proprioceptive reflexes of the eye and head in rabbits.) *Fiziologičeski Zhurnal*, **31**, 62

KONDZIALLA, W. (1983) Zervikales Globusgefühl – Ursache und Behandlung. *Manuelle Medizin*, **21**, 51

KORR, I. M. (1948) The emerging concept of the osteopathic lesion. *Journal of the American Osteopathic Association*, **47**, 127

KORR, I. M. (1975) Proprioceptors and somatic dysfunction. *Journal of the American Osteopathic Association*, **74**, 638

KORR, I. M. (1978) Sustained sympathicotonia as a factor in disease. In *Neurobiologic Mechanisms in Manipulative Therapy*, p.229. Ed. Korr, I. M. New York and London: Plenum Press

KORR, I. M. and CHASE, J. A. (1964) Cutaneous patterns of sympathetic activity in clinical abnormalities of the musculoskeletal system. *Acta Neurovegetativa*, **25**, 589

KORR, I. M., THOMAS, P. E. and WRIGHT, H. M. (1955) Symposium of the functional implications of segmental facilitation. *Journal of the American Osteopathic Association*, **54**, 1

KORR, I. M., WRIGHT, H. M. and THOMAS, P. E. (1962) Effects of experimental myofascial insults on cutaneous patterns of sympathetic activity in man. *Acta Neurovegetativa*, **23**, 331

KORR, I. M., WILKINSON, P. N. and CHORNOCK, F. W. (1967) Axonal delivery of neuroplasmic components to muscle cells. *Science*, **135**, 342

KOS, J. (1968) Contribution à l'étude de l'anatomie de la vascularisation des articulations intervertébrales. *Bulletin de l'Association des Anatomistes*, **53**, 1088

KOS, J. and WOLF, J. (1972) Die 'Menisci' der Zwischenwirbelgelenke und ihre mögliche Rolle bei Wirbelblockierung. *Manuelle Medizin*, **10**, 105

KOTTKE, F. J. and MUNDALE, M. O. (1959) Range of mobility of the cervical spine. *Archives of Physical Medicine*, **40**, 379

KOUTNÝ, J. (1975) Inzidenz vertebragener Störungen unter Betriebsangestellten. *Manuelle Medizin*, **13**, 61

KOVÁZC, A. (1955) Subluxation of the cervical apophyseal joints. *Acta Radiologica*, **43**, 1

KRAEFF, T. (1983) Muskuläre Dysbalance bei Menschen im fortgeschrittenen Alter. *Manuelle Medizin*, **21**, 71

KRÄMER, J. (1973) Biomechanische Veränderungen im lumbalen Bewegungssegment. *Wirbelsäule in Forschung und Praxis*, vol.58. Stuttgart: Hippokrates

KRAUSOVÁ, L., KREJČOVÁ, H., NOVOTNÝ, Z., STARÝ, O., ŠIROKÝ, A. and JIROUT, J. (1968) Otoneurologische Symptomatologie bei dem Cervicocranialsyndrom vor und nach der Manipulationstherapia. *Manuelle Medizin*, **6**, 25

KRAUSS, H. (1980) *Atemtherapie*. Berlin: VEB Verlag Volk und Gesundheit

KRAUSS, H. (1982) Reflextherapie in der Physiotherapie. *Manuelle Medizin*, **20**, 85

KRUEGER, R. K. and OAZAKI, H. (1980) Vertebro-basilar distribution infarction following cervical manipulation. *Mayo Clinic Proceedings*, **55**, 322

KUBIS, E. (1969) Iliosakralverschiebung und Muskelfunktion im Beckenbereich als Diagnostikum. *Manuelle Medizin*, **7**, 52

KUBIS, E. (1970) Manualtherapeutische Erfahrungen am Becken. *Manuelle Medizin*, **8**, 63

KUNC, Z., STARÝ, O. and ŠETLÍK, L. (1955) Výsledky chirurgické léčby výhřezu meziobratlových destiček se zřetelem posuzování pracovní schopnosti. (The result of herniated disc operation with regard to working capacity.) *Časopis lékařů českých*, **94**, 1186

KUNERT, W. (1975) *Wirbelsäule und Innere Organe*. Stuttgart: F. Enke

LA BAN, M. M., MEERSCHAERT, J. R. and TAYLOR, R. S. (1979) Breast pain: a symptom of cervical radiculopathy. *Archives of Physical Medicine and Rehabilitation*, **60**, 315

LÁNIK, V. (1971) Poznámky ku kinetike a dynamike chrbtice. (Contribution to spinal kinetics and dynamics.) *Acta Chirurgiae Orthopedicae et Traumatologicae čechoslovacae*, **38**, 67

LAVEZZARI, R. (1948) *L'Osteopathie*. Paris: Doin

LEICHSENRING, F. (1964) Pathologisch-anatomische Befunde in der Halswirbelsäulenregion bei verstorbenen Patienten mit Schädeltrauma. *Deutsche Medizinische Wochenschrift*, **89**, 1469

LEUBE, H. and DICKE, E. (1951) *Massage reflektorischer Zonen im Bindegewebe*. Jena: Fischer

LEWIS, Th. (1942) *Pain*. New York: Macmillan

LEWIT, K. (1955) Trakční test. (Traction test.) *Časopis lékařů českých*, **94**, 60

LEWIT, K. (1959) Migréna a krční páteře. (Cervical spine and migraine.) *Ceskoslovenská Neurologie*, **22**, 61

LEWIT, K. (1962) Komoce a Krční páteř. (Concussion and the cervical spine.) *Rozhledy v Chirurgii*, **41**, 258

LEWIT, K. (1963) Méniersche Krankheit und die Halswirbelsäule. (Menier's disease and the cervical spine.) *Wirbelsäule in Forschung und Praxis*, **26**, 92

LEWIT, K. (1964) Die schmerzhafte Wirbelblockierung als Zeichen eines Spinaltumors. *Hippokrates*, **35**, 843

LEWIT, K. (1965) Sakroiliakalverschiebung und Muskelfehlsteuerung. *Asklepios*, **6**, 269

LEWIT, K. (1967) Steissbein und Kreuzschmerz. *Manuelle Medizin*, **5**, 93

LEWIT, K. (1968) Beitrag zur reversiblen Gelenksblockierung. *Zeitschrift für Orthopädie und ihre Grenzgebiete*, **105**, 150

LEWIT, K. (1969) Vertebral artery insufficiency and the cervical spine. *British Journal of Geriatric Practice*, **6**, 37

LEWIT, K. (1970) Blockierung von Atlas-Axis und Atlas-Okziput in Röntgenbild und Klinik. *Zeitschrift für Orthopädie und ihre Grenzgebiete*, **108**, 43

LEWIT, K. (1971) Ligament pain and anteflexion headache. *European Neurology*, **5**, 365

LEWIT, K. (1972) Funktionsdiagnose als Grundlage der Manuellen Therapie. *Manuelle Medizin*, **10**, 37

LEWIT, K. (1973) X-ray criteria of spinal statics. *Agressologie*, **6(14)**, 41

LEWIT, K. (1975) Ein Fall von Auffahrunfall. *Manuelle Medizin*, **13**, 71

LEWIT, K. (1976) On Dalseth's paper: Anatomic studies of the osseous craniovertebral joints. *Manuelle Medizin*, **14**, 9

LEWIT, K. (1978) Impaired joint function and entrapment syndromes. *Manuelle Medizin*, **16**, 45

LEWIT, K. (1979) The needle effect in the relief of myofascial pain. *Pain*, **6**, 83

LEWIT, K. (1979) 2 Fälle von Rotations-Dislokation zwischen Atlas und Axis. Ihre Behandlung in Narkose. *Manuelle Medizin*, **17**, 84

LEWIT, K. (1980) Relation of faulty respiration to posture with clinical implication. *Journal of the American Osteopathic Association*, **79**, 525

LEWIT, K. (1981) Muskelfazilitations – und Inhibitionstechniken in der Manuellen Medizin, Teil II. Postisometrische Muskelrelaxation. *Manuelle Medizin*, **19**, 12, 40

LEWIT, K. (1982) Röntgenologische Kriterien statischer Störungen der Wirbelsäule. *Manuelle Medizin*, **20**, 26

LEWIT, K. (1983) Die postisometrische Relaxation in der Diagnose des Scalenus-Syndroms. *Manuelle Medizin*, **21**, 27

LEWIT, K. (1984) *Manuelle Medizin im Rahmen der medizinischen Rehabilitation*, 4th edn. Leipzig: Barth

LEWIT, K. (1984) Schmerzen bei Funktionsstörungen des Bewegungssystems. In *Schmerzstudien 6. Schmerz und Bewegungssystem*, p. 43. Eds Berger, M., Gerstenbrand, F. and Lewit, K. Stuttgart, New York, Gustav Fischer

LEWIT, K. (1984) Muskelfehlsteuerung und Schmerz. In *Schmerzstudien 6. Schmerz und Bewegungssystem*, p. 88. Eds Berger, M., Gerstenbrand, F. and Lewit, K. Stuttgart, New York, Gustav Fischer

LEWIT, K. (1984) Mobilization mit Hilfe muskulärer Fazilitation und Inhibition. In *Schmerzstudien 6. Schmerz und Bewegungssystem*, p. 203. Eds Berger, M., Gerstenbrand, F. and Lewit, K. Stuttgart, New York, Gustav Fischer

LEWIT, K. and ABRAHAMOVIČ, M. (1976) Kopfgelenksblockierungen und chronische Tonsillitis. *Manuelle Medizin*, **14**, 106

LEWIT, K. and BERGER, M. (1983) Zervikales Störungsmuster bei Schwindelpatienten. *Manuelle Medizin*, **21**, 15

LEWIT, K. and GAYMANS, F. (1980) Muskelfazilitations und Ihnibitionstechniken in der Manuellen Medizin, Teil I. Mobilisation. *Manuelle Medizin*, **18**, 102

LEWIT, K. and JANDA, V. (1963) Entwicklung von Gefügestörungen der Wirbelsäule im Kindesalter und die Grundlagen einer Prävention vertebragener Beschwerden. *Hippokrates*, **34**, 308

LEWIT, K. and KRAUSOVÁ, L. (1962) Beitrag zur Flexion der Halswirbelsäule. *Fortschritte auf dem Gebiete der Röntgenstrahlen*, **97**, 38

LEWIT, K. and KRAUSOVÁ, L. (1963) Messungen von Vor- und Rückbeuge in den Kopfgelenken. *Fortschritte auf dem Gebiete der Röntgenstrahlen*, **99**, 538

LEWIT, K. and KRAUSOVÁ, L. (1967) Mechanismus und Bewegungsausmass in den Kopfgelenken bei passiven Bewegungen. *Zeitschrift für Orthopädie und ihre Grenzgebiete*, **103**, 323

LEWIT, K. and KUNCOVÁ, Z. (1971) Anteflexní bolest hlavy v dětském věku. (Anteflexion headache in children.) *Československá pediatrie*, **26**, 233

LEWIT, K. and SIMONS, D. G. (1984) Myofascial pain: Relief by post-isometric relaxation. *Archives of Physical Medicine and Rehabilitation*, **65**, 452

LEWIT, K., KNOBLOCH, V. and FAKTOROVÁ, Z. (1970) Vertebragene Störungen und Entbindungsschmerz. *Manuelle Medizin*, **8**, 79

LICHT, S. (Ed.) (1976) *Massage, Manipulation and Traction*. New York: Robert E. Krieger

LISÝ, L. (1983) Propriozeptive und exterozeptive Reflexe in den Nackenmuskeln. *Manuelle Medizin*, **21**, 23

LIVINGSTON, M. C. P. (1971) Spinal manipulation causing injury. *Clinical Orthopaedics*, **81**, 82

LOBECK, G. (1982) Zur Wechselwirkung zwischen Funktionsstörungen des Bewegungsapparates und Neurose. *Manuelle Medizin*, **20**, 140

LORENZ, R. and VOGELSANG, H. G. (1972) Thrombose der Arteria basilaris nach chiropraktischen Manipulationen an der Halswirbelsäule. *Deutsche Medizinische Wochenschrift*, **97**, 36

LOVETT, R. (1907) *Lateral Curvature of the Spine and Round Shoulders.* Philadelphia: Blakiston

McCOUCH, G. P., DEERING, I. D. and LING, T. H. (1951) Location of receptors for tonic neck reflexes. *Journal of Neurophysiology*, **14**, 191

MACDONALD, A. J. R. (1980) Abnormally tender muscle regions and associated painful movements. *Pain*, **8**, 197

McKENZIE, R. A. (1981) *The Lumbar Spine – Mechanical Diagnosis and Therapy.* Upper Hutt, New Zealand: Spinal Publications

MACNAB, I. (1964) Acceleration injury of the cervical spine. *Journal of Bone and Joint Surgery*, **46A**, 1797

MACNAB, I. (1972) The mechanism of spondylogenic pain. In *Cervical Pain*, p.89. Eds. Hirsch, C. and Zotterman, Y. Oxford: Pergamon Press

McRAE, D. L. (1956) Asymptomatic intervertebral disc protrusion. *Acta Radiologica*, **46**, 9

McRAE, D. L. (1960) The significance of abnormalities of the cervical spine. Caldwell lecture 1959. *American Journal of Roentgenology*, **84**, 3

MAEX, L. (1970) New Factors in migraine, motion sickness and equilibrium. A cybernetic study of equilibrium. *Headache*, **10**, 24

MAGNUS, R. (1924) *Körperstellung.* Berlin: Springer

MAGOUN, H. I. (1966) *Osteopathy in the Cranial Field*, 2nd edn. Kirksville: Journal Printing Company

MAIGNE, R. (1957) Le traitement des épicondylites. *Rheumatologie*, **6**, 293

MAIGNE, R. (1964) L'algie interscapulo-vertébrale, forme fréquente de dorsalgie bénigne. Son origine cervicale. *Annales de Médecine Physique*, **7**, 1

MAIGNE, R. (1968) *Douleurs d'origine vertébrale et traitements par Manipulations.* Paris: Expansion Scientifique

MAIGNE, R. (1972) *Orthopedic Medicine.* Springfield: Charles C Thomas

MAIGNE, R. (1974) Die klinischen Zeichen der geringfügigen intervertebralen Störung. *Manuelle Medizin*, **12**, 102

MAIGNE, R. and LE CORRE, F. (1969) Donnés nouvelles sur le méchanisme des dorsalgies communes de l'adulte. *Manuelle Medizin*, **7**, 73

MAINZER, F. (1960) Diagnostic differentiation of coexisting pseudoanginal root syndrome and angina pectoris. *American Heart Journal*, **59**, 191

MAITLAND, G. D. (1974) *Vertebral Manipulation.* London: Butterworths

MARKUSKE, H. (1971) *Untersudhungen zur Statik und Dynamik der kindlichen Halswirbelsäule: Der Aussagewert seitlicher Röntgenaufnahmen. Wirbelsäule in Forschung und Praxis*, vol.50. Stuttgart: Hippokrates

MARKUSKE, H. (1983) Röntgenologische Halswirbelsäulendiagnostik im Kindesalter. *Psychiatrie, Neurologie und medizinische Psychologie*, **35**, 257

MATTHIASCH, H. (1956) Arbeitshaltung und Bandscheibenbelastung. *Archiv für Orthopädie und Unfalls-Chirurgie*, **48**, 147

MAYOUX, R., GIRARD, P. and CHIPPAT, P. (1952) Les signes objectives dans le syndrome sympathique postérieure de Barré. *Revue Oto-neuro-ophthalmologique*, **24**, 51

MED, M. (1972) Articulations of the thoracic vertebrae and their variability. *Folia Morphologica*, **20**, 217

MED, M. (1973) Articulations of the cervical vertebrae and their variability. *Folia Morphologica*, **21**, 324

MEIER, B. (1975) Der Schmerz im Bewegungsapparat – Manuelle Therapie in einer Betriebspoliklinik. *Zeitschrift für Ärztliche Fortbildung*, **69**, 599

MELZACK, R. (1975) Prolonged relief of pain by brief intense transcutaneous somatic stimulation. *Pain*, **1**, 357

MELZACK, R. and WALL, P. D. (1965) Pain mechanisms. *Science*, **150**, 971

MELZACK, R., STILLWELL, D. M. and FOX, E. J. (1977) Trigger points and acupuncture points for pain: correlations and implications. *Pain*, **3**, 3

MENEGAZ, A. and FASOLI, M. (1970) Die Innervation der vertebralen interapophysären Gelenke in verschiedenen Abschnitten der Wirbelsäule. In *Manuelle Medizin und Ihre Wissenschaftlichen Grundlagen*, p.69. Ed. Wolff, H. D. Heidelberg: Physikalische Medizin

MENNELL, J. (1952) *The Science and Art of Joint Manipulation*, vol. II. *The Spinal Column.* London: Churchill

MENNELL, J. McM. (1964) *Joint Pain.* London: Churchill

MENSOR, M. C. and DUVAL, G. (1959) Absence of motion at the fourth and fifth lumbar interspace in patients with and without low back pain. *Journal of Bone and Joint Surgery*, **41A**, 1047

MESDACH, H. (1976) Morphological aspects and biomechanical properties of the vertebroaxial joint (C2–C3). *Acta Morphologica Neerlando Scandinavica*, **14**, 19

METZ, E. G. (1971) Die Manuelle Therapie, ihre Möglichkeiten und Grenzen des Einsatzes in der Sportmedizin. *Sport und Medizin*, **11**, 353

METZ, E. G. (1976) Manuelle Therapie in der inneren Medizin. *Zeitschrift für Physiotherapie*, **28**, 83

METZ, E. G. and BADTKE, G. (1975) Beckentypen im Kindesalter, Konsequenzen für Belastbarkeit. In *Functional Pathology of the Motor System, Rehabilitácia*, Supplementum 11–12, p.205. Eds. Lewit, K. and Gutmann, G. Bratislava: Obzor

METZ, E. G. and BADTKE, G. (1980) *Manuelle Therapie. Tagunsbericht, Potsdam 28.1–31.1.1980, Wissenschaftlich-Technisches Zentrum der Pädagogischen Hochschule.* Potsdam: Karl Liebnecht

METZ, E. G., KNÄBLICH, C., FRÖHLING, P. and LEMKE, E. (1980) Die Bedeutung vertebragener Funktionsstörungen für den Beschwerdekomplex bei Nephroptose. *Zeischrift für Physiotherapie*, **32**, 405

MEYERMANN, R. (1982) Möglichkeiten einer Schädigung der Arteria vertebralis. *Manuelle Medizin*, **20**, 105

MICHELS, A. A. (1962) *Iliopsoas.* Springfield: Charles C Thomas

MILDENBERGER, F. (1979) Indikationen zur Röntgenuntersuchung der Wirbelsäule. *Manuelle Medizin*, **17**, 99

MILNE, R. J., FOREMAN, R. D., GIESLER, G. J., Jr. and WILLIS, W. D. (1981) Convergence of cutaneous and pelvic visceral nociceptive inputs onto primate spinothalamic neurons. *Pain*, **11**, 163

MITCHELL, F. Jr., MORAN, P. S. and PRUZZO, N. A. (1979) *An Evaluation of Osteopathic Muscle Energy Procedures.* Valley Park: Pruzzo

MOHR, U. (1977) Kopfgelenksblockierungen beim Kleinkind. *Manuelle Medizin*, **15**, 45

MOHR, U. and SCHIMEK, J. J. (1984) Fusionsstörungen des Auges als Folge vertebragener Funktionsstörungen. *Manuelle Medizin*, **22**, 2

MONTGOMERY, C. et al. (1976) Pre-employment back X-rays. (Review article) *Journal of Occupational Medicine*, **19**,

MORRIS, J. M. (1973) Biomechanics of the spine. *Archives of Surgery*, **107**, 418

MORRIS, J. M., LUCAS, D. B. and BRESSLER, B. (1961) Role of the trunk in stability of the spine. *Journal of Joint and Bone Surgery*, **43A**, 327

MORRISON, M. C. T. (1975) Manipulation for backache. *Orthopaedics*, **8**, 19

MOSER, M. (1974) Zervikalnystagmus und seine diagnostische Bedeutung, HNO, **22**, 350

MOSER, M. and SIMON, H. (1977) Der Cervikalnystagmus als objektiver Befund beim HWS-Syndrom und seine Beeinflussbarkeit durch Manualtherapie. *HNO*, **25**, 265

MOSER, M., CONRAUX, C. and GREINER, G. F. (1972) Der Nystagmus zervikalen Ursprungs und seine statische Bewertung. *Ohrenheilkunde, Laringo-Rhinologie*, **106**, 259

MÜLLER, D. (1960) Zur Frage der kompensatorischen Hypermobilität bei anatomschem und funktionellen Block der Wirbelsäule. *Radiologia Diagnostica*, **1**, 345

MÜLLER, E. (1963) *Commotio čerebri und Halswirbelsäule. Wirbelsäule in Forschung und Praxis*, vol.26, p.36. Ed. Schuler, B. Stuttgart: Hippokrates

MUMENTHALER, M. (1980) *Der Schulter-Arm-Schmerz.* Bern: Huber

MUSIOL, A. (1976) Vertebragene Beschwerden bei Bergleuten. *Zeitschrift für Physiotherapie*, **28**, 117

MUSIOL, A. (1984) Neuro-orthopädischer Untersuchungsbefund bei Schmerzen im Bewegungsapparat, In *Schmerzstudien 6. Schmerz und Bewegungssystem*, p. 139. Eds Berger, M., Gerstenbrand, F., and Lewit, K. Stuttgart, New York, Gustav Fischer

NACHEMSON, A. (1959) Measurements of intradiscal pressure. *Acta Orthopaedica Scandinavica*, **28**, 269

NACHEMSON, A. (1980) A critical look at conservative treatment of low back pain. In *The Lumbar Spine and Back Pain*, 2nd edn., p.453. Ed. Jayson, M. I. V. London: Pitman Medical

NAEGELI, O. (1954) *Nervenleiden und Nervenschmerzen*, 3rd edn. Ulm: Haug

NASH, C. L. and MOE, J. E. (1969) A study of vertebral rotation. *Journal of Bone and Joint Surgery*, **51A**, 233

NELSON, M. A. (1973) Manual correction of sciatic scoliosis. *Journal of Bone and Joint Surgery*, **55B**, 194

NESIT, V. and HORINOVÁ, M. (1975) Funktionsstörungen der Wirbelsäule in der ambulanten gynäkologischen Praxis. *Manuelle Medizin*, **13**, 31

NEUMANN, H. D. (1981) Die manualmedizinische Behandlung des akuten Schiefhalses. *Zeitschrift für Orthopädie und ihre Grenzgebiete*, **119**, 693

NEUMANN, H. D. (1983) *Manuelle Medizin, eine Einführung in theorie, Diagnostik und Therapie.* Berlin, Heidelberg, New York, Tokyo, Springer

NEUMANN, H. D. and WOLFF, H. D. (Eds) (1979) Theoretische Fortschritte und Praktische Erfahrungen der Manuellen Medizin. 6. *Internationaler Kongress der FIMM, Baden-Baden.* Bühl: Konkordia

NIBOYET, J. E. H. (1967) *La Pratique de la Médicine Manuelle.* Paris: Maisonneuve

NORDEMAR, R. and THÖRNER, C. (1981) Treatment of acute cervical pain – a comparative group study. *Pain*, **10**, 93

NORRÉ, M., STEVENS, A. and DEGEYTER, P. (1976) Der Zervikal-Nystagmus und die Gelenksblockierung. *Manuelle Medizin*, **14**, 45

NOVOTNÝ, A. and DVOŘÁK, V. (1972) Funktionsstörungen der Wirbelsäule in der Gynäkologischen Praxis. *Manuelle Medizin*, **10**, 84

ONDERKA, W. and MÜLLER-STEPHAN, H. (1973) Die manuelle Extension der Halswirbelsäule. *Zeitschrift für Physiotherapie*, **25**, 461

PALMER, S. G. (1933) *The Subluxation Specific, the Adjustment Specific.* Davenport, Iowa

PANDYA, S. K. (1972) Atlantoaxial Dislocation (review). *Neurology (Bombay)*, **20**, 13

PARADE, G. W. (1956/57) Wirbelsäule und Herz. *Therapiewoche*, **7**, 295

PAROW, J. (1953) *Funktionelle Atmungstherapie.* Stuttgart: Thieme

PATTERSON, J. (1976) A model mechanism for spinal segmental facilitation. *Journal of the American Osteopathic Association*, **76**, 62

PENNING, L. (1968) *Functional Pathology of the Cervical Spine.* Amsterdam: Excerpta Medica

PENNING, L. (1978) Normal movements of the cervical spine. *American Journal of Roentgenology*, **130**, 317

PEPER, W. (1953) *Technik der Chiropraktik.* Saulgau: Haug

PEPER, W. (1978) *Der Chiropraktische Report.* Heidelberg: Haug

PERL, E. R. (1972) Mode of action of nociceptors. In *Cervical Pain*, p.157. Eds. Hirsch, C. and Zottermann, Y. Oxford: Pergamon Press

PFEIFFER, J., BAUER, J., BERKOVÁ, L. and SÜSSOVÁ, J. (1964) Elektromyografie zádových a břišních svalu u iniciálních poruch dynamiky páteře. (EMG examination of back and abdominal muscles in the initial stage of disturbed spinal function.) *Československá Neurologie*, **27**, 229

PHILLIPS, R. B. (1980) The use of X-rays in spinal manipulative therapy. In *Modern Developments in the Principles and Practice of Chiropractic*, p.189. Ed. Haldemann, S. New York: Appleton-Century-Crofts

PINDER, H. E. (1970) Über den Beckenschiefstand im Sitzen. *Beiträge zur Orthopädie und Traumatologie*, **17**, 220

PIŤHA, V. and DROBNÝ, M. (1972) Klbové a periostálne reflexné zony krčcnej chrbtice. (Articular and periostal reflex zones of the cervical spine.) *Československá Neurologie*, **35**, 113

POHL, D. (1974) Die manuelle Mobilisation des Akromioklavikulargelenkes beim Schulter-Arm-Syndrom. *Heilberufe*, **25**, 5

POPELYANSKI, Ya. Yu. (1966) *Sheyni Osteokhondroz.* (Cervical Osteochondrosis.) Moscow: Medicina

POPELYANSKI, Ya. Yu. (1974) Vertebralniye sindromi poyasnitshnovo osteokhondrosa. (Vertebrogenic syndromes in lumbar osteochrondrosis.) Izdatelstvo Kazanskovo Universiteta

POPELYANSKI, Ya, Yu (1983) *Vertebrogennye zabolevanya nervnoi sistemy (vertebrogenic affections of the nervous system.)* Ioshkar-Ola, Mariiskoye knizhnoye izdatelstvo

PORTER, R. W., HIBBERT, C. and WELLMAN, P. (1980) Backache and the lumbar spinal canal. *Spine*, **5**, 99

RASH, P. J. and BURKE, R. K. (1971) *Kinesiology and Applied Anatomy.* Philadelphia: Lea and Febiger

RASMUSSEN, G. G. (1979) Manipulation in treatment of low back pain – a randomized clinical trial. *Manuelle Medizin*, **17**, 8

REFIOR, H. and ZENKER, H. (1970) Wirbelsäule und Leistungsturnen. *Münchner Medizinische Wochenschrift*, **112**, 463

RENOULT, C. and DE WINTER, E. (1961) Technique des manipulations ostéoarticulaires du système lumbopelvien. *Vie Médicale*, **42**, 115

REYNOLDS, M. D. (1981) Myofascial trigger point syndromes in the practice of rheumatology. *Archives of Physical Medicine and Rehabilitation*, **62**, 111

REYNOLDS, M. (1983) The development of the concept of fibrositis. *Journal of the History of Medicine and Allied Sciences*, **38**, 5

RICHTER, R. (1971) Die Bedeutung der 'entrapment neuropathy' für die Differentialdiagnose vertebragener Schmerzzustände. *Manuelle Medizin*, **9**, 101

ROESSLER, H. *et al.* (1972) Beinlängendifferenz und Verkürzungsausgleich. *Zeitschrift für Orthopädie und ihre Grenzgebiete*, **110**, 623

ROGERS, J. T. and ROGERS, J. G. (1976) The role of osteopathic manipulative therapy in the treatment of coronary artery disease. *Journal of the American Osteopathic Association*, **76**, 71

ROHDE, J. (1975; 1976)) Die Automobilisation der Extremitätengelenke. *Zeitschrift für Physiotherapie*, **27**, 57; **28**, 51, 121

ROSS, E. (1964) Verschiebungsphänomen und Wirbelblockierung an der Hals und Lendenwirbelsäule. *Fortschritte auf dem Gebiet der Röntgenstrahlen*, **100**, 367

RUBIN, D. (1981) Myofascial trigger points syndromes: an approach to management. *Archives of Physical Medicine and Rehabilitation*, **62**, 107

RUDDY, T. J. (1961) Osteopathic rhythmic resistant duction therapy. *Academy of Applied Osteopathy Yearbook*, p.58. Colorado Springs: AAO

RUDDY, T. J. (1962) Osteopathic rapid rhythmic resistive technique. *Academy of Applied Osteopathy Yearbook*, p.23. Colorado Springs: AAO

RYAN, G. M. S. (1955) Cervical vertigo. *Lancet*, **ii**, 1355

RYCHLÍKOVÁ, E. (1974) Schmerzen im Gallenblasenbereich auf Grund vertebragener Störungen. *Deutsches Gesundheitswesen*, **29**, 2092

RYCHLÍKOVÁ, E. (1975) Vertebragene funktionelle Störungen bei chronischer ischämischer Herzkrankheit. *Münchner Medizinische Wochenschrift*, **117**, 127

RYCHLÍKOVÁ, E. (1975) *Vertebrokardiální Syndrom*. (The vertebrocardial syndrome.) Praha: Avicenum

SACHSE, J. (1969) Die Hypermobilität des Bewegungsapparates als potentieller Krankheitsfaktor. *Manuelle Medizin*, **7**, 77

SACHSE, J. (1973) *Manuelle Mobilisationsbehandlung der Extremitätengelenke. Leitfaden der Untersuchungs-und Behadnlungstechnik*, 2nd edn. Berlin: Volk und Gesundheit

SACHSE, J. (1976) Neurologie und Bewegungsapparat – Aspekte der Manuellen Therapie. *Psychiatrie, Neurologie und Medizinische Psychologie*, **28**, 193

SACHSE, T. and SACHSE, J. (1975) Muskelbefunde bei chronisch obstruktiven Atemwegserkrankungen. In *Functional Pathology of the Motor System, Rehabilitácia*, Suppl. 10–11, p.98. Eds. Lewit, K. and Gutman, G. Bratislava: Obzor

SACHSE, T. and SACHSE, J. (1976) Verspannungsbefunde am M.levator scapulae. *Zeitschrift für Physiotherapie*, **28**, 149

SACHSE, J., WIECHMANN, J. and GOMOLKA, U. (1976) Vorschlag für einen gestuften Test zur Beurteilung des Bewegungssystems. *Zeitschrift für Physiotherapie*, **28**, 95

SACHSE, J., ECKARDT, E., LIESS, A. and SACHSE, T. (1982) Reflextherapie bei Migränekranken. *Manuelle Medizin*, **20**, 59

SÄKER, G. (1955) Schädeltrauma und Halswirbelsäule. *Deutsche Medizinische Wochenschrift*, **79**, 547

SÄKER, G. (1957) Die Morbidität an Lumbago-Ischias. *Münchner Medizinische Wochenschrift*, **104**, 1151

SANDBERG, L. B. (1955) *Atlas und Axis*. Stuttgart: Hippokrates

SAUTIER, P. (1979) Stellungnahme zum Memorandum zur Verhütung von Zwischenfällen bei gezielter Handgrifftherapie an der Halswirbelsäule. *Manuelle Medizin*, **17**, 103

SCHALTENBRAND, G. (1938) Der hintere Bandscheibenprolaps in seinen klinischen Auswirkungen. *Frankfurter Zeitschrift für Pathologie*, **52**, 363

SCHILDT, K. (1975) Untersuchungen zum Entwicklungsstand der Motorik bei Kindergartenkindern. In *Functional Pathology of the Motor System. Rehabilitácia*, Suppl. 10–11, p.166. Eds. Lewit, K. and Gutmann, G. Bratislava: Obzor

SCHILDT, K. (1982) Funktionelle Therapie von Sprunggelenkfrakturen unter manualtherapeutischen Gesichtspunkten. *Manuelle Medizin*, **20**, 137

SCHMORL, G. and JUNGHANNS, H. (1953) *Die Gesunde und die Kranke Wirbelsäule in Röntgenbild und Klinik*. Stuttgart: Thieme

SCHOENIG, H. A. (1963) A radiological study of the changes of the cervical articular mass with age. *Archives of Physical Medicine and Rehabilitation*, **44**, 303

SCHÖN, D. (1956) Röntgenologische Untersuchungen über die Morbidität der Halswirbelsäule und deren klinische Wertigkeit. *Klinische Wochenschrift*, **897**

SCHRÖTER, G. (1971) Die Bedeutung von aussergewöhnlicher Haltung und Belastung für die Entstehung von Abnützungsschäden der Wirbelsäule. *Beiträge zur Orthopädie und Traumatologie*, **18**, 250

SCHULZE, A. J. (1962) Über die Fehlanwendung chiropraktischer Behandlungs-massnahmen. *Medizinische Welt*, **45**, 2379

SCHWARZ, E. (1970) Internistische Indikationen der manipulativen Therapie. *Manuelle Medizin*, **8**, 25

SCHWARZ, E. (1973) Herz und Wirbelsäule. *Schweizer Rundschau für Medizin Praxis*, **63**, 837

SCHWARZ, E. (1976) Manual-therapeutische Kasuistik aus einer internistischen Praxis. *Manuelle Medizin*, **14**, 52

SCHWARZ, E. (1978) Zur Frage des Epikondylitis-humeri-Syndroms. *Manuelle Medizin*, **16**, 17

SEIDEL, A. (1969) Beckenstellung, Wirbelsäulenstatik und Körpergewichtsverteilung. *Manuelle Medizin*, **7**, 100

SEIDEL, K. (1976) Wert und Grenzen der funktionellen Röntgendiagnostik der Wirbelsäule. *Orthopäde*, **5**, 217

SEIFERT, I. (1975) Kopfgelenksblockierung bei Neugeborenen. In *Functional Pathology of the Motor System; Rehabilitácia*, Suppl. 10–11, p.53. Eds. Lewit, K. and Gutmann, G. Bratislava: Obzor

SEIFERT, I. (1981) Manualtherapeutische Aspekte bei der Hüftdysplasie. *Beiträge zur Orthopädie und Traumatologie*, **28**, 161

SEIFERT, K. (1981) Cervical-vertebragene Schluckschmerzen in der Hals-Nasen-Ohren-Heilkunde – Die Zungenbeintendopathie. *Manuelle Medizin*, **19**, 85

SELECKI, B. R. (1969) The effect of rotation of the atlas on the axis. *Medical Journal of Australia*, **1**, 1012

SELL, K. (1969) Spezielle manuelle Segment-Technik als Mittel zur Abklärung spondylogener Zusammenhangsfragen. *Manuelle Medizin*, **7**, 99

SEYFARTH, H. (1965) Überlastungskrankheiten im Skelettmuskelsystem. *Physikalisch-Diätetische Therapie*, **6**, 51

DE SÈZE, S. (1960; 1961) Étude sur l'epaule douloureuse I, II, III. *Revue du Rheumatisme*, **27**, 323, 443; **28**, 85

DE SÈZE, S. and WELFLING, J. (1957) Interprétation et intérêt du signe de Lasègue dans les sciatiques par hernie discale avec attitude antalgique laterale. *Semaine des Hôpitaux de Paris*, **33**, 1013

SHIN-HO CHUNG and DICKENSON, A. (1980) Pain, enkephalin and acupuncture. *Nature (London)*, **283**, 243

SIMON, H., MOSER, M. and HOLZER, M. (1975) Der Zervikalnystagmus. In *Functional Pathology of the Motor System, Rehabilitácia*, Suppl. 10–11, p.132. Eds. Lewit, K. and Gutmann, G. Bratislava: Obzor

SIMON, H. and MOSER, M. (1977) Der Zervikalnystagmus aus manual-medizinischer Sicht. *Manuelle Medizin*, **15**, 47

SIMONS, D. G. (1975; 1976) Muscle pain syndromes. *American Physical Medicine*, **54**, 289; **55**, 15

SIMONS, D. G. (1981) Myofascial trigger points: a need for understanding. *Archives of Physical Medicine and Rehabilitation*, **62**, 97

SIMONS, D. G. and TRAVELL, J. (1981) Re: Myofascial trigger points, a possible explanation. (Letter to the editor.) *Pain*, **10**, 106

SIMONS, D. G. and TRAVELL, J. G. (1983) Myofascial origin of low back pain. *Postgraduate Medicine*, **73**, 66

SIMS-WILLIAMS, H. (1979) Controlled trial of mobilisation and manipulation for low back pain: hospital patients. *British Medical Journal*, **2**, 1318

SIMS-WILLIAMS, H., JAYSON, M. I. V., YOUNG, S. M. S. *et al.* (1978) Controlled clinical trial of mobilisation and manipulation for patients with low back pain in general practice. *British Medical Journal*, **2**, 1338

SKLÁDAL, J., ŠKAVRAN, K., RUTH, C. and MIKULENKA, V. (1970) Posturální funkce bránice. (The postural function of the diaphragm.) *Československá Fysiologie*, **19**, 279

SMITH, R. A. and ESTRIDGE, M. V. (1962) Neurologic complications of head and neck manipulation. *Journal of the American Medical Association*, **182**, 5

SOLLMANN, A. H. and BREITENBACH, H. (1961) Röntgenanalyse und Klinik von 1000 seitlichen Röntgenganzaufnahmen. *Fortschritte auf dem Gebiete der Röntgenstrahlen*, **94**, 704

SOLONEN, K. A. (1957) The sacroiliac joint in the light of anatomical, roentgenological and clinical studies. *Acta Orthopaedica Scandinavica*, Suppl. 27

SPIŠÁK, J. (1972) Bedeutung des Segments C2–3 im klassischen Bild des akuten Torticollis. *Manuelle Medizin*, **10**, 133

ŠRÁČEK, J. and ŠKRABAL, J. (1975) Neurasthenie und Funktionsstörungen der Wirbelsäule. *Manuelle Medizin*, **13**, 106

STAPEL, R. (1976) Erfahrungen mit der manuellen Therapie in der Sportmedizin. *Zeitschrift für Physiotherapie*, **28**, 145

STARÝ, O. (1970) Die Reflexwirkingen nozizeptiver Reize im Bewegungsapparat. In *Manuelle Medizin und ihre Wissenschaftlichen Grundlagen*, p.84. Ed. Wolff, H. D. Heidelberg: Physikalische Medizin

STARÝ, O. and LEWIT, K. (1958) Polyrheografické reakce u sensitivních radikotomií při diskogenní nemoci. (Polyrheographic reactions after sensory root section in discogenic disease.) *Acta Universitatis Carolinae Medica*, **1–3**, 236

STEGLICH, H. D. (1972) In: Lewit, K.: Wirbelsäule und innere Organe (Bericht uber ein Symposium der Tschechosl. Sektion für Manuelle und Reflextherapie, Karlovy Vary vom 16, 19. Juni 1971). *Manuelle Medizin*, **10**, 37

STEINBRÜCK, K. and ROMPE, G. (1980) Hochleistungssport – planmässig erworbene Hypermobilität. *Manuelle Medizin*, **18**, 62

STEINBRÜCK, K. and TILSCHER, H. (1983) Manuelle Medizin und Sport. *Manuelle Medizin*, **21**, 38

STEINRÜCKEN, H. (1980) *Chirotherapeutisch Beeinflussbare Krankheitsbilder*. Stuttgart: Hippokrates

STEINRÜCKEN, H., SACHER, I. and BETZ, P. (1984) Untersuchungen über das Costovertebralsyndrom mit pseudoanginöser Symptomatik bei Patienten einer kardiologischen Spezialklinik. *Manuelle Medizin*, **22**, 54

STEJSKAL, L. (1967) L'influence facilitative et l'influence inhibitive de la respiration sur l'activité musculaire. *Europa Mediophysica*, **3**, 1

STEJSKAL, J. (1972) *Postural Reflexes in Theory and Motor Re-education*. Praha: Academia

STENWERS, H. W. (1918) Un 'Stellreflex' du bassin chez l'homme. *Archives Néerlandais de Physiologie de L'homme et de L'animal,* **2,** 669

STEVENS, A. and GIELEN, E. (1975) Manual medicine and miners. In *Functional Pathology of the Motor System. Rehabilitácia,* Suppl. 10–11, p.240. Eds. Lewit, K. and Gutmann, G. Bratislava: Obzor

STODDARD, A. (1961) *Manual of Osteopathic Technique.* London: Hutchinson

STODDARD, A. (1969) *Manual of Osteopathic Practice.* New York: Harper and Row

STOFFT, E. (1979) Bau und Funktion der Iliosakralgelenke. In *Theoretische Fortschritte und Praktische Erfahrungen der Manuellen Medizin,* p.318. Eds. Neumann, H. D. and Wolff, H. D. Bühl: Konkordia

SUNDERLAND, S. (1978) Traumatized nerves, roots and ganglia; musculo-skeletal factors and neuropathological consequences. In *The Neurobiologic Mechanisms in Manipulative Therapy,* p.137. Ed. Korr, I. M. New York and London: Plenum Press

SUTTER, M. (1975) Wesen, Klinik und Bedeutung spondylogener Reflexsyndrome. *Schweizerische Rundschau für Medizin (Praxis),* **64,** 1351

SUTTER, M. (1977) Rücken-Kreuz- und Beinschmerzen beim funktionell instabilen Becken. *Therapeutische Umschau (Revue Thérapeutique),* **34,** 452

SUTTER, M. (1983) Diagnostische Weichteilpalpation des Bewegungsapparates. *Manuelle Medizin,* **21,** 120

TEPE, H. J. (1956) Die Häufigkeit der Osteochondrose im Röntgenbild der Halswirbelsäule bei 400 beschwerdefreien Erwachsenen. *Fortschritte auf dem Gebiete der Röntgenstrahlen,* **85,** 659

TERRIER, J. C. (1968) Indikationen und Kontraindikationen der Manipulativen Therapie. *Orthopädische Praxis,* **4,** 128

TESAŘOVÁ, A. (1969) Diagnostik der Beweglichkeitsstörungen der Wirbelsäule durch Inspektion der Wirbelsäule während der Atmung. *Manuelle Medizin,* **7,** 29

THABE, H. (1982) Die Elektromyographie als Befunddokumentation bei der Therapie von Kopfgelenks- und Kreuzdarmbeingelenksblockierungen. *Manuelle Medizin,* **20,** 131

THALHEIM, W. (1975) Die Differentialdiagnose wichtiger Funtionsstörungen im Beckenbereich. *Beiträge zur Orthopädie und Traumatologie,* **22,** 430

TILSCHER, H. (1984) Möglichkeiten der Rehabilitation bei Funktionsstörungen des Achsenorgans. In *Schmerzstudien 6. Schmerz und bewegungssystem,* p. 225, Eds Berger, M., Gerstenbrand, F., Lewit, K. Stuttgart, New York, Gustav Fischer

TILSCHER, H. (1984) Zweckmässiger Aufbau des klinischen Untersuchungsganges bei neuroorthopädischen Erkrankungen im Bereich der Lenden-Becken-Hüftregion. In *Neuroorthopädie 2, Lendenwirbelsäulenerkrankungen mit Beteiligung des Nervensystems,* p. 63, Eds Hohmann, D., Kügelgen, B. and Schirmer, M. Berlin, Heidelberg, New York, Tokyo, Springer

TILSCHER, H. (1984) Indikationen und Erfolgsaussicht der Manualtherapie bei Funktionsstörung des Iliosakralgelenkes. In *Neuroorthopädie 2, Lendenwirbelsäulenerkrankungen mit Beteiligung des Nervensystems,* p. 573. Eds Hohmann, D., Kügelgen, B. and Schirmer, M. Berlin, Heidelberg, New York, Tokyo, Springer

TILSCHER, H. and OBLAK, O. (1974) Untersuchungen von ehemaligen Jugendleistungssportlern. *Orthopädische Praxis,* **16,** 100

TILSCHER, H. and BOGNER, G. (1975) Pain syndromes involving the locomotor apparatus – a possible manifestation of masked depression. In *Diagnostik und Therapie der Depression in der ambulaten Praxis,* p.292. Ed. Kielholz, P. Bern: Huber

TILSCHER, H. and STEINBRÜK, K. (1980) Symptomatik und manualmedizinische Befunde bei der Hypermobilität. *Orthopädische Praxis,* **16,** 100

TILSCHER, H., BOGNER, G. and LANDSIEDL, F. (1977) Viszerale Erkrankungen als Ursache von Lumbalsyndromen. *Zeitschrift für Rheumatologie,* **36,** 161

TILSCHER, H., WESSELY, P. and EDER, M. (1982) Die topischen Zusammenhänge zwischen Gesichtsschmerz und subokzipitalen Maximalpunkten. *Manuelle Medizin,* **20,** 127

TKAČENKO, S. S. (1973) O zakrytom odnomomentnom vpravlenii ostrovo vypadeniya mezpozvonotshno-vo diska. (The bloodless single reposition of an acute disc prolapse.) *Ortopedia, travmatologia, protezirovanye,* **8,** 46

TLUSTEK, H. and METZ, E. G. (1980) Karpaltunnelsyndrom und Reflextherapie. In *Manuelle Medizin, Tagungsbericht, Potsdam 28–31.1.1980,* p.187. Eds. Metz, E. G. and Badtke, G. Potsdam: Wissenschaftlich-Technisches Zentrum der Pädagogischen Hochschule

TÖNDURY, G. (1948) Beitrag zur Kenntnis der kleinen Wirbelgelenke. *Zeitschrift für Anatomische Entwicklungsgeschichte,* **110,** 568

TORKLUS, D. (1979) Zervikaler Kopfschmerz – Typenbildung I bis III. *Orthopädische Praxis,* **15,** 730

TORKLUS, D. and GEHLEN, W. (1970) *Die obere Halswirbelsäule.* Stuttgart: Thieme

TORRES, F. and SHAPIRO, S. E. (1961) EEG in whiplash injury. *Archives of Neurology,* **5,** 28

TOWNSEND, E. H. (1952) Mobility in the upper cervical spine in health and disease. *Pediatrics*, **10**, 567

TRACEY, D. (1978) Joint receptors – changing ideas. *Trends in Neurosciences*, **1**, 63

TRAVELL, J. (1976) Myofascial trigger points: clinical view. In *Advances in Pain Research and Therapy*, vol. 1, p.919. Eds. Bonica, J. J. and Albe-Fessard, D. New York: Raven Press

TRAVELL, J. (1981) Identification of myofascial trigger point syndromes: a case of atypical facial neuralgia. *Archives of Physical Medicine and Rehabilitation*, **62**, 100

TRAVELL, J. and RINZLER, S. H. (1952) Myofascial genesis of pain in the neck and shoulder girdle. *Postgraduate Medicine*, **11**, 425

TRAVELL, J. and SIMONS, D. G. (1983) Myofascial pain and dysfunction. *The Trigger Point Manual.* Baltimore: Williams and Wilkins

UNTERHARNSCHEIDT, F. (1956) Das synkopale cervicale. *Vertebralsyndrome Nervenarzt*, **27**, 481

UPTOM, A. R. M. and McCOMAS, A. J. (1973) The double crush in nerve entrapment syndromes. *Lancet*, **ii**, 359

USHIO, N., HINOKI, M., HINE, S., OKADA, S., ISHADA, Y., KOIKE, S. and SHIZUKU, S. (1973) Studies on ataxia of lumbar origin in cases of vertigo due to whiplash injury. *Agressologie*, **6(14)D**, 73

UTTL, K. (1964) Přízpěvek ke studiu výskytu vertebrogenních poruch. (On the incidence of vertebrogenic disorders.) *Československé zdravotnictví*, **12**, 317

UTTL, K. (1966) On the incidence of discogenic disease (vertebrogenic disorders) with regard to work capacity. *Review of Czechoslovak Medicine*, **12**, 116

VALEANU, C. (1972) Contribution à l'étude de l'anatomie fonctionelle de la colonne vértébrale cervicale. *Timisoara Medicala*, **17**, 367

VECAN, T. and LEWIT, K. (1980) Plurisegmentale Funktionsstörung der Wirbelsäule als pathogenetischer Faktor bei einem Fall von Überleitungsstörung mit stenokardischen Beschwerden. *Manuelle Medizin*, **18**, 79

VÉLE, F. (1968) Wirbelgelenk und Bewegungssegment innerhalb des Steuerungssystems der Haltemuskulatur. *Manuelle Medizin*, **6**, 94

VÉLE, F. (1984) Muskelspannung und Schmerz. In *Schmerzstudien 6. Schmerz und Bewegungssystem*, p. 80. Eds Berger, M., Gerstenbrand, F. and Lewit, K. Stuttgart, New York, Gustav Fischer

VÉLE, F. and GUTMANN, G. (1971) Die Beeinflussung der Posturalreflexe über die Gelenke. *Zeitschrift für Physiotherapie*, **23**, 383

VERBIEST, H. (1954) A radicular syndrome from developmental narrowing of the lumbar vertebral canal. *Journal of Bone and Joint Surgery*, **36**, 230

VERBIEST, H. (1955) Further experiences on the pathological influence of a developmental narrowness of the bony lumbar vertebral canal. *Journal of Bone and Joint Surgery*, **37**, 576

VESELSKÝ, J., HUDEČKOVÁ, I. and MAYZLÍK, J. (1968) Zkušenosti s manipulační léčbou lumbosakralgií v denní praxi závodní polokliniky. (Experience with manipulative therapy of low back pain in daily practice in a works clinic.) *Acta Chirurgiae Orthopaedicae Traumatologicae Čechoslovacae*, **35**, 421

VISHNYEVSKI, A. V. (1956) *Miestnoye Obezbolivanye po Metodu Polzushtshevo Infiltrata.* (Local anaesthesia in the form of surface infiltration.) Moscow: Medgiz

VÍTEK, J. (1970) Das zervikokraniale Syndrome des hinteren Halssympathicus und die Arteriosklerose des Gehirns. *Manuelle Medizin*, **8**, 13

VOLEJNÍK, V. *et al.* (1984) Rentgenové nálezy na krční páteři u 14–17ti letých mladistvých (X-ray findings of the cervical spine in adolescents of 14–17) *Československá neurologie a neurochirurgie*, **47** (80), 169

VOSS, D. E. (1967) Proprioceptive neuromuscular facilitation. *American Journal of Physical Medicine*, **64**, 838

VOGLER, P. and KRAUSS, H. (1975) *Periostbehandlung*, 2nd edn. Leipzig: Thieme

WACKENHEIM, A. (1968) Céphalées, insertion orbito-oculaire asymmétrique et dislocation transversale de la charnière cervico-occipitale. *Semaine des Hôpitaux*, **44**, 1233

WACKENHEIM, A. (1974) *Roentgendiagnosis of the Cranio-vertebral Region.* Berlin, Heidelberg, New York: Springer

WACKENHEIM, A. and LOPEZ, F. (1969) Étude radiographique des mouvements des C1 et C2 lors de la flexion et de l'extension de la tête. *Journal Belge de Radiologie*, **52**, 117

WACKENHEIM, A., BABIN, E., THIÉBAUT, M. S. D. and LOPEZ, F. (1969) Une nouvelle épreuve fonctionelle pour l'exploration de la dynamique cervico-occipitale. *Concours Médicale*, **11**, 7130

WAERLAND, A. (1950) *Die Chiropraktik und ihre Erfolge im Lichte der Menschheitsentwicklung.* Bern: Humafa

WAGHEMAKER, R., DUMOULINET, J. and SPY, E. (1963) Le facteur musculaire dans la coxarthrose. *Annales de Médicine Physique*, **6**, 263

WALL, P. D. (1972) The mechanism of pain associated with cervical vertebral disease. In *Cervical Pain*, p.201. Eds. Hirsch, C. and Zottermann, Y. Oxford: Pergamon Press

380   References

WALTHER, G. (1963) Zur Physiologie und Pathophysiologie der Rippenwirbelgelenke. *Ärztliche Praxis*, **15,** 1806

WALTHER, G. (1963) Halswirbelsäule und Herz. *Therapiewoche*, **13,** 469

WALTHER, G. (1971) Brustschmerzen und Brustkorbwandschmerzen. *Manuelle Medizin*, **9,** 56

WALTON, J. (Ed.) (1981) Inflammatory myopathies (polymyositis) In *Disorders of Voluntary Muscle*, p.525. Ed. Walton, J. Edinburgh: Churchill Livingstone

WEBER, E. (1974) Die Anwendung der manuellen Extension bei der konservativen Koxarthrosebehandlung. *Beiträge zur Orthopädie und Traumatologie*, **21,** 351

WEISL, H. (1954) The movements of the sacroiliac joint. *Acta Anatomica*, **23,** 80

WELLS, K. F. and LUTTGENS, K. (1976) *Kinesiology*, 6th edn. Philadelphia, London, Toronto: W. B. Saunders

WERNE, S. (1957) Studies in spontaneous atlas dislocation. *Acta Radiologica*, Suppl. 23

WESSELY, B., TILSCHER, H. (1984) Atypische Gesichtsschmerzen bei Funktionsstörungen des cervikookzipitalen Überganges. In *Schmerzstudien 6. Schmerz und Bewegungssystem*, p. 154. Eds. Berger, M., Gerstenbrand, F. and Lewit, K. Stuttgart, New York, Gustav Fischer

WHITE, A. M. and PANJABI, M. (1978) *Clinical Biomechanics of the Spine*. Philadelphia: Lippincott

WICKSTRÖM, G. (1974) Effect of work on degenerative back disease. *Scandinavian Journal of Work, Environment and Health*, **4,** Suppl. 1, 1

WINDHORST, Ch. B. and STEGER, E. (1973) Beschwerden im Kopfbereich bei veränderter Bisshöhe. *Münchner Medizinische Wochenschrift*, **115,** 1385

WINTER, E. DE (1963) Manipulations lombo-pelviennes. II. Bases physio-pathologiques. *Vie Médicale*, **44,** M.T.3, 117

WINTER, E. DE (1963) Manipulations lombo-pelviennes. III. Sémiologie. *Vie Médicale*, **44,** M.T6, 81

WINTER, E. DE (1963) Manipulations lombo-pelviennes. IV. Clinique. *Vie Médicale*, **44,** M.T7, 59

WINTER, E. DE and RENOULT, C. (1961) Techniques des manipulations ostéoarticulaires due système lombo-pelvien. I. Anatomie physiologique. *Vie Médicale*, **42,** M.T3, 115

WINTER, E. DE and RENOULT, C. (1963) Manipulations lombo-pelviennes. V. Technique. *Vie Médicale*, **44,** M.T8, 81

WOLF, J. (1970) Die Chondrosynovialmembran als einheitliche Auskleidungshaut der Gelenkhöhle mit Gleit- und Barrierefunktion. In *Manuelle Medizin und Ihre Wissenschaftlichen Grundlagen*, p.16. Ed. Wolff, H. D. Heidelberg: Physikalische Medizin

WOLF, J. (1975) The reverse deformation of the joint cartilage surface and its possible role in joint blockage. In *Functional Pathology of the Motor System. Rehabilitaácia*, Suppl. 10–11, p.30. Eds. Lewit, K. and Gutmann, G. Bratislava: Obzor

WOLFF, H. D. (1968) Die Rotation des Wirbels. *Manuelle Medizin*, **6,** 37

WOLFF, H. D. (1974) Wandlungen theoretischer Vorstellungen über die Manuelle Medizin. *Manuelle Medizin*, **12,** 121

WOLFF, H. D. (1978) Komplikationen bei manueller Therapie der Halswirbelsäule. *Manuelle Medizin*, **16,** 89

WOLFF, H. D. (1978) *Neurophysiologische Aspekte der Manuellen Medizin (Chirotherapie). Schriftenreihe Manuelle Medizin*. Heidelberg: E. Fischer.

WOLFF, H. D. (1980) Kontra-Indikationen gezielter Handgriffe an der Wirbelsäule. *Manuelle Medizin*, **18,** 39

WOLFF, H. D. (1984) Die Stellung der manuellen Medizin in der Schmerztherapie. In *Schmerzstudien 6. Schmerz und Bewegungssystem*, p. 192, Eds Berger, M., Gerstenbrand, F. and Lewit, K. Stuttgart, New York, Gustav Fischer

WOLFF, H. G. (1948) *Headache and other Head Pain*. New York University Press

WOOD, P. H. N. and BADLEY, E. M. (1980) Epidemiology of back pain. In *The Lumbar Spine and Back Pain*, 2nd edn. p.29. Ed. Jayson, M. I. V. London: Pitman Medical

WORZMAN, G. and DEWAR, F. P. (1968) Rotatory fixation of the atlantoaxial joint. *Radiology*, **90,** 479

WRIGHT, H. M. (1962) Progress in osteopathic research. A review of investigation in the division of physiological sciences. *Journal of the American Osteopathic Association*, **61,** 347

WRIGHT, H. M., KORR, I. M. and THOMAS, P. E. (1960) Local and regional variations in cutaneous vasomotor tone of the human trunk. *Acta Neurovegetativa*, **22,** 33

WRIGHT, V. (1981) Hypermobile states. *Manuelle Medizin*, **19,** 78

WYKE, B. D. (1979) Neurology of the cervical spine joints. *Physiotherapy*, **65,** 72

WYKE, B. D. (1979) Reflexsysteme in der Brustwirbelsäule. In *Theoretische Fortschritte und Praktische Erfahrungen der Manuellen Medizin*, p.99. Eds. Neumann, H. D. and Wolff, H. D. Bühl: Konkordia

WYKE, B. D. (1980) The neurology of low back pain. In *The Lumbar Spine and Back Pain*, p.265. Ed. Jayson, M. I. V. London: Pitman Medical

WYKE, B. D. (1972) Articular neurology. *Physiotherapy*, **58,** 94

WYKE, B. D. (1975) Morphological and functional features of the innervation of the costovertebral joints. *Folia Morphologica, Prague,* **23,** 296

WYKE, B. D. and POLÁČEK, P. (1975) Articular neurology – the present position. *Journal of Bone and Joint Surgery,* **57B,** 401

YATES, C. A. H. (1981) Spinal stenosis. *Journal of the Royal Society of Medicine,* **74,** 334

YERUSALEMSKII, A. P. (1983) *Teoreticheskie osnovy reabilitacii pri osteokhondroze pozvonochnika.* (Theoretical principles of rehabilitation in osteochondrosis of the spinal column.) Novokuznetsk, Izdatelstvo 'Nauka'

ZBOJAN, L. (1981) Antigravitational postisometric relaxation. (Personal communication.)

ZEITLER, E. (1963) Röntgenologische Differenzierung kompensierter und dekompensierter Bewegungseinschränkungen. *Zeitschrift für Orthopädie und ihre Grenzgebiete,* **97,** 218

ZEITLER, E. and MARKUSKE, P. (1962) Röntgenologische Bewegungsanalysen der Halswirbelsäule bei gesunden Kindern und Jugendlichen. *Fortschritte auf dem Gebiete der Röntgenstrahlen,* **96,** 87

ZICHA, K. (1970) Manuelle Therapie bei der Spondylitis ankylopoetica. *Manuelle Medizin,* **8,** 97; **9,** 117

ZICHA, K. and ZABEL, M. (1979) Proliferationstherapie bei Enthesopathien. *Manuelle Medizin,* **17,** 101

ZICHA, K. and RUHRMANN, W. (1980) Erfahrungen mit isometrischen Übungen bei lumbosakralem Insuffizienz- und Schmerzsyndrom. *Manuelle Medizin,* **18,** 110

ZUCKSCHWERDT, L., BIEDERMANN, F., EMMINGER, E. and ZETTEL, H. (1960) *Wirbelgelenk und Bandscheibe,* 2nd edn. Stuttgart: Hippokrates

Index